Housing to Optimize Comfort, Health, and Productivity of Dairy Cattle

Editor

NIGEL B. COOK

VETERINARY CLINICS OF NORTH AMERICA: FOOD ANIMAL PRACTICE

www.vetfood.theclinics.com

Consulting Editor
ROBERT A. SMITH

March 2019 • Volume 35 • Number 1

ELSEVIER

1600 John F. Kennedy Boulevard ● Suite 1800 ● Philadelphia, Pennsylvania, 19103-2899

http://www.vetfood.theclinics.com

VETERINARY CLINICS OF NORTH AMERICA: FOOD ANIMAL PRACTICE Volume 35, Number 1
March 2019 ISSN 0749-0720, ISBN-13: 978-0-323-67803-2

Editor: Colleen Dietzler
Developmental Editor: Meredith Madeira

Veterinary Clinics of North America: Food Animal Practice (ISSN 0749-0720) is published in March, July, and November by Elsevier Inc., 360 Park Avenue South, New York, NY 10010-1710. Subscription prices are $256.00 per year (domestic individuals), $434.00 per year (domestic institutions), $100.00 per year (domestic students/residents), $283.00 per year (Canadian individuals), $572.00 per year (Canadian institutions), $335.00 per year (international individuals), $572.00 per year (international institutions), and $165.00 per year (international and Canadian students/residents). To receive student/resident rate, orders must be accompanied by name of affiliated institution, date of term, and the signature of program/residency coordinator on institution letterhead. *Clinics* subscription prices. All prices are subject to change without notice. **POSTMASTER:** Send address changes to *Veterinary Clinics of North America: Food Animal Practice*, Elsevier Health Sciences Division, Subscription Customer Service, 3251 Riverport Lane, Maryland Heights, MO 63043. Customer Service (orders, claims, online, change of address): Elsevier Health Sciences Division, Subscription **Customer Service, 3251 Riverport Lane, Maryland Heights, MO 63043. Tel: 1-800-654-2452 (U.S. and Canada); 314-447-8871 (ouside U.S. and Canada). Fax: 314-447-8029. E-mail: journalscustomerservice-usa@elsevier.com (for print support); journalsonlinesupport-usa@elsevier.com (for online support).**

Reprints. For copies of 100 or more, of articles in this publication, please contact the Commercial Reprints Department, Elsevier Inc., 360 Park Avenue South, New York, NY 10010-1710. Tel.: 212-633-3874; Fax: 212-633-3820; E-mail: reprints@elsevier.com.

Veterinary Clinics of North America: Food Animal Practice is covered in *Current Contents/Agriculture, Biology and Environmental Sciences, MEDLINE/PubMed (Index Medicus), and Excerpta Medica.*

Contributors

CONSULTING EDITOR

ROBERT A. SMITH, DVM, MS
Diplomate, American Board of Veterinary Practitioners; Veterinary Research and Consulting Services, LLC, Greeley, Colorado, USA

EDITOR

NIGEL B. COOK, BSc, BVSc, Cert CHP, DBR, MRCVS
Professor in Food Animal Production Medicine, Chair, Department of Medical Sciences, School of Veterinary Medicine, University of Wisconsin-Madison, Madison, Wisconsin, USA

AUTHORS

NEIL G. ANDERSON, DVM, MSc
(Retired) Lead Veterinarian, Disease Prevention, Ruminants, Animal Health and Welfare Branch, Ontario Ministry of Agriculture and Food and Ministry of Rural Affairs, Elora, Ontario, Canada

ANNABELLE BEAVER, MA, PhD
Animal Welfare Program, Faculty of Land and Food Systems, University of British Columbia, Vancouver, British Columbia, Canada

KARL BURGI
Owner, Sure Step Consulting International LLC, Baraboo, Wisconsin, USA

NIGEL B. COOK, BSc, BVSc, Cert CHP, DBR, MRCVS
Professor in Food Animal Production Medicine, Chair, Department of Medical Sciences, School of Veterinary Medicine, University of Wisconsin-Madison, Madison, Wisconsin, USA

TREVOR J. DEVRIES, BSc (Agr), PhD
Professor, Department of Animal Biosciences, University of Guelph, Guelph, Ontario, Canada

COURTNEY E. HALBACH, MBA
Associate Outreach Specialist, The Dairyland Initiative, School of Veterinary Medicine, University of Wisconsin-Madison, Madison, Wisconsin, USA

HAROLD K. HOUSE, MSc, PEng
DairyLogix, Goderich, Ontario, Canada

VIRPI HUOTARI, MSc
4dBarn Oy, Oulu, Finland

DAVID W. KAMMEL, PhD
Professor, Biological Systems Engineering, University of Wisconsin-Madison, Madison, Wisconsin, USA

PETER D. KRAWCZEL, PhD
Associate Professor, Department of Animal Science, The University of Tennessee, Knoxville, Knoxville, Tennessee, USA

VIRPI KURKELA, DVM
4dBarn Oy, Oulu, Finland

AMANDA R. LEE, MS
PhD Student, Department of Animal Science, The University of Tennessee, Knoxville, Knoxville, Tennessee, USA

JIM LEWIS
Owner, Stepright Stockmanship Solutions LLC, Colfax, Wisconsin, USA

MARIO R. MONDACA, PhD
Research Associate, Department of Medical Sciences, School of Veterinary Medicine, University of Wisconsin-Madison, Madison, Wisconsin, USA

KENNETH V. NORDLUND, DVM
Emeritus Clinical Professor in Food Animal Production Medicine, Department of Medical Sciences, Food Animal Production Medicine, School of Veterinary Medicine, University of Wisconsin-Madison, Madison, Wisconsin, USA

JOUNI PITKÄRANTA, MSc
Architect, 4dBarn Oy, Seinäjoki, Finland

MARJO POSIO, MSc
4dBarn Oy, Oulu, Finland

KATHRYN L. PROUDFOOT, MS, PhD
Assistant Professor, Veterinary Preventive Medicine, College of Veterinary Medicine, The Ohio State University, Columbus, Ohio, USA

CAROLINE RITTER, DVM, PhD
Animal Welfare Program, Faculty of Land and Food Systems, University of British Columbia, Vancouver, British Columbia, Canada

JENNIFER M.C. VAN OS, PhD
Assistant Professor and Extension Specialist in Animal Welfare, Department of Dairy Science, College of Agricultural and Life Sciences, University of Wisconsin-Madison, Madison, Wisconsin, USA

MARINA A.G. VON KEYSERLINGK, MSc, PhD
Animal Welfare Program, Faculty of Land and Food Systems, University of British Columbia, Vancouver, British Columbia, Canada

Contents

times, and increases social stress. This article reviews the relevant literature to establish the recommended stocking density with freestall systems.
Novel housing systems and the considerations of transition cows are also
reviewed.

The feeding behavior of dairy cows, including how, when, and what cows
eat of the feed provided to them, has a significant impact on cow health
and productivity. The design and management of the feeding area impact
the feeding behavior of dairy cows. To ensure good eating patterns, dairy
cows need sufficient space to eat simultaneously, and a bunk design that
minimizes competition, ensures good feed access, and minimizes risk of
injury. Continuous feed access throughout the day, through adequate
feeding levels, and frequent feed delivery and push-ups, also contribute
to ensuring good eating behavior.

It is important to maximize tiestall comfort by designing and building for the
cow. Optimizing cow comfort improves cow health and productivity, leading to greater producer satisfaction. Tiestall housing is the name given to
dairy cattle housing where the cows are individually tethered in distinct
stalls. Stalls must be designed to accommodate the size of the cow and
to provide freedom of movement to reduce hock lesions while maintaining
clean stalls. The stall also must accommodate easy access to feed and
water as part of the stall design.

This article provides information necessary to assist in creation of freestall
facilities in which cows thrive through designs that optimize the resting
behavior of dairy cattle and provide a safe, comfortable, clean, and dry
place to lie down with easy access to feed and water. Comfortable stalls
require a deep-bedded surface, affording cows the cushion they need to
lie down for 12 hours per day and the traction necessary to facilitate rising
and lying movements. Stalls should be sized to accommodate cows using
them and prevent obstructions to lunge and bob areas and impediments to
normal rising and lying movements.

Labor is likely a painful and stressful experience for dairy cows. Understanding maternal behavior can help inform the design of maternity pens
that best accommodate the cow. The maternity pen should provide the
cow an opportunity to seclude from other cows and barn activity. It should
also be well-bedded, dry, and cleaned regularly to create a comfortable

environment and minimize the spread of pathogens to the cow and her calf. Management of the maternity pen should aim to reduce environmental and social stressors to encourage a smooth transition for cows into the lactating herd.

Improvements during transition, following a blueprint that allows for all cows to eat from the feedbunk simultaneously and have access to a comfortable soft bed, avoiding regrouping stress 2 to 7 days before calving. Approaches to prefresh cow housing have incorporated dedicated pens for cows and heifers, sequential fill approaches in larger herds and all-in-all-out pens to maintain social stability throughout the prefresh or dry period. This blueprint has improved postpartum health and early lactation milk performance.

Ventilation systems for adult dairy cattle can be divided into natural and mechanical systems. Mechanical systems include tunnel and cross ventilation. Hybrid systems incorporate both mechanical and natural ventilation design elements. All systems need to provide appropriate airspeeds at the stalls, adequate ventilation rates, and a methodology to operate year-round. Typically, mechanical ventilation systems cost double to operate compared with natural systems, and the differences between mechanical systems are modest. Selection of high-efficiency fans and regular maintenance are higher priorities for proper fan operation than the choice between ventilation systems, which can be herd size, location, and owner preference dependent.

Heat stress results in substantial economic losses to the dairy industry and is problematic for animal welfare. Soaking cattle with water is an effective form of heat abatement. This technique cools cattle when water evaporates from the skin and drips from the animal, and cools the microclimate. To evaluate cooling effectiveness and make appropriate adjustments to heat abatement, animal-based indicators should be recorded in addition to environmental measures. Ideally, heat abatement should be provided to all life stages of dairy cattle and soakers should be combined with shade.

As automatic milking systems grow in popularity in North America, questions about how to design the barn to improve labor efficiency arise.

Multiple considerations such as cow flow traffic type, robot positioning within the pen, the number of cows per pen, and how cows are managed around the robots must be discussed during the barn planning period. This article focuses on barn design and pen layout to maximize labor efficiency in herds with single-box automatic milking systems.

 Video content accompanies this article at http://www.vetfood. theclinics.com.

The design and management of proper handling systems for dairy cows begin with a cow handling management plan that considers the cow and the stock person's behavior. The safety of the cow and stock person is important to the plan and design decisions. Cow welfare can be addressed in a proper cow handling system design. Key components of a handling system are the skills of the stock person, the cow handling management plan, and the design of the handling facility. Good design enhances stockmanship ability and minimizes stress for cows and stock persons, lowering the risk of injury to both.

VETERINARY CLINICS OF NORTH AMERICA: FOOD ANIMAL PRACTICE

SERIES OF RELATED INTEREST

Veterinary Clinics of North America: Equine Practice
Available: https://www.vetequine.theclinics.com/

THE CLINICS ARE NOW AVAILABLE ONLINE!
Access your subscription at:
www.theclinics.com

Preface

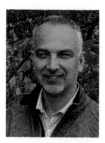

Nigel B. Cook, BSc, BVSc,
Cert CHP, DBR, MRCVS
Editor

Globally, as the dairy industry has consolidated into fewer larger herds, there has been a shift from grazing to confinement housing, predominantly in freestall facilities. When I arrived in Wisconsin at the turn of the century, herd expansions were in full flow and barns were being constructed with little thought to the needs of the cow.

I recall attending several veterinary meetings and listening to a Canadian veterinarian with a dry sense of humor tell stories of cows in barns, motivating producers to improve their facilities with the power of video recording. At that time, I realized that a lack of cow comfort was having a significant negative impact on health, particularly lameness, and inspired by Dr Neil Anderson, we set out to video cows in commercial dairy herds, and for the first time determined individual cow time budgets and began to question how facilities were being constructed. By 2003, I had convinced the first dairy producers to remodel their barns, working with some intrepid construction professionals, converting mattress beds to sand, extending side walls to allow greater lunge space, choosing dividers that did not injure the cow, redesigning brisket locators, and giving cows the resting space they needed. Soon, inspired by Dr Ken Nordlund's passion for ventilation, we were designing new barns with comfortable beds and fresh air for calves and heifers. Along this remarkable journey, we were joined in our efforts by colleagues from the Animal Welfare Program in British Columbia, who were able to perform controlled experiments to test working hypotheses, and later still, with the advent of low-cost and accurate dataloggers that facilitated data gathering, more joined in to question current dogma and dare to challenge the industry to improve facility design. In 2010, we developed the Dairyland Initiative (https://thedairylandinitiative.vetmed.wisc.edu/), a Web-based resource to facilitate information transfer, to ensure that every dairy producer worldwide had access to the most up-to-date information on the housing of dairy cattle of all ages. We trained over 1000 workshop attendees and have seen cow-friendly facilities constructed all around the world, from the United States, Canada, and Europe to Australia. Of course, there were the industry nay-sayers. They questioned the economics of building from the cow up; they said it wouldn't work, producers couldn't afford it. What did veterinarians

Vet Clin Food Anim 35 (2019) xi–xii
https://doi.org/10.1016/j.cvfa.2018.11.004
0749-0720/19/© 2018 Published by Elsevier Inc.

know about building barns anyway? They were wrong. Unsurprisingly, facilities in which cows thrive did rather well, with increases in health and production more than offsetting increases in cost. Even today, the nay-sayers still try to have their way, which is why I agreed to edit this issue of the *Veterinary Clinics of North America: Food Animal Practice* on Housing to Optimize Comfort, Health, and Productivity of Dairy Cattle. Anyone who works with the dairy industry knows that the half-life of information is around 15 years, and we have a propensity to forget what we have learned in the pursuit of a "new idea." In this collection of authors, I took the opportunity to document what we have collectively learned, and I thank them for their efforts in putting this issue together.

It has been the privilege of my life to live through a time whereby we discovered so many amazing things to improve cow comfort and welfare. It will likely never be repeated. The convergence of new technology and like-minded inquisitive researchers, working with dairy producers that were willing to take a chance on something new, created a seismic change in facility design. I rest easily knowing that this knowledge has been passed on and cattle have benefited from it.

Nigel B. Cook, BSc, BVSc, Cert CHP, DBR, MRCVS
Department of Medical Sciences
University of Wisconsin-Madison
School of Veterinary Medicine
2015 Linden Drive
Madison, WI 53706, USA

E-mail address:
nigel.cook@wisc.edu

Introduction: Building from the Cow Up

Neil G. Anderson, DVM, MSc

KEYWORDS

- Dairy cattle • Behavior • Freestall • Tiestall • Comfort • Welfare

KEY POINTS

- The cow, and her behavior, comfort, health, safety, and performance, are the foundations for building a barn.
- Caregivers must know what is going on with the fitness of their cows, barns, and management.
- A cow's welfare is impaired if she cannot cope successfully with her environment.
- Cow comfort is judged by assessing her injuries, lameness, and behaviors while she occupies stalls, rests, eats, drinks, and walks.
- Stall designs and dimensions are based on body measurement, and the space a cow uses for natural resting postures and lying and rising motions.

INTRODUCTION

This introductory article aims to familiarize readers with the terminology and concepts needed to build a cow-friendly dairy barn. To comply with the editor's directive, it also introduces scant historical background of this writer's involvement and my personal journey carrying the message of improving facility design to the industry.

Heritage knowledge for cow housing has been questioned, challenged, complemented, and/or replaced over the past 20 years. The pace of discovery seemed to speed up in the 1980s to 1990s. By the early 2000s, there were dramatic changes in stall designs and other stabling. Adoption of new ideas has been widespread, in large part due to the combined efforts of the authors of the articles in this issue, to their mentors and students, and to a wealth of practical national and international research and empirical experiences. Dairy producers have been very successful at finding what does and does not work in their barns, innovators have shown alternative ways to husband cows, and welcomed guests have shared their knowledge and made a difference. Many veterinarians, feed company consultants, milking equipment dealers,

Disclosure Statement: The author has nothing to disclose.
14789 Creditview Road, Cheltenham, Ontario L7C 3G6, Canada
E-mail address: nganderson@rogers.com

Vet Clin Food Anim 35 (2019) 1–9
https://doi.org/10.1016/j.cvfa.2018.10.001
0749-0720/19/© 2018 Elsevier Inc. All rights reserved.

barn builders, and dairy industry advisors also have become excellent resources and advocates. Good designs and construction do several things brilliantly. First and foremost, they build from the cow up.

COW ERGONOMICS

Cow ergonomics concerns the improvement of cow health and performance through the careful design of her work environment. Building from the cow up alludes to building a house from the ground up with the footings and foundations. For a cow house, the footings and foundations are the cow and her behavior, comfort, health, safety, and performance. Barn design must meet the needs of the cow and the farmer because these choices determine success or failure for both. Recognition of challenges in vintage designs has resulted in an evolution to features in new barns that give cows, owners, and farm workers better lives and put fun into going to the barn. To build ergonomically correct housing requires basic and advanced understanding about

- Body dimensions
- Natural resting positions and space requirements
- Natural rising and lying motions, and space requirements
- Natural walking motions
- Natural feeding, estrus, and calving behavior, and social interactions
- Comfort, health, and safety.

Familiarity with cow ergonomics has come from assessments of cows, facilities, and management performed by the author on dairy farms in Ontario, Canada, and by several other groups around the world represented in this edition.

COMFORT, HEALTH, BEHAVIOR, AND SAFETY

The author's local milk transporter gave a nickname to almost everyone on his route. One dairy producer was given the moniker "Misty" because he always appeared to be in a foggy state of mind, unaware of what was happening around him. Preoccupation with barn chores may be why one misses things.

Characteristics of comfort may not be obvious, whereas signs of discomfort may be very noticeable. Stable blindness, desensitization to animal suffering, or unawareness may limit a persons' ability to see comfort, discomfort, natural behavior, or unnatural behavior. Misinterpretation of cause and effect may misdirect a person's remedies:

- Comfort is a state of ease and freedom from pain, want, other afflictions, or unpleasant conditions.
- Health, sometimes referred to as well-being, is optimal functioning and freedom from disease or abnormality.
- Behavior refers to actions or reactions under specified circumstances.
- Safety is freedom from danger, risk, or injury.
- Fear or apprehension refers to feelings of alarm or disquiet caused by the expectation of danger, pain, or disaster.

Injury, pain, fear, frustration, and stress alter behavior. Cows have feelings, sensations, and emotions. Cows may become fearful from pain caused by injections, bruising, or pressure, and then show signs of unusual or unwanted behavior. Pain from lameness alters behavior in stalls and walk alleys. Fear from intrusion on their comfort zones or from design features may alter their use of stalls, water troughs, floors, or dark passages.

Behavior is useful to judge a cow's feelings about her housing and to reveal the consequences of choices a caregiver made for her workplace. Behavior has been monitored over the years: at first, through direct visual observations; subsequently, through video monitoring; and, most recently, through the use of activity loggers and trackers. Studies using these approaches have greatly added to knowledge of cow behavior in cow barns over the last 2 decades.

AWARENESS: KNOWING WHAT IS GOING ON

Awareness is knowledge about the fitness of cows, their barns, and their management. Because all 3 are subject to change, one must continually update one's understanding about them. My happiness at work came from discoveries in barns and communicating them using the newer technologies of video and digital images, and PowerPoint presentations, which became available in the 1990s.

I did not get it. Although researchers were telling us about the needs of the cow, vintage barns were built without paying attention to these findings. For example, prevention of environmental mastitis focused on the cleanliness of a cow's workplace and the cleanliness of the cow. Yet, in vintage barns, cows chose to lie in walkways and narrow, slurry-laden alleys led to dirtiness of feet, legs, udders, and teats. Reasons may have included slowness of knowledge transfer, stubbornness, saving costs when building barns, a lack of workspace awareness, or not knowing what to do. Today, there is greater awareness of housing features or management practices that contribute to cow cleanliness,[1] and barns are finally being built accordingly.

In my early extension days, color slides and cheekiness may have helped my messages stick. I showed images of discomfort in stalls, gutter queens, alley queens, dog sitters, perchers, and tail amputations. Good images of deep-bedded tie stalls also were in my spiel and I praised farmers who provided a good mattress for their cows. In 1991, an inventor, motivated by my mattress analogy and the ribbed pattern on a tea cozy at his home, invented the multicelled, rubber-filled cow mattress. Producers reacted by inviting me to see their uncomfortable stalls and to facilitate on-farm workshops to audit cow comfort. People were listening and interested.

Timing is everything in teaching and learning. For example, during a workshop, a large Holstein cow's attempt to rise in her tie stall ended with her trapped beneath the tie rail. Workshop attendees watched and then discussed this. Her bed provided excellent traction and she was not lame. Most suggestions were to prevent her from going forward by lowering the tie rail, shortening the tie chain, and adding a board to the top of the manger curb. However, when she got onto the walkway, she stood with ease, showing the group that she needed more freedom, not less, for forward lunging and rising. There were many similar examples in vintage freestalls. Seeing is believing, sometimes.

On-farm study groups, demonstrations, open-houses, and bus tours are educational when one knows what to look for or at, and how to interpret what one sees. Guided tours are most valuable when guides point out the lessons before the group. Attendees learn from their hosts when the hosts reveal what worked, what did not, and what they would do differently. Regrettably, some attendees wander off in self-guided exploration and miss the sage advice. In other events, the hosts simply walk groups around to view aspects of the farm without any critique, leaving attendees to come to their own conclusions based solely on what they see at the time. Some astutely ask questions, take photos, make notes, return to their farms, and implement change. In Ontario, Canada, Jack Rodenburg and Harold House taught practical dairy housing courses from 1993 to 2015, and I enjoyed participating with them for several years.

More recently, other educational initiatives have begun. Close to home, in 2016, the Ontario Veterinary College established the Saputo Dairy Care Program,[2] a dairy cattle welfare rotation, as an elective for veterinary students in their final year of study. The main learning objectives are to recall existing dairy welfare standards and recognize contraventions, practice on-farm dairy cattle welfare assessments, and master communication with clients and colleagues about animal welfare. These sessions facilitate discussions about Canada's proAction animal care program. In the United States, similar approaches, such as the DairyFARM program provided by the US National Milk Producers Federation, have been used to prepare producers.

Believe it or not, in the past 20 years, video recordings may have been the greatest contributor to changing knowledge, attitudes, opinions, and actions about barn designs. Data loggers have facilitated collection of resting and standing data for research projects but video opened eyes to what cows do in barns. I found video to be useful for research, consultation, diagnosis, and outreach programs. Video clips of natural actions, struggles, unwanted behavior, and cow responses to stall modifications were used in my cow behavior and comfort talks, starting about 1999. By accepting national and international speaking requests, my local awareness campaign took on a new life. I would like to believe that my video clips were educational and increased awareness. Images of cows performing the hesitation waltz; that is, making multiple aborted attempts to lie down because of poor stall design, became the highlight of a conference, and consultants and producers took notice and began to use my terminology in common vernacular.

Undoubtedly, one cannot see everything, even when one is looking. Teaching what is going on may be essential to prepare for building from the cow up.

BEYOND COPING

The welfare of a cow is impaired if she is unable to cope successfully with her environment. Assessments of cows allow caregivers to score how well they are coping. Caregivers do their best to help cows manage in their workplaces. For example, sand bedding provides excellent traction for rising and provides cushioning to prevent hock sores. It may have helped cows manage in short, narrow stalls with obstructions to natural lunging motions and resting postures. To many stockpersons, that is not good enough. When one build from the cow up, one assures that cows have the freedom for natural actions and that they do not have to cope by adopting uncharacteristic or unwanted behavior.

To build from the cow up, one needs to observe and understand so-called nature's way.

NATURAL RESTING POSITIONS AND FREEDOMS

Cows rest in wide, narrow, short or long positions, or completely on their side (dead cow position). To allow for natural resting positions, the resting area must provide cows with 6 freedoms:

- To stretch their front legs forward
- To lie on their sides, with unobstructed space for their neck and head
- To rest their heads against their sides without hindrance from a partition
- To rest with their legs, udders, and tails on the platform
- To stand or lie without pain or fear from neck rails, partitions, or supports
- To rest on a clean, dry, and soft bed,

The daily time budget of cows includes resting time. This measure of stall comfort only became available as a herd metric with the development of activity and positional data loggers. Before this, daily resting times were unknown. Although known for decades, natural rising and reclining motions seemed to be ignored when vintage stalls were built.

NATURAL RISING AND RECLINING MOTIONS

To rise or lie down, a cow needs space for vertical, forward, and lateral movement without obstruction, injury, or fear:

- The rising motion includes the freedom to lunge forward, to bob the head down and up, and to stride forward.
- The resting motion also includes the freedom to lunge forward, to bob the head, and to shuffle the foreleg knees on the bed.
- Both rising and resting motions include lateral and vertical movements.

The space needed for the lunge and stride can be seen using video images of cows rising and lying on pasture, and by superimposing a grid on the images. Cows may adopt unwanted behaviors to cope with discomfort in stalls.

UNWANTED OR ABNORMAL OUTCOMES

Cows do not lie. Caregivers must have the ability to see the truths that cows are telling us. Management can be judged by cows' actions or reactions and interpreted through desirable, unwanted, or abnormal outcomes. Examples of unwanted results include

- Idle standing in stalls
- Perching with front feet in the bed and rear feet in the alley
- Lying backwards in stalls
- Diagonal standing and lying
- Alternate occupancy
- Dog sitting or rising like a horse (front-end first)
- Nose pressing behavior
- Restlessness while lying (frequent, repetitive leg movements over the bed)
- Kneeling to eat (in tie stalls)
- Injuries to legs, necks, and other body parts
- Lameness
- Dirtiness.

The caregiver's job is to unzip each of the truths and to find out what is initiating the actions or reactions. In many cases, there may be obstructions to nature's way. For example, freestall brisket boards bracketed to the lower pipe of loops prevent cows from resting with their legs outstretched, promote restlessness, and lead to hock abrasions (in stalls with scant bedding). The height of brisket boards and mounds of concrete or bedding at the front of the stall interfere with the natural stride while rising. Solid fronts, boards, pipes, facing cows, or piles of bedding interfere with forward lunging motions and encourage lying backwards or diagonally. Neck rail location may discourage standing with all feet in the stall, encourage perching, and predispose to lameness.

The basic elements of a stall have useful purposes when matched with cow dimensions and natural behavior.

COW DIMENSIONS

In the early 1970s, a dairy farmer I will call Art raised the top rail in his stanchion barn for the third time in his career. Because of genetic selection and good heifer husbandry, his cattle were taller and he matched their stabling to their stature. Another dairy farmer, David, replaced his freestall stabling in 2003 within a few years of entering his new barn and after losing most of his original herd to lameness or injuries. His cows perched because of neck-rail location, obstructions to forward lunging, discomfort from high brisket boards, and scant bedding. Lameness and other outcomes associated with mismatching cows and stalls[3] had been published a half decade before his barn was built. Yet another, Joe, raised the top rail of the angle feed fronts at his feed bunk after seeing injuries to the supraspinous processes of cows' necks in his new freestall barn. Through happenstance, the feed fronts were mismatched for his tall cattle. Art was aware; David knew very little about freestalls and accepted out-of-date advice; and Joe missed comparing his cow height to his choice of stabling during his planning.

Freestalls (cubicles) appeared in the 1960s. Before the mid-1980s, designers may not have paid much attention to cow behavior. Vintage stall dimensions aimed to provide for the needs of the cow and the caregiver. However, based on outcomes and critical appraisal, they may have missed the target, interfered with natural behavior, or caused harm. Although the use of cow body measurements and movements was being promoted for stall design in 1988,[4] mismatching was obvious in barns constructed thereafter and throughout the 1990s. Outdated cow dimensions and misjudging the actual space requirements for natural motions are possible explanations. In 1996, Faull and colleagues[5] published the following list of cow measurements needed to establish stall dimensions for Friesian/Holsteins in the United Kingdom. These still apply to cows and barns:

- Nose to tail-head length
- Imprint width while resting
- Imprint length while resting
- Length of head-lunging space
- Length of front-leg stride to rise.

After measuring some cows and studying records from Holstein Canada and a private research farm, it was apparent that Canadian Holsteins had increased in stature and body weight over a few decades. Clearly, the cows had outgrown their stalls or stalls were not being built to meet the cows' needs. Extension activities in Ontario throughout the 1990s and 2000s increased awareness about cow dimensions, cow behavior, and cow-friendly stall designs. Many dairy producers saw that their cows did not fit the stalls. They wanted to know how to fix it and several manufacturers and contractors stepped up to the plate to help.

SEEING IS BELIEVING OR BELIEVING ENABLES SEEING

The reason one cannot see what is in front of one may be a belief or mental blind spot that one has built. Although seeing is believing may be true, it is likely that believing enables seeing. Sometimes responses to suggestions are followed with the response, "That will not work on my farm." A useful tactic to continue the conversation toward changing beliefs is "I used to believe that too but I do not anymore." Dairy barns are set in concrete and difficult to modify. However, to test concepts in existing barns in the 1990s and early 2000s, reformers undertook the ordeal of experiment, altered stalls, and changed beliefs. Galileo would have been proud of them.

Several Ontario dairy producers with tie stall barns were fed up with tramped-on teats, gutter queens, and dumb heifers. General instructions to open the lunge space, install a higher tie rail, and lengthen the tie chain resulted in unique modifications to stalls. A producer I will call Dan built a few test stalls and used his box-stall cattle (dumb heifers and crampy or lame cows) as experimental subjects. Within a day of entry, the once-coddled cows stood up and lay down with ease. His comment was, "Makes you wonder who was dumb?" Others modified a few stalls, saw a positive difference, and told everyone who would listen. Milk truck drivers, nutritionists, and veterinarians carried their testimonials. Action and improvisation became rampant. To allow for flexibility in an evolving environment, local manufacturers produced stabling with tie rails adjustable in height and forward location.

While studying cow behavior in tie stalls, it was apparent that electric trainers could be ineffective or abusive. Part of the problem may have been a local manufacturer's installation instructions and/or the location of milk and vacuum pipe lines. European research[6] showed that trainers helped to keep stalls and cows clean when properly installed. Studies at a local farm with new stall dimensions showed that eliminations accurately entered the gutter when a cow's hind feet were situated just in front of the gutter curb. To assure training and humane use, the trainer had to be located where the cow's back begins to arch (when she is humped-up to eliminate) relative to the gutter curb. For mature Holsteins, the location was 48 inches forward of the gutter curb. Placement of the hind feet, location of the chine (beginning of an arched back), and cow dimensions determined the forward location and vertical height of the trainers. It took a bit of convincing but milking equipment dealers now give precedence to trainer location. Electric trainer location and height adjustment are checklist items in the Canadian proAction animal care assessment program.

In freestalls, the neck rail could be ineffective, restrictive, and abusive. The problem seemed to be the height above the bed and the forward location relative to the alley curb. The forward location of the neck rail had to allow a cow to stand straight in her stall with her hind feet placed at the alley curb. The height had to be a few inches below the top line. The measurements were horizontal and vertical, not the hypotenuse of the imaginary triangle as commonly used by installers.

During an evening barn check in 1999, a dairy farmer I will call Deb rushed to examine 2 cows that appeared dead in the stalls that she had modified that morning. To her surprise, they were very much alive, just resting on their sides in deep sleep. She had never seen cows sleeping in their barn. During a consultation with her for lameness, hock sores, and mastitis, I saw stall refusals, idle standing, perching, and restlessness while lying.[7] Nothing could be done about the short (15-ft head-to-head platform) and narrow (45 in) stalls or the transverse lower mounting pipe for the loops. With cameras rolling, they workers raised the neck rail and moved it forward, and removed the brisket board and its brackets to a harmless position outside the barn wall. After they went to lunch, the first cow stepped into a stall, looked over the bed (with no brisket board), moved her head and mouth as if shouting across the pen, and promptly lay down in the long position with front legs stretched out, and hind feet and tail on the bed. The next cow did a similar inspection and called out to others. Soon the stalls were fully occupied with resting cows. In the unmodified facing stalls, cows perched or stalls were empty. Also, I had an entertaining video showing that cows talk.

In 2003, a dairy producer built the first Ontario freestall barn for Holsteins with an 18-ft head-to-head platform, loops on 50-in centers, a floor-mounted brisket locator 70 in forward of the curb, and a neck rail at 68 in forward of the curb and 50 inches above the bed. Video from this barn confirmed predictions that natural behaviors happened when cows were given more space in freestalls.

SUMMARY

A revolution has occurred in cow comfort in the past 20 years. The tipping point may have come in the early 2000s when Dr Ken Nordlund and Dr Nigel Cook accumulated considerable practical knowledge through personal experiences and experimentation and spread their findings far and wide. They boldly challenged existing recommendations in the United States, provided practical guides for assessments, and offered solid recommendations for new dimensions. The increase in research about cattle in their natural habitat and in confinement housing has been remarkable since the 2000s. Noteworthy among the sources of this knowledge is the University of British Columbia Animal Welfare Program, where resources were available for controlled experiments that had not occurred elsewhere. Moreover, the Internet has made the information readily available. Producers can no longer build facilities in a vacuum or without knowledge, which is readily available to inform better decision-making.

The good choices that I have seen in many new barns this past year have given me great joy. However, the inescapable realities are that sometimes what salespersons sell, owners choose, equipment dealers insist on, contractors build, or what experts recommend may run counter to what they should. Cow advocates and educators cannot rest on their laurels and pat themselves on the back for a job well done. Bad ideas make a habit of returning when enough people forget. For example, the stalls that I saw in the last new freestall barn that I visited were flashbacks to the dimensions used in the 1980s and 1990s. Thankfully, the owners chose sand for bedding and the cows were coping. At some other farms, a loop-mounted plastic pipe seems to be the modern equivalent of vintage brisket boards. New ideas seem to have been forgotten and, again, I do not get it. Certainly, education about workspace awareness must be ongoing to refresh old memories and to inform those new to the industry.

Examinations of the limitations and failures within cow barns leads to discoveries of better practices. In the past 20 or more years, reformers have turned specific features of dairy barn design upside down. These designs ensure that cows' wants or needs are not sacrificed. What has been leaned along this journey of discovery should not be forgotten. The ultimate goal is to provide a good life for cattle, from birth all the way to the end of their productive lives.

REFERENCES

1. Anderson NG. Cow houses and udders: challenges and opportunities. Proc. National Mastitis Council Regional Conference. Charlottetown, Prince Edward Island, Canada. August 9–10, 2006.
2. Saputo Dairy Care Program. Ontario Veterinary College, University of Guelph, Guelph, ON. Available at: https://www.uoguelph.ca/ccsaw/sites/uoguelph.ca.ccsaw/files/public/Saputo%20Dairy%20Care%20Program%20Annual%20Report%202018_0.pdf. Accessed November 16, 2018.
3. Philipot JM, Pluvinage P, Cimarosti I, et al. Risk factors of dairy cow lameness associated with housing conditions. Vet Res 1994;25:244–8.
4. Cermak J. Cow comfort and lameness - design of cubicles. The Bovine Practitioner 1988;23:79–83.
5. Faull WB, Hughes JW, Clarkson MJ, et al. Epidemiology of lameness in dairy cattle: the influence of cubicles and indoor and outdoor walking surfaces. Vet Rec 1996;139:130–6.

6. Oswald T. Der Kuhtrainer. 1992. Is the cow trainer compatible with proper stock keeping? ISSN 0257-9200, ISBN 3-9520182-3-6.
7. Anderson N. Dairy cattle behavior: cows interacting with their workplace. Volume 36. Proc. 36th Annual Convention Am. Assoc. Bovine Pract. Columbus, OH. September 18–20, 2003. p. 10–22.

The Dairy Cattle Housing Dilemma

Natural Behavior Versus Animal Care

Annabelle Beaver, MA, PhD, Caroline Ritter, DVM, PhD,
Marina A.G. von Keyserlingk, MSc, PhD*

KEYWORDS

- Tie-stalls • Calf feeding • Maternal behavior • Artificial rearing • Natural behavior

KEY POINTS

- The intensification of indoor housing systems has led to an increased ability to provide individualized care for farm animals, but this sometimes results in the thwarting of natural behaviors.
- Indoor housing systems can be modified to better allow the expression of important behaviors.
- Motivation tests can be used to understand the relative importance of natural behaviors and associated resources in dairy cattle.

INTRODUCTION

Over the last few decades, a broad array of stakeholders has raised concerns about the quality of life for dairy cattle.[1] This growing interest in animal welfare has motivated policymakers to consider the sufficiency of current legislation, with global regions, such as the European Union and New Zealand, developing additional requirements to improve welfare on farm.[2,3] In other regions, such as in North America, changes in animal care have largely been driven by growing pressure from corporations,[4] resulting in the development of producer-led quality-control programs (eg, Dairy Farmers Assuring Responsible Management program[5] and ProAction[6]).

Individuals vary in how they conceive of animal welfare. For example, farmers and their advisors working in farm animal industries often focus on production and health,[7] whereas others place more importance on the animal's affective state (eg, Ref.[8]). Affective states may be negative, such as the feelings of pain, hunger, and stress, or

Disclosure Statement: The authors have nothing to disclose.
Animal Welfare Program, Faculty of Land and Food Systems, University of British Columbia, 2357 Main Mall, Vancouver, British Columbia V6T 1Z6, Canada
* Corresponding author.
E-mail address: marina.vonkeyserlingk@ubc.ca

Vet Clin Food Anim 35 (2019) 11–27
https://doi.org/10.1016/j.cvfa.2018.11.001
0749-0720/19/© 2018 Elsevier Inc. All rights reserved.

vetfood.theclinics.com

positive, such as those associated with play (reviewed by Boissy and colleagues[9]). Some individuals also place considerable importance on whether an animal can live a natural life or express natural behavior.[10] This construct can be considered conceptually or practically difficult for those working with intensive production systems,[7,11] but concerns pertaining to naturalness are frequently voiced by those external to the livestock industry (eg, Ref.[12]).

In this article, the authors introduce the concept of natural behavior and summarize the viewpoints of different stakeholders. They then focus on the housing sector by examining shortfalls of current systems and describing how modern dairy husbandry might foster natural behavior.

WHAT IS "NATURAL BEHAVIOR"?

The concept of "naturalness" (as one of the 3 spheres of animal welfare; **Fig. 1**) is the most conceptually ambiguous and, arguably, the most challenging for animal agriculture. Definitions and interpretations of the term have been advanced by veterinarians, animal behaviorists, and philosophers, with somewhat contradictory conclusions (see Ref.[13]). It is a common misconception that "natural living" universally contributes to good welfare and is therefore synonymous with the development of positive affective states.[14] At one extreme, "natural" stimuli, such as predation or inclement weather conditions, cannot reasonably be considered to enhance welfare. The ability of the animal to perform its full behavioral repertoire (eg, fleeing a predator or huddling to stay warm) is therefore not essential to good welfare; of greater importance is the extent to which behaviors are feasible when circumstances compel them.[10]

Nevertheless, domestic farm animals, such as dairy cattle, benefit from a diverse repertoire of natural behaviors, many of which do provide both short- and long-term welfare advantages. Identification of the behaviors that are of importance to the animal is a critical step in improving housing systems for captive species.[15] One complexity that arises in understanding natural behavior is the extent to which

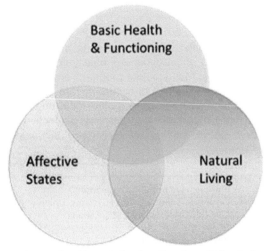

Fig. 1. The 3 spheres of animal welfare. Animal welfare is optimized where health and functioning, positive affective states, and natural living overlap. (*Adapted from* Fraser D. Understanding animal welfare. Acta Vet Scand 2008;50(1):S1; with permission.)

"naturalness" shifts alongside domestication and many generations of artificial selection; what once constituted a natural behavior for the wild ancestors of modern dairy cattle may have little relevance to animals in existing dairy systems. Some research has indicated that many natural behaviors remain constant following domestication. For example, Stolba and Wood-Gush[16] observed a group of domestic pigs in a semi-natural environment and recorded a wide range of behaviors reminiscent of feral counterparts, including grazing, rooting, wallowing, and nest building. Similarly, Keeling and Duncan[17] noted that domestic fowl released in semi-natural conditions exhibited a behavioral repertoire that evoked that of wild ancestors.

Although natural behavior appears to persist across time and even withstands genetic selection, it is also characterized by a high degree of plasticity. Thus, somewhat paradoxically, natural behaviors are flexible as well as enduring. Farm animals are known to implement a diverse array of strategies to meet their behavioral needs, dependent in part on contextual cues. Segerdahl[13] suggests viewing the animal as an amalgam of its nature and its current environment, not defined solely by its nature or phylogeny but rather demonstrating adaptability in a variety of conditions, and in response to ontogenic experiences. The interaction between the animal and its environment becomes important when evaluating the role of agricultural housing systems in shaping natural behavior. Several investigators (see Refs.[15,16,18]) highlight the distinction between intrinsically and extrinsically motivated behaviors. That is, the value of a given behavior often depends on the interaction between the internal state of the animal and environmental stimuli. These different sources of motivation can dictate the relative importance of a behavior; for example, if a behavior is extrinsically driven and prompted exclusively by "opportunity,"[19] the animal's inability to perform it in captivity is unlikely to compromise welfare. This insight has perhaps led to the incorporation of intrinsic motivation in several definitions of "natural behavior" as a prerequisite for its relevance to welfare (eg, Ref.[20]).

The lack of consensus as to what constitutes natural behavior leads one to consider the role of humans in nature, and indeed, the question of whether humans should be seen as part of, or separate from, nature (see, eg, Ref.[21]). The notion that humans must minimize interaction with cattle in order to restore (or at least approximate) the natural order is arguably misplaced. For one, technology such as automated milking systems that allow farmers to reduce their contact with animals may be considered to deviate even further from naturalness. Consumers and producers of organic food cite the concept of "naturalness" as a foundational aspect of organic agriculture,[22] yet organic compared with conventional producers often demonstrate *greater* involvement with the animals in their care.[23] Segerdahl[13] attempts to resolve this apparent contradiction by clarifying that "natural living" for farm animals may now be thought to encompass interactions with humans, as a consequence of the domestication process.

The plasticity of natural behavior, influenced by a variety of feedback mechanisms, represents a critical advantage in finding practical methods for improving living conditions for farmed animals.[15] There is often a range of refinements that may not involve "natural" stimuli but still offer animals the opportunity to express behaviors that satisfy their motivational needs. It is not the "naturalness" of the environment per se that affects animal welfare, but the ability of the environment to afford animals the opportunity to express natural tendencies.[24] Thus, there is perhaps a distinction to be made between "natural living" and "natural behavior," with the former not necessarily a precondition for the latter.

PERCEPTIONS OF ANIMAL WELFARE AND NATURAL LIVING BY DIFFERENT STAKEHOLDERS

Recent studies demonstrate that different stakeholders have varying attitudes and priorities regarding animal welfare. People working in the dairy industry often define animal welfare by good health, and conventional farms are primarily designed to maximize animal health and production.[7,25] Whereas some farmers regard natural living as a prerequisite for good animal welfare, others view naturalness either as a luxury or as a welfare risk (eg, harsh weather conditions for outdoor-housed animals; Ref.[26]). Unlike outdoor living, indoor housing systems provide the opportunity to "keep a close eye" on the animals, allowing farmers to react quickly to any problems. Therefore, modern indoor housing systems may allow farmers to better fulfill their caretaking role.[27]

Veterinarians are often seen as important influencers regarding animal welfare (eg, Refs.[28,29]) and seem to place considerable weight on biological functioning and affective concerns associated with animal welfare.[30,31] Less is known regarding veterinarians' concerns about naturalness,[32] but research to date suggests that views are likely to be diverse. For example, although veterinarians in Norway thought that keeping calves with their mothers provided welfare advantages on organic dairy farms,[33] North American veterinarians seemed to support early separation of cow and calf.[34]

Citizens' views often reflect the importance of naturalness for farm animals. For example, citizens sometimes view tie-stall housing as too restrictive[35] and suggest that cows should have access to pasture (which is perceived to provide space to "roam," access to fresh air and grass, and the ability to interact socially; Refs.[1,12,36]). Premium (higher-priced) milk products that include the term "pasture" or "meadow" have been established in several countries (eg, the Netherlands, Switzerland, United States), providing an incentive for farmers to implement pasture-based farming.[37] Overall, consumers' ethical considerations translate into increased willingness to pay for products associated with high animal welfare, although this shows great variation associated with sociodemographic factors (see Ref.[38]).

Although citizens appear to value outdoor access for dairy cows, this concern can sometimes be outweighed. For example, in a recent study, survey participants were presented with scenarios describing different housing systems for dairy cows.[39] Participants responded more favorably to scenarios with cows on pasture, but only when these cows were provided shade. These results suggest that citizens hold diverse welfare concerns and balance these in relation to the case at hand. In this instance, they clearly valued the naturalness of pasture, but not to the extent that this eclipsed health and affective-state concerns associated with heat stress.

In several US states, citizens used petitions and governmental intervention strategies to reform existing practices for animal confinement.[2,40] The public has an increased interest in animal welfare issues, believes that animal welfare should be considered for food production, and has the power to motivate changes in legislation. It is therefore indisputable that (future) developments must account for societal concerns to ensure that proposed solutions become common practice and are sustainable.[41,42]

WHAT IS THE ANIMAL TELLING US?

The lack of consensus on the definition of "natural behavior" does not preclude the integration of this concept into housing for dairy cattle. Empirical research directed toward understanding preferences and motivations can inform us as to what behaviors are important to the animal, and what modifications facilitate behavioral expression.[43]

Several strategies for assessing the importance of various behaviors have gained traction in the literature. One simple method involves the construction of time budgets to determine behavioral durations and frequencies (eg, see Ref.[44]). A limitation of this method centers on the notion that a behavior is only valuable to the extent that it is continuously performed; however, animals may spend relatively little time engaging in behaviors that are critical for their welfare. For example, calves direct only 2% of their daily time budget to social interactions within the first weeks of life,[45] but they are highly motivated to initiate social contact[46] and show strong preferences for known conspecifics.[47]

Preference tests are also useful for assessing the relative importance of behaviors, but these tests do not provide information about inherent value of the behavior or associated resource (eg, animals may consistently select one of 2 food options, but both options may be nutritionally inadequate, or the preference may be very slight; Ref.[48]). Motivation tests can be used to determine how hard animals are willing to work for a given resource (or behavioral freedom), and this motivation can then be compared with that for other resources (see Refs.[49,50]).

The continued development of motivation tests in the context of indoor housing systems is particularly important in assessing animals' priorities. In one compelling example, new research using a weighted gate has indicated that dairy cattle are highly motivated to access rotating brushes, as much as they are motivated to access a "necessity": fresh feed.[51] In nature, cows can use the bark of trees or other rough surfaces as a grooming substrate to remove dirt and external parasites, and the presence of rotating brushes indoors may alleviate some of the frustration and discomfort of not being able to effectively groom. This example points to the usefulness of continued evaluation of animals' motivations, which can be directed toward constructive housing modifications.

One important element of dairy cattle housing is the extent to which animals are provided agency in their living environment. The ability to exert control over one's environment has been shown be advantageous to welfare in a variety of domestic and captive animal species. Providing animals with choices is one effective method of affording such agency. Some experimental research has shown that cows are highly motivated to access pasture,[52] yet a 2013 census of dairy cattle housing in the United States reported that upwards of 80% of lactating dairy cattle are housed permanently indoors.[53] Dairy cattle preference for pasture, however, is strongest during the nighttime and is influenced by temperature, humidity, and level or rainfall (see review by Charlton and Rutter[54]). When cows are kept permanently outdoors, heat stress can have an important negative impact on animal welfare, and heat waves are associated with higher mortalities in older cows.[55] Housing systems that are exclusively indoors or outdoors provide control for farm personnel, but the effects of pasture access or shelter may differ in important ways for the animals when it is free versus forced.

CHALLENGES TO NATURAL BEHAVIOR IN MODERN DAIRY HOUSING SYSTEMS

In the last half century, the global dairy industry has undergone considerable intensification, with North American systems moving away from more naturalistic environments toward more confined indoor housing options.[56] Such intensification can offer benefits, including the ability to invest in more specialized care[57] and to more closely monitor the health and feed intake of individual animals, for which farmers feel responsible.[58] Conversely, these systems may limit animals' freedom of movement and restrict the expression of natural behavior.

Restriction of Movement

Tie-stall housing, in which animals are typically chained to the head rail at the front of the stall, comprise nearly 39% and 74% of US and Canadian dairy farms, respectively.[53,59] This type of housing permits individualized care and rationing and reduces the risk of agonistic behavior. However, tie-stalls also prevent animals from interacting with one another; such social interactions are considered by US citizens to be the single most important factor to ensure the welfare of cattle.[60]

Some research has demonstrated that physiologic parameters (eg, β-hydroxybutyrate and nonesterified fatty acids) are unchanged in cows housed in tie-stalls versus free-stalls.[35] This finding could lead some to suggest that the welfare of animals kept in more restrictive housing types is unimpaired. Tie-stall systems may thus provide an example of the prioritization of health and maintenance over behavioral freedom (see Refs.[25,30]), and the insufficiency of physiologic parameters to provide a complete picture of animal welfare. The thwarting of natural behavior can lead to negative experience while failing to impact biological functioning.[10] Furthermore, although the comparison of health in tie-stall versus free-stall systems is conflicting at best (eg, Refs.[61–63]), there is ample evidence in support of behavioral benefits in less restrictive housing types (eg, Refs.[64,65]). In one study, cows transferred from pasture to tie-stall housing exhibited irregular patterns of lying behavior and a temporary deterioration of locomotor ability, which was still apparent 4 days after their return to pasture.[66] Moreover, when permitted access to outdoor spaces, cows typically housed in tie-stalls devote large portions of their time budget to romping and exploring the environment.[67,68]

Aggressive behavior is predictably reduced in tie-stalls compared with open housing types, because, in addition to freedom of movement, social interactions themselves are constrained.[69] To the authors' knowledge, no research has been conducted to investigate how cattle housed in tie-stalls are affected when they are released onto pasture and potentially have to reestablish a social hierarchy. In any case, temporary release into outdoor spaces and regular exercise opportunities are beneficial from the perspective of both behavior and health.[61,66,69] Temporary pasture access also reduced tongue playing in cows normally kept in tie-stalls,[70] whereas tethering after a period of grazing on pasture resulted in more oral stereotypies.[71] It is important to note that tie-stall housed dairy farms often provide pasture access for at least part of the year (eg, 73% in the United States; Ref.[53]), and this might be viewed as compensation for close indoor confinement.

Flooring Substrates and Stall Design

Dairy cattle exhibit a wide variety of behaviors associated with estrus, including standing to be mounted (primary estrus), restlessness, anogenital sniffing, flehmen, chin resting, and mounting attempts (secondary signs). Social behaviors, such as licking, rubbing, and head butting, have also been associated with estrus expression.[72] Tie-stall housing systems greatly impair the expression of estrus behaviors, because cows are restricted to individual stalls. Free-stalls provide greater opportunity for the realization of these behaviors, but slippery flooring in many of these facilities is considered inhibitory.[73] Certain open housing types and floor substrates may partially offset this concern; cattle housed on pasture, on dirt surfaces, and in bedded-pack barns often express comparatively higher levels of estrus behavior.[73–75] Efforts to improve cow fertility (eg, timed artificial insemination programs such as

Ovsynch; Pursley and colleagues[76]) may be perceived as diverting from a natural-living conception of welfare. Rather than modifying floor substrate to facilitate natural estrus behaviors, such as mounting, the solutions to such problems have shifted into a highly artificial domain, a solution that has also been questioned by some veterinarians[77] and researchers.[41]

Bedding substrate and housing design also factor greatly into the expression of other natural behaviors of dairy cattle. Deep sawdust bedding affords flexibility in lying patterns and leads to an increase in lying bouts and durations.[78] Similarly, lying time increases when free-stalls are more appropriately sized and less restrictive, bedding is cleaner, and stocking densities are lower.[79–81] Nevertheless, more time spent recumbent is not always synonymous with improved comfort and welfare; high lying times have previously been associated with lameness.[82] Cattle on pasture spend less time lying down than cows kept indoors,[83] which perhaps reflects a combination of increased comfort standing on grass, a greater portion of the time-budget devoted to grazing,[84] and a heightened vigilance toward potential predators.[85] Daily lying time per se is therefore a poor behavioral predictor of good welfare.[86]

Grouping and Regrouping Management

In a study of feral cattle in Mexico, animals were observed to form small groups of up to 20 animals; domestic cattle in the same region generally lived in larger groups.[87] In indoor housing systems for adult cattle, where there is an abundance of food, herd size varies greatly, but the space that each animal has available is substantially smaller than what the animals would naturally experience.[88] This space restriction can lead to increased aggression and social licking (potentially as a means of reducing social tension) when animals are kept indoors compared with on pasture.[89] In free-stall barns, these negative effects can, for example, be reduced by limiting overstocking, providing enough feeding space, and designing alleys so that animals can avoid each other.

The feral cattle observed in Mexico generally remained in the same small group.[87] Consistent social groups likely reduce social distress for the animals; Proudfoot and colleagues[90] found that housing dairy cattle in predictable and noncompetitive social environments provided health and behavioral benefits. Other studies of both feral and domestic cattle have demonstrated social preferences based on attachment between individuals.[91,92] However, dairy cattle are often regrouped based on factors, such as age, pregnancy status, or nutritional requirements.[93] Mixing unfamiliar animals can lead to undesired behavior, such as aggression,[94] decreased feeding time, and a reduction in affiliative behaviors, such as allogrooming.[95] Developing management practices that allow cattle to familiarize themselves gradually with other cattle could potentially reduce these negative effects.[93]

Feed and Nutrition Management

One substantive benefit to indoor housing is the ability to provide rations tailored to the nutritional needs of individual animals or groups of animals in differing lactation stages.[96] However, despite the fulfillment of nutritional requirements, the deviation from a naturalistic diet may compromise welfare. For example, if cattle are not provided with adequate roughage, feeding time and rumination are shown to decrease, and oral stereotypies, such as tongue rolling, may also develop.[97] Tongue rolling is observably similar to the natural oral manipulation of grass required in grazing, and the stereotypy may thus have developed out of an attempt to realize a thwarted behavior.[98] Indeed, tongue rolling is almost never observed in pasture-based systems.[71]

Cow and Calf Separation

In nature, the dam finds a secluded area in which to calve, and the neonate remains hidden in shrubs for the first few days after parturition while the dam grazes nearby. During suckling bouts, both calf and dam reciprocally lick and sniff one another. These affiliative behaviors most commonly manifest as the calf sniffing the udder of the dam, and the dam grooming the calf in areas the calf would not otherwise be able to reach.[55]

On commercial dairies, calves are typically separated from the dam within the first 24 hours postpartum and housed individually through weaning.[99] Immediate separation is frequently motivated by an effort to prevent the immunologically naive calf from acquiring pathogens from the dam or calving environment and to control the delivery of colostrum, although a recent systematic review has found little health-related evidence to support the practice.[100]

Cow-calf rearing within the context of the dairy farm environment appears to diversify the behavioral repertoire of calves, permitting higher levels of exploratory behaviors in social tests, including sniffing, mounting, and play-fighting.[101] The range of social behaviors of dam-reared calves has also been shown to be more varied when exposed to an unfamiliar calf, including head butting, rubbing, and tail wagging[102] and other social play.[103]

In addition to increasing the inventory of positive behaviors, the literature is generally in agreement that cow-calf suckling reduces the frequency of abnormal behaviors in calves. Dam-rearing mitigates cross-sucking of other calves and nonnutritive sucking of objects within the pen[104,105] and is associated with a reduction in calf stereotypies, including tongue rolling.[106] Many facets of cow-calf suckling likely interact to produce this reduction in stereotypies, including higher milk volumes, fulfillment of the sucking reflex, and increased frequency of milk meals associated with nursing the dam. Calves offered high volumes of milk throughout the day are still extremely motivated to suck,[107] pointing to the multidimensional nature of milk-feeding behavior. Further research will be necessary to disentangle these elements (ie, method, volume, and frequency) and assess their relative contributions toward mitigating oral stereotypies.

Longer-term effects of cow-calf contact have been identified, with cows nursed by the dam (as calves) displaying greater involvement with their own calves, and devoting a higher percentage of their time budget to licking and nursing.[108] Other long-term effects on behavior are less clear, with some studies demonstrating higher herd dominance rankings for cows that had been nursed,[109,110] and others indicating higher submission in these animals when integrated into the herd.[111]

Colostrum Management

Successful immunoglobulin transfer to newborn dairy calves, which hinges on the timely feeding of sufficient high-quality colostrum, is widely seen as the most important management factor for future calf health and productivity.[112] Difficulties in cow-calf rearing systems have arisen when calves fail to suckle the dam within the first few hours of life.[113] Where the "natural system" is seen to fail, producers may be inclined to think it is their duty to intervene. In the case of colostrum feeding, efforts at individualized care associated with the current practice of separating the calf from the dam at birth involve feeding colostrum by bottle, bucket, or tube, rather than permitting suckling. Of course, feeding calves colostrum by artificial means is not contingent on dam-calf separation; calves can be fed colostrum while in the presence of the dam.

Results of a large-scale study[114] indicate that nearly 94% of calves on US dairy operations are hand-fed colostrum. On these operations, 23.6% of calves are fed by esophageal tube, an increase from the 13.7% reported in 2007.[115] Esophageal tube feeding is more time efficient, but it may increase the risk of aspiration-related complications[116] and cause temporary injury or pain that makes swallowing more difficult; in fact, routine tube feeding of colostrum is controversial in Europe and is even prohibited in several European countries (see Refs.[117,118]). Some calves (eg, those that do not possess a suckling reflex) may still benefit from tube feeding, but for healthy calves, this method circumvents the opportunity to express natural suckling behavior.

Individual Housing for Calves

In feral cattle, beginning at 4 to 5 days after parturition, the mother rejoins the grazing herd, with distance and time away from the calf gradually increasing as the calf matures (see review by von Keyserlingk and Weary[119]). In turn, the calf begins to spend time interacting with conspecifics. The calf engages in a variety of social play behaviors, including frontal pushes, play mounting, and "runs and gambols," punctuated by short vocalizations.[55]

Thus, for the dairy calf (but not for the dam), some of the behavioral benefits afforded by dam-rearing may also be realized through other forms of social contact. Compared with individual housing, social housing from birth improves cognition and solid feed intake before weaning[120,121] and mitigates the effects of weaning and regrouping.[122,123] Socially reared calves are generally less fearful (reviewed by Bøe and Færevik[124]), which may be viewed as a social buffering effect when in the presence of conspecifics. Neophobic responses are reduced in socially housed calves,[125] and calves are less reactive to being startled.[126] Recent work on pair housing in modified hutches provides a practical, low-cost example of how natural behavior expression can be easily facilitated on commercial farms.[127]

Restricted Milk Feeding

When given the opportunity, calves are observed to nurse the dam between 8 and 12 times per day for the first week after parturition. The number of suckling bouts and total time spent suckling typically decrease as the calf ages, with the duration of each bout increasing in parallel.[55] In most conventional herds, individual housing is commonplace, and calves are provided milk twice per day by bucket at approximately 10% of body weight, a much lower volume than would be obtained via nursing the dam. Even when fed artificially, calves provided ad libitum milk throughout the day consume substantially more (eg, 89% more; Ref.[128]) than calves fed traditional allotments. Although some farms now provide calves higher milk rations, most calves in commercial herds are still provided restricted amounts of milk (**Fig. 2**).

Promising research has been conducted into the effects of feeding dairy calves high milk rations. Work comparing groups of calves with either ad libitum or restricted access to a milk feeder has shown that restricted-fed calves are more competitive and spend a higher portion of their daily time-budget standing. These calves also spent twice as long at the teat, consuming their full milk meal in a single bout and continuing to suckle unrewarded, perhaps indicative of both frustration and hunger.[129] When calves are provided continuous access to milk, they consume their milk meals rather randomly,[107] reminiscent of suckling bouts in nature. Moreover, as previously discussed, bucket-fed calves remain motivated to suck even when receiving high quantities of milk: calves fed ad libitum by bucket sucked a sham teat 13 minutes per day, compared with 1 minute for calves fed ad libitum by artificial teat.[107] Offering milk by teat versus bucket and providing more regular access to milk in higher volumes can also lead to a reduction in cross-sucking of pen mates (see review by Costa and colleagues[130]). This method of milk allowance is a preferred management adaptation for

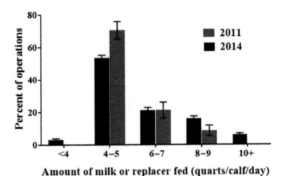

Fig. 2. The amount of milk or milk replacer fed per calf per day in 2011 and 2014 expressed as a percent of dairy operations; data were collected as part of the 2011 Heifer raiser study[109] and the 2014 Dairy National Animal Health Monitoring Survey.[53] Farms reported volumes in US quarts. In 2014, there was a 16% increase in the number of dairy operations feeding more than 8 quarts of milk per day compared with 2011. Error bars represent ± 1 standard error of the mean.

paired or group-raised calves in order to avoid the negative behaviors historically associated with social rearing.

Abrupt Weaning

In nature, the calf begins grazing and ruminating at approximately 3 weeks of age. At this time, the calf is still dependent on the dam and older conspecifics for social cues, such as learning to identify a suitable diet. The weaning process in nature is gradual, with calves consuming some quantity of milk from the dam for approximately 10 months.[91] Conversely, commercial farms typically initiate weaning when calves are 2 months of age, with the entire weaning process lasting several days. Until recently, early provision of forage to dairy calves was considered inadvisable[131]; however, recent findings indicate that providing forage to preweaned calves (that are also fed higher milk rations and starter) can improve calf weight gain and gut microbial maturation (see review by Khan and colleagues[132]).

In commercial settings, in the absence of the dam, calves may be housed with an older conspecific to promote social facilitation, encourage feeding behavior, and reduce neophobic responses to novel feed.[122,133] Early and rapid weaning can result in cross-suckling, increased vocalizations, and other signs of hunger.[134] In addition to raising the weaning age and moving toward a more natural weaning process (such as gradually reducing the milk volume; see review by Khan and colleagues[135]), the social learning afforded by older pen mates (akin to the diverse social groups formed by feral cattle) may also help mitigate weaning distress.[122]

SUMMARY

In this review, the authors have attempted to summarize some of the challenges created by the housing environment on the desire to provide cattle the opportunity to exercise natural behavior. When there is a conflict between naturalness and perceived best practice, there is often a tendency among conventional dairy farmers to prioritize health and biological functioning of the animal, sometimes by highly artificial means. Examples of such processes and systems include tie-stall housing, individual housing of calves, and tube feeding of colostrum. Nevertheless, in many cases, individualized animal care may be preserved while fostering an environment conducive to the expression of natural behavior.

ACKNOWLEDGMENTS

C. Ritter is a Banting Fellow hosted by the Animal Welfare Program and supported through the Banting Postdoctoral Fellowships program, administered by the Government of Canada. The authors extend their gratitude to Dr Jason Lombard of USDA-APHIS for providing summary data on the US dairy industry. In addition, the authors thank Dr Dan Weary of the Animal Welfare Program for his comments on a previous draft and Anne-Marieke Smid of the Animal Welfare Program for sharing her knowledge. M.A.G. von Keyserlingk is supported by Canada's Natural Sciences and Engineering Research Council Industrial Research Chair Program with industry contributions from the Dairy Farmers of Canada (Ottawa, ON, Canada), British Columbia Dairy Association (Burnaby, BC Canada), Westgen Endowment Fund (Milner, BC, Canada), Intervet Canada Corporation (Kirkland, QC, Canada), Novus International Inc (Oakville, ON, Canada), Zoetis (Kirkland, QC, Canada), BC Cattle Industry Development Fund (Kamloops, BC, Canada), Alberta Milk (Edmonton, AB, Canada), Valacta (St. Anne-de-Bellevue, QC, Canada), and CanWest DHI (Guelph, ON, Canada).

REFERENCES

1. Clark B, Stewart GB, Panzone LA, et al. A systematic review of public attitudes, perceptions and behaviours towards production diseases associated with farm animal welfare. J Agr Environ Ethic 2016;29(3):455–78.
2. Centner TJ. Limitations on the confinement of food animals in the United States. J Agr Environ Ethic 2010;23(5):469–86.
3. von Keyserlingk MAG, Hötzel MJ. The ticking clock: addressing farm animal welfare in emerging countries. J Agr Environ Ethic 2015;28(1):179–95.
4. Fraser D. Animal welfare assurance programs in food production: a framework for assessing the options. Anim Welf 2006;15(2):93–104.
5. NMPF (National Milk Producers Federation). Animal care reference manual 2016. Available at: http://www.nationaldairyfarm.com/sites/default/files/Version-3-Manual.pdf. Accessed October 2, 2018.
6. Dairy Farmers of Canada. ProAction: Leading the way for sustainable dairy farming; providing assurance to customers about farm practices. Dairy Farmers of Canada, Ottawa, Ontario, Canada 2015. Available at: https://www.dairyfarmers.ca/Media/Files/proaction/proaction_ang_lr15.pdf. Accessed November 30, 2018.
7. Benard M, de Cock Buning T. Exploring the potential of Dutch pig farmers and urban-citizens to learn through frame reflection. J Agr Environ Ethic 2013;26(5):1015–36.
8. Duncan IJ. A concept of welfare based on feelings. The well-being of farm animals: challenges and solutions. Ames (IA): Blackwell Publishing; 2004. p. 85–101.
9. Boissy A, Manteuffel G, Jensen MB, et al. Assessment of positive emotions in animals to improve their welfare. Physiol Behav 2007;92(3):375–97.
10. Fraser D, Weary DM, Pajor EA, et al. A scientific conception of animal welfare that reflects ethical concerns. Anim Welf 1997;6:187–205.
11. von Keyserlingk MAG, Weary DM. A 100-year review: animal welfare in the Journal of Dairy Science—The first 100 years. J Dairy Sci 2017;100(12):10432–44.
12. Cardoso CS, Hötzel MJ, Weary DM, et al. Imagining the ideal dairy farm. J Dairy Sci 2016;99(2):1663–71.

13. Segerdahl P. Can natural behavior be cultivated? The farm as local human/animal culture. J Agr Environ Ethic 2007;20(2):167–93.

14. Ross M, Mason GJ. The effects of preferred natural stimuli on humans' affective states, physiological stress and mental health, and their potential implications for well-being in captive animals. Neurosci Biobehav Rev 2017;83:46–62.

15. Spinka M. How important is natural behaviour in animal farming systems? Appl Anim Behav Sci 2006;100(1-2):117–28.

16. Stolba A, Wood-Gush D. The behaviour of pigs in a semi-natural environment. Anim Sci 1989;48(2):419–25.

17. Keeling L, Duncan IJ. Social spacing in domestic fowl under seminatural conditions: the effect of behavioural activity and activity transitions. Appl Anim Behav Sci 1991;32(2):205–17.

18. Bracke MB, Hopster H. Assessing the importance of natural behavior for animal welfare. J Agr Environ Ethic 2006;19(1):77–89.

19. Fraser D, Duncan IJ. 'Pleasures', 'pains' and animal welfare: toward a natural history of affect. Anim Welf 1998;7(4):383–96.

20. Hughes BO, Duncan IJ. The notion of ethological 'need', models of motivation and animal welfare. Anim Behav 1988;36(6):1696–707.

21. Costanza R, Graumlich L, Steffen W, et al. Sustainability or collapse: what can we learn from integrating the history of humans and the rest of nature? Ambio 2007;36(7):522–7.

22. Verhoog H, Matze M, Van Bueren EL, et al. The role of the concept of the natural (naturalness) in organic farming. J Agr Environ Ethic 2003;16(1):29–49.

23. Vaarst M, Wemelsfelder F, Seabrook M, et al. The role of humans in the management of organic herds. In: Vaarst M, Roderick S, Lund V, et al, editors. Animal health and welfare in organic agriculture. Wallingford (United Kingdom): CABI Publishing, CAB International; 2004. p. 205–26 (ISBN 0-85199-668-X).

24. Musschenga AW. Naturalness: beyond animal welfare. J Agr Environ Ethic 2002; 15(2):171–86.

25. Te Velde H, Aarts N, Van Woerkum C. Dealing with ambivalence: farmers' and consumers' perceptions of animal welfare in livestock breeding. J Agr Environ Ethic 2002;15(2):203–19.

26. Spooner JM, Schuppli CA, Fraser D. Attitudes of Canadian beef producers toward animal welfare. Anim Welf 2012;21(2):273–83.

27. Engster D. Care ethics and animal welfare. J Soc Philos 2006;37(4):521–36.

28. Jansen J, Steuten C, Renes R, et al. Debunking the myth of the hard-to-reach farmer: effective communication on udder health. J Dairy Sci 2010;93(3):1296–306.

29. Wolf C, Tonsor G, McKendree M, et al. Public and farmer perceptions of dairy cattle welfare in the United States. J Dairy Sci 2016;99(7):5892–903.

30. Heleski CR, Mertig AG, Zanella AJ. Results of a national survey of US veterinary college faculty regarding attitudes toward farm animal welfare. J Am Vet Med Assoc 2005;226(9):1538–46.

31. Ventura BA, von Keyserlingk MAG, Weary DM. Animal welfare concerns and values of stakeholders within the dairy industry. J Agr Environ Ethic 2015; 28(1):109–26.

32. Sumner CL, von Keyserlingk MAG, Weary DM. Perspectives of farmers and veterinarians concerning dairy cattle welfare. Anim Frontiers 2018;8(1):8–13.

33. Ellingsen K, Mejdell CM, Hansen B. Veterinarians' and agricultural advisors' perception of calf health and welfare in organic dairy production in Norway. Org Agr 2012;2:67–77.

34. Ventura BA, von Keyserlingk MAG, Schuppli CA, et al. Views on contentious practices in dairy farming: the case of early cow-calf separation. J Dairy Sci 2013;96(9):6105–16.
35. Giuliotti L, Benvenuti MN, Lai O, et al. Welfare parameters in dairy cows reared in tie-stall and open-stall housing systems. Anim Sci Pap Rep 2017;35(4):379–86.
36. Schuppli CA, von Keyserlingk MAG, Weary DM. Access to pasture for dairy cows: responses from an online engagement. J Anim Sci 2014;92(11):5185–92.
37. Weinrich R, Kühl S, Zühlsdorf A, et al. Consumer attitudes in Germany towards different dairy housing systems and their implications for the marketing of pasture raised milk. Int Food Agribus Man 2014;17(4):205–22.
38. Clark B, Stewart GB, Panzone LA, et al. Citizens, consumers and farm animal welfare: a meta-analysis of willingness-to-pay studies. Food Pol 2017;68:112–27.
39. Cardoso C, von Keyserlingk MAG, Hötzel MJ, et al. Hot and bothered: public attitudes towards heat stress and outdoor access for dairy cows. PLoS One 2018;13(10):e0205352.
40. Shields S, Shapiro P, Rowan A. A decade of progress toward ending the intensive confinement of farm animals in the United States. Animals (Basel) 2017; 7(5):40.
41. von Keyserlingk MAG, Martin NP, Kebreab E, et al. Invited review: sustainability of the US dairy industry. J Dairy Sci 2013;96:5405–25.
42. Weary DM, Ventura BA, von Keyserlingk MAG. Societal views and animal welfare science: understanding why the modified cage may fail and other stories. Animal 2016;10(2):309–17.
43. Lidfors L, Berg C, Algers B. Integration of natural behavior in housing systems. Ambio 2005;34(4):325–30.
44. Gomez A, Cook N. Time budgets of lactating dairy cattle in commercial freestall herds. J Dairy Sci 2010;93(12):5772–81.
45. Chua B, Coenen E, van DJ, et al. Effects of pair versus individual housing on the behavior and performance of dairy calves. J Dairy Sci 2002;85(2):360–4.
46. Holm L, Jensen MB, Jeppesen LL. Calves' motivation for access to two different types of social contact measured by operant conditioning. Appl Anim Behav Sci 2002;79(3):175–94.
47. Duve LR, Jensen MB. The level of social contact affects social behaviour in pre-weaned dairy calves. Appl Anim Behav Sci 2011;135(1–2):34–43.
48. Broom DM. Animal welfare: concepts and measurement. J Anim Sci 1991; 69(10):4167–75.
49. Olsson I, Keeling L. The push-door for measuring motivation in hens: laying hens are motivated to perch at night. Anim Welf 2002;11(1):11–9.
50. Petherick JC, Rutter SM. Quantifying motivation using a computer-controlled push-door. Appl Anim Behav Sci 1990;27(1):159–67.
51. McConnachie E, Smid AMC, Thompson AJ, et al. Cows are highly motivated to access a grooming substrate. Biol Lett 2018;14(8) [pii:20180303].
52. von Keyserlingk MAG, Cestari AA, Franks B, et al. Dairy cows value access to pasture as highly as fresh feed. Sci Rep 2017;7:44953.
53. USDA. 2016. Dairy 2014, "Dairy Cattle Management Practices in the United States, 2014" USDA–APHIS–VS–CEAH–NAHMS. Fort Collins (CO). #692.0216. Available at: https://www.aphis.usda.gov/animal_health/nahms/dairy/downloads/dairy14/Dairy14_dr_PartI.pdf. Accessed September 27.
54. Charlton GL, Rutter SM. The behaviour of housed dairy cattle with and without pasture access: a review. Appl Anim Behav Sci 2017;192:2–9.

55. Vitale A, Tenucci M, Papini M, et al. Social behaviour of the calves of semi-wild Maremma cattle, Bos primigenius taurus. Appl Anim Behav Sci 1986;16(3):217–31.

56. Barkema HW, von Keyserlingk MAG, Kastelic J, et al. Invited review: changes in the dairy industry affecting dairy cattle health and welfare. J Dairy Sci 2015; 98(11):7426–45.

57. Robbins J, von Keyserlingk MAG, Fraser D, et al. Invited review: farm size and animal welfare. J Anim Sci 2016;94(12):5439–55.

58. Taylor GB. One man's philosophy of welfare. Vet Rec 1972;91:426–8.

59. CDIC (Canadian Dairy Information Centre). Dairy barns by type in Canada 2017. Available at: http://www.dairyinfo.gc.ca/index_e.php?s1=dff-fcil&s2=farm-ferme&s3=db-el. Accessed September 27, 2018.

60. Widmar NO, Morgan CJ, Wolf CA, et al. US resident perceptions of dairy cattle management practices. Agri Sci 2017;8(07):645.

61. Regula G, Danuser J, Spycher B, et al. Health and welfare of dairy cows in different husbandry systems in Switzerland. Prev Vet Med 2004;66(1–4):247–64.

62. Sogstad Å, Fjeldaas T, Østerås O. Lameness and claw lesions of the Norwegian red dairy cattle housed in free stalls in relation to environment, parity and stage of lactation. Acta Vet Scand 2005;46(4):203.

63. Valde JP, Hird DW, Thurmond MC, et al. Comparison of ketosis, clinical mastitis, somatic cell count, and reproductive performance between free stall and tie stall barns in Norwegian dairy herds with automatic feeding. Acta Vet Scand 1997; 38(2):181–92.

64. Haley D, De Passille A, Rushen J. Assessing cow comfort: effects of two floor types and two tie stall designs on the behaviour of lactating dairy cows. Appl Anim Behav Sci 2001;71(2):105–17.

65. Higashiyama Y, Nashiki M, Narita H, et al. A brief report on effects of transfer from outdoor grazing to indoor tethering and back on urinary cortisol and behaviour in dairy cattle. Appl Anim Behav Sci 2007;102(1–2):119–23.

66. Enriquez-Hidalgo D, Teixeira DL, Lewis E, et al. Behavioural responses of pasture based dairy cows to short term management in tie-stalls. Appl Anim Behav Sci 2018;198:19–26.

67. Krohn CC, Munksgaard L, Jonasen B. Behaviour of dairy cows kept in extensive (loose housing/pasture) or intensive (tie stall) environments I. Experimental procedure, facilities, time budgets—diurnal and seasonal conditions. Appl Anim Behav Sci 1992;34(1):37–47.

68. Loberg J, Telezhenko E, Bergsten C, et al. Behaviour and claw health in tied dairy cows with varying access to exercise in an outdoor paddock. Appl Anim Behav Sci 2004;89(1–2):1–16.

69. Popescu S, Borda C, Diugan EA, et al. Dairy cows welfare quality in tie-stall housing system with or without access to exercise. Acta Vet Scand 2013;55(1):43.

70. Dovier S, Piasentier E, Corazzin M, et al. Effect of summer grazing on welfare of dairy cows reared in mountain tie-stall barns. Italian Journal of Animal Science 2010;9(3):304–12.

71. Redbo I. Stereotypies and cortisol secretion in heifers subjected to tethering. Appl Anim Behav Sci 1993;38(3–4):213–25.

72. Roelofs J, López-Gatius F, Hunter R, et al. When is a cow in estrus? Clinical and practical aspects. Theriogenology 2010;74(3):327–44.

73. Palmer MA, Olmos G, Boyle LA, et al. Estrus detection and estrus characteristics in housed and pastured Holstein–Friesian cows. Theriogenology 2010;74(2):255–64.

74. Britt JH, Scott RG, Armstrong JD, et al. Determinants of estrous behavior in lactating Holstein cows. J Dairy Sci 1986;69(8):2195–202.

75. Phillips C, Schofield S. The effect of cubicle and straw yard housing on the behaviour, production and hoof health of dairy cows. Anim Welf 1994;3(1):37–44.
76. Pursley JR, Wiltbank MC, Stevenson JS, et al. Pregnancy rates per artificial insemination for cows and heifers inseminated at a synchronized ovulation or synchronized estrus. J Dairy Sci 1997;80(2):295–300.
77. Higgins HM, Ferguson E, Smith RF, et al. Using hormones to manage dairy cow fertility: the clinical and ethical beliefs of veterinary practitioners. PLoS One 2013;8(4):e62993.
78. Tucker CB, Weary DM, Fraser D. Effects of three types of free-stall surfaces on preferences and stall usage by dairy cows. J Dairy Sci 2003;86(2):521–9.
79. Fregonesi J, von Keyserlingk MAG, Tucker C, et al. Neck-rail position in the free stall affects standing behavior and udder and stall cleanliness. J Dairy Sci 2009; 92(5):1979–85.
80. Tucker CB, Weary DM, Fraser D. Free-stall dimensions: effects on preference and stall usage. J Dairy Sci 2004;87(5):1208–16.
81. Tucker CB, Zdanowicz G, Weary DM. Brisket boards reduce freestall use. J Dairy Sci 2006;89(7):2603–7.
82. Ito K, von Keyserlingk MAG, LeBlanc S, et al. Lying behavior as an indicator of lameness in dairy cows. J Dairy Sci 2010;93(8):3553–60.
83. Hernandez-Mendo O, von Keyserlingk MAG, Veira D, et al. Effects of pasture on lameness in dairy cows. J Dairy Sci 2007;90(3):1209–14.
84. Kennedy E, McEvoy M, Murphy JP, et al. Effect of restricted access time to pasture on dairy cow milk production, grazing behavior, and dry matter intake. J Dairy Sci 2009;92(1):168–76.
85. Kluever BM, Breck SW, Howery LD, et al. Vigilance in cattle: the influence of predation, social interactions, and environmental factors. Rangeland Ecol Manage 2008;61(3):321–8.
86. Ito K, Chapinal N, Weary DM, et al. Associations between herd-level factors and lying behavior of freestall-housed dairy cows. J Dairy Sci 2014;97(4):2081–9.
87. Hernández L, Barral H, Halffter G, et al. A note on the behavior of feral cattle in the Chihuahuan Desert of Mexico. Appl Anim Behav Sci 1999;63(4):259–67.
88. Kondo S, Sekine J, Okubo M, et al. The effect of group size and space allowance on the agonistic spacing behavior of cattle. Appl Anim Behav Sci 1989; 24:127–35.
89. Tresoldi G, Weary DM, Pinheiro Machado Filho LC, et al. Social licking in pregnant dairy heifers. Animals (Basel) 2015;5(4):1169–79.
90. Proudfoot K, Weary DM, LeBlanc S, et al. Exposure to an unpredictable and competitive social environment affects behavior and health of transition dairy cows. J Dairy Sci 2018;101(10):9309–20.
91. Reinhardt V, Reinhardt A. Cohesive relationships in a cattle herd (Bos indicus). Behaviour 1981;77(3):121–50.
92. Val-Laillet D, Guesdon V, von Keyserlingk MAG, et al. Allogrooming in cattle: relationships between social preferences, feeding displacements and social dominance. Appl Anim Behav Sci 2009;116(2–4):141–9.
93. Patison KP, Swain DL, Bishop-Hurley GJ, et al. Changes in temporal and spatial associations between pairs of cattle during the process of familiarisation. Appl Anim Behav Sci 2010;128(1–4):10–7.
94. Kondo S, Hurnik J. Stabilization of social hierarchy in dairy cows. Appl Anim Behav Sci 1990;27(4):287–97.
95. von Keyserlingk MAG, Olenick D, Weary DM. Acute behavioral effects of regrouping dairy cows. J Dairy Sci 2008;91(3):1011–6.

96. Grant R, Albright J. Effect of animal grouping on feeding behavior and intake of dairy cattle. J Dairy Sci 2001;84:E156–63.
97. Redbo I, Nordblad A. Stereotypies in heifers are affected by feeding regime. Appl Anim Behav Sci 1997;53(3):193–202.
98. Jensen P. Diurnal rhythm of bar-biting in relation to other behaviour in pregnant sows. Appl Anim Behav Sci 1988;21(4):337–46.
99. Vasseur E, Borderas F, Cue RI, et al. A survey of dairy calf management practices in Canada that affect animal welfare. J Dairy Sci 2010;93(3):1307–16.
100. Beaver A, Meagher RK, von Keyserlingk MAG, et al. Invited review: a systematic review of the effects of early separation on dairy cow and calf health. J Dairy Sci, in press.
101. Jensen MB, Munksgaard L, Mogensen L, et al. Effects of housing in different social environments on open-field and social responses of female dairy calves. Acta Agr Scand A-An 1999;49(2):113–20.
102. Flower FC, Weary DM. Effects of early separation on the dairy cow and calf: 2. separation at 1 day and 2 weeks after birth. Appl Anim Behav Sci 2001;70(4):275–84.
103. Wagner K, Barth K, Hillmann E, et al. Mother rearing of dairy calves: reactions to isolation and to confrontation with an unfamiliar conspecific in a new environment. Appl Anim Behav Sci 2013;147(1–2):43–54.
104. Roth BA, Barth K, Gygax L, et al. Influence of artificial vs. mother-bonded rearing on sucking behaviour, health and weight gain in calves. Appl Anim Behav Sci 2009;119(3–4):143–50.
105. Veissier I, Caré S, Pomiès D. Suckling, weaning, and the development of oral behaviours in dairy calves. Appl Anim Behav Sci 2013;147(1–2):11–8.
106. Fröberg S, Lidfors L. Behaviour of dairy calves suckling the dam in a barn with automatic milking or being fed milk substitute from an automatic feeder in a group pen. Appl Anim Behav Sci 2009;117(3–4):150–8.
107. Hammell KL, Metz J, Mekking P. Sucking behaviour of dairy calves fed milk ad libitum by bucket or teat. Appl Anim Behav Sci 1988;20(3):275–85.
108. Le Neindre P. Influence of cattle rearing conditions and breed on social relationships of mother and young. Appl Anim Behav Sci 1989;23(1):117–27.
109. Le Neindre P. Influence of rearing conditions and breed on social behaviour and activity of cattle in novel environments. Appl Anim Behav Sci 1989;23(1):129–40.
110. Le Neindre P, Sourd C. Influence of rearing conditions on subsequent social behaviour of Friesian and Salers heifers from birth to six months of age. Appl Anim Behav Sci 1984;12(1):43–52.
111. Wagner K, Barth K, Palme R, et al. Integration into the dairy cow herd: long-term effects of mother contact during the first twelve weeks of life. Appl Anim Behav Sci 2012;141(3–4):117–29.
112. Godden S. Colostrum management for dairy calves. Vet Clin North Am Food Anim Pract 2008;24(1):19–39.
113. Edwards SA, Broom DM. The period between birth and first suckling in dairy calves. Res Vet Sci 1979;26(2):255–6.
114. USDA. Special tabulation—Colostrum management: dairy 2014, Dairy Cattle Management Practices in the United States, 2014. Fort Collins (CO): USDA-APHIS-VS, CEAH; 2016.
115. USDA. 2010. Dairy 2007, Heifer Calf Health and Management Practices on U.S. Dairy Operations, 2007 USDA:APHIS:VS, CEAH. Fort Collins (CO). Available at: https://www.aphis.usda.gov/animal_health/nahms/dairy/downloads/dairy07/Dairy07_ir_CalfHealth.pdf. Accessed September 27, 2018.

116. Bradley JA, Niilo L. Immunoglobulin transfer and weight gains in suckled beef calves force-fed stored colostrum. Can J Comp Med 1985;49(2):152.
117. Bonk S, Nadalin A, Heuwieser W, et al. Lying behaviour and IgG-levels of newborn calves after feeding colostrum via tube and nipple bottle feeding. J Dairy Res 2016;83(3):298–304.
118. Lorenz I, Mee JF, Earley B, et al. Calf health from birth to weaning. I. General aspects of disease prevention. Ir Vet J 2011;64(1):10.
119. von Keyserlingk MAG, Weary DM. Maternal behavior in cattle. Horm Behav 2007;52(1):106–13.
120. Gaillard C, Meagher RK, von Keyserlingk MAG, et al. Social housing improves dairy calves' performance in two cognitive tests. PLoS One 2014;9(2):e90205.
121. Meagher RK, Daros RR, Costa JH, et al. Effects of degree and timing of social housing on reversal learning and response to novel objects in dairy calves. PLoS One 2015;10(8):e0132828.
122. de Paula Vieira A, von Keyserlingk MAG, Weary DM. Presence of an older weaned companion influences feeding behavior and improves performance of dairy calves before and after weaning from milk. J Dairy Sci 2012;95:3218–24.
123. de Paula Vieira A, von Keyserlingk MAG, Weary DM. Effects of pair versus single housing on performance and behavior of dairy calves before and after weaning from milk. J Dairy Sci 2010;93(7):3079–85.
124. Bøe KE, Færevik G. Grouping and social preferences in calves, heifers and cows. Appl Anim Behav Sci 2003;80(3):175–90.
125. Jensen MB, Vestergaard KS, Krohn CC, et al. Effect of single versus group housing and space allowance on responses of calves during open-field tests. Appl Anim Behav Sci 1997;54(2):109–21.
126. Veissier I, Chazal P, Pradel P, et al. Providing social contacts and objects for nibbling moderates reactivity and oral behaviors in veal calves. J Anim Sci 1997;75(2):356–65.
127. Whalin L, Weary DM, von Keyserlingk MAG. Pair housing dairy calves in modified calf hutches. J Dairy Sci 2018;101(6):5428–33.
128. Jasper J, Weary D. Effects of ad libitum milk intake on dairy calves. J Dairy Sci 2002;85(11):3054–8.
129. de Paula Vieira A, Guesdon V, De Passille AM, et al. Behavioural indicators of hunger in dairy calves. Appl Anim Behav Sci 2008;109(2–4):180–9.
130. Costa J, von Keyserlingk MAG, Weary DM. Invited review: effects of group housing of dairy calves on behavior, cognition, performance, and health. J Dairy Sci 2016;99(4):2453–67.
131. Žitnan R, Voigt J, Schönhusen U, et al. Influence of dietary concentrate to forage ratio on the development of rumen mucosa in calves. Arch Anim Nutr 1998; 51(4):279–91.
132. Khan MA, Bach A, Weary DM, et al. Invited review: transitioning from milk to solid feed in dairy heifers. J Dairy Sci 2016;99(2):885–902.
133. de Paula Vieira A, de Passillé AM, Weary DM. Effects of the early social environment on behavioral responses of dairy calves to novel events. J Dairy Sci 2012; 95(9):5149–55.
134. Nielsen PP, Jensen MB, Lidfors L. Milk allowance and weaning method affect the use of a computer controlled milk feeder and the development of cross-sucking in dairy calves. Appl Anim Behav Sci 2008;109(2–4):223–37.
135. Khan MA, Weary DM, von Keyserlingk MAG. Invited review: effects of milk ration on solid feed intake, weaning, and performance in dairy heifers. J Dairy Sci 2011;94:1071–81.

Calf Barn Design to Optimize Health and Ease of Management

Kenneth V. Nordlund, DVM[a], Courtney E. Halbach, MBA[b],*

KEYWORDS

- Calf barn • Nursing calves • Ventilation • Positive-pressure tube systems
- Individual and group housing

KEY POINTS

- Size the calf barn to accommodate calving surges and allow for an "all-in, all-out" system so that the barn can rest between uses to minimize the spread of disease.
- Natural ventilation supplemented with a positive pressure tube system improves calf health in most barn systems.
- Building features that contribute to calf health and maximize natural ventilation include drainage beneath the bedding, plenty of bedding and space, narrow barns with open sidewalls and low permanent walls, and open calf pens.

INTRODUCTION

This article describes the authors' concepts of an ideal calf barn. Our opinions are based on a variety of experiences, including clinical investigations of calf health problems and field research projects[1] conducted on dairies by the University of Wisconsin School of Veterinary Medicine, as well as dairy housing and ventilation advisory services performed by The Dairyland Initiative. We work in a continental climate in which summers are warm and winters are very cold, and that range in weather conditions has a major influence on our impression of nursery calf barn design. Although calf hutches can provide excellent housing for calves, the working conditions for calf caregivers can be miserable at times. With careful design and management, we believe that calf barns can provide an optimal environment for calves that is equivalent to that in hutches while offering superior working conditions for the caregivers.

The authors have nothing to disclose.
[a] Department of Medical Sciences, Food Animal Production Medicine, University of Wisconsin-Madison, School of Veterinary Medicine, Madison, WI, USA; [b] The Dairyland Initiative, University of Wisconsin-Madison, School of Veterinary Medicine, 2015 Linden Drive, Madison, WI 53706-1102, USA
* Corresponding author.
E-mail address: Courtney.halbach@wisc.edu

Essential features of ideal calf barns include the provision of fresh air at all times, dry and comfortable beds, opportunities for social interactions between calves, and some protection from temperatures outside of a calf's thermoneutral zone. Other features of an ideal nursery system include having enough barn capacity to avoid overstocking, limiting the age range of nursing calves within a single room or barn to a maximum of 2 to 3 weeks, and allowing time for an entire room or barn to be cleaned and let dry between uses.

Excellent calf barn design can contribute much to successful calf rearing, but consistently good results also require good maternity pen management, colostrum programs, and careful and consistent nursery care.

SIZING THE NURSERY SYSTEM

In designing nursing calf facilities, the first priority is to avoid overstocking, both to avoid the immediate adverse effects on calf health and to avoid risks to future groups of calves that may be exposed to chronic infections that began during a prior period of overstocking.

Calculating the capacity needed in a calf nursery system is complex. The first of 3 steps to calculating the size of the nursery system is to estimate the average number of calves that will enter the nursery per week based on the herd size. In this industry, there are usually more calves born per year than the number of cows in the herd due to the number of heifers freshening and cull cows leaving the herd without completing a full lactation. Typically, this number is 110% of the total herd size, including lactating and dry cows. From this number, the expected percentage of stillborn calves are subtracted. If the male calves do not enter the nursery, the total number of live calves born are multiplied by the percentage of female calves. The use of sexed semen will increase this percentage from the traditional 50% assumption. The resulting number of nursing calves can be divided by 52 weeks to estimate the average number of calves to enter the nursery per week.

The second step in sizing the nursery system is sizing to accommodate variation in calving throughout the year. Sizing the calf barn based on the assumption that calving will be uniform throughout the year can lead to significant overcrowding for 2 to 3 months of a year.[2] The simplest approach is to place a fixed number of calves per week into the nursery and sell any extras, male or female. If the dairy prefers to admit all calves born alive, it needs to build extra capacity into the nursery to accommodate the surges in numbers. Assuming a nursing barn cycle length of about 10 weeks, a cushion of about 10% will handle most calving surges. From these calculations, multiply the number of calves entering the nursery per week by 1.1 or 110%.

The third step to sizing is to determine the calf barn cycle length; this depends on several management decisions. The major item to be determined is the age at weaning, usually 7 or 8 weeks. Ideal calf nurseries will have all-in-all-out groupings in separate barns, meaning that the barns will start empty and fill over a planned period of time, preferably over a period of 3 weeks or less. Although called "all-in, all-out", a more accurate description would be "trickle-in, small groups-out". Pedersen and colleagues[3] showed that stable groups are preferable to dynamic groups because calves that were continuously introduced and removed from groups had a higher incidence of disease and lower daily gain than those housed in stable groups.

In an example situation in which each individual barn fills over a period of 3 weeks, we would add 3 weeks to the weaning age. Following weaning, many dairies may want to leave the weaned calf in place for a few days before moving to another barn, commonly 3 to 4 days. After the last calf exits the barn, the barn is cleaned and disinfected and allowed a period of time to dry or rest before another barn cycle begins. Although general recommendations for the length of the rest phase vary widely in the livestock industries, a peer-reviewed trial has not been conducted. We offer the general recommendation of 1 to 1.5 weeks, provided that the barn remains ventilated during the rest period, preferably with positive-pressure ventilation tubes. So, a 13-week barn cycle may plan for a calf to be on milk for 8 weeks with a postweaning acclimation of 0.5 weeks, and for the barn to fill in 3 weeks and be cleaned and allowed to rest for 1.5 weeks.

The "all-in, all-out" systems provide at least 2 significant health benefits. First, very young calves are not directly exposed to older calves that may be shedding infectious pathogens. Second, the ability to clean and let a barn dry out for a week between uses seems to be a powerful tool for breaking infectious disease cycles.

A less desirable approach is to have a continuous flow system in which new calves enter and weaned calves leave the barn almost every day. Continuous flow systems do not allow for facility cleaning and rest, and there is some exposure of younger calves to older calves within the same space. Although there are health disadvantages, the advantages are that the overall nursery system can be smaller and building costs will be less.

In summation, to determine the overall capacity needed for the nursery system, multiply the number of calves entering the nursery per week times the seasonal overstocking factor times the number of weeks in the nursery barn cycle. This value provides the total capacity to be accommodated in the nurseries. For "all-in, all-out" systems, this total number should be divided into a fixed number of individual barns. The optimal systems seem to have 4 or more individual calf nurseries that allow for "all-in, all-out" management.

INDIVIDUAL VERSUS PAIR VERSUS GROUP RAISING SYSTEMS

Calves raised in the North American dairy industry have typically been raised in individual pens or hutches, largely because of a perception of higher weight gains, a lower incidence of disease, and a reduction of behavioral problems such as cross-sucking.[4] However, those assumptions have been challenged and it now seems that raising nursing calves in pairs is preferable because calves raised individually tend to have poorer learning abilities, show deficient social skills, and have difficulty coping with novel situations, whereas calves raised socially have improved solid feed intakes preweaning and improved weight gains before and after weaning.[5] With equivalent growth rates through the nursing period, paired calves go through the weaning phase with less setback than calves raised alone.[5,6] Costa and colleagues[7] showed that pairs established at 6 days of age outperformed calves raised as singles and pairs established at 43 days of age, whereas Jensen and colleagues[8] found the growth rate advantage to be found in pairs over singles only at higher rates of milk feeding.

More recently, the development of automated group feeders has raised interest in housing nursing calves in larger groups. Earlier literature tended to examine relationships between group size and health,[9] whereas more recent studies have examined group size as 1 of several risk factors associated with calf health.[10] A consistent finding is that larger groupings of calves are associated with an increased risk of disease, especially respiratory disease. But grouping calves per se does not necessarily mean higher incidences of respiratory disease and diarrhea. Hänninen and colleagues[11] and Babu and colleagues[12] found that calves housed in groups had lower incidences of diarrhea and were less likely to have respiratory disease compared with individually housed calves.

Svensson and Liberg[9] recommended that group-housed calves be maintained in pens of fewer than 10 calves. In contrast, industry consultants currently suggest that excellent health and growth performance can be achieved in groups of 20 to 25; however, the maximum number would be interrelated with other on-farm management factors. There is a consensus that increasing group size presents an increased risk of calf disease and deaths. Other factors associated with the success of group housing include colostrum management, age at entry into the pen, age range within the pen, bedding and drainage, air quality and ventilation, milk quality and quantity, hygiene of feeding equipment, and disease detection and treatment practices, among others. The farm management should be confident that each of these risk factors can be managed consistently at an excellent level before constructing barns to hold 20 or more calves per pen.

STOCKING DENSITY

Stocking density is the single most important determinant of air quality in a calf barn,[13] and has a major impact on the quality and moisture of the bedded surface on which the calves lie. Based on airborne bacterial density studies,[1] we recommend that calf pens should provide a minimum of 35 ft^2 (3.3 m^2) of bedded area per calf.

Although density discussions usually focus on area, the volume of the barn is also a critical factor. In a survey of naturally ventilated calf barns in Wisconsin, the average barn volume per calf was about 1300 ft^3 (36.8 m^3), with a range of 600 to 3000 ft^3 (17–85 m^3).[1] It is our clinical opinion that if the barn volume is less than 600 ft^3 (17 m^3) per calf, efforts should be made to reduce calf density in the barn.

VENTILATION

Proper ventilation design can have a major preventive effect of minimizing calf respiratory disease. Buildings can be ventilated successfully using either natural or mechanical ventilation. However, the authors' preference is for natural ventilation supplemented with a positive-pressure tube ventilation system.

Natural Ventilation

Natural ventilation has obvious advantages in that natural forces are used to ventilate buildings, reducing costs for both fans and electrical power. Natural forces include wind moving through, against, and over buildings, as well as thermal buoyancy of warmed air rising inside of the building. Wind roses that summarize wind conditions are available for most parts of the United States, and can be accessed through the US Department of Agriculture at the following Web site: http://www.wcc.nrcs.usda. gov/ftpref/downloads/climate/windrose/. When the wind is still, naturally ventilated barns depend on thermal buoyancy and the stack effect for ventilation (**Fig. 1**). Because calves do not generate sufficient heat to effectively create thermal buoyancy, ventilation becomes insufficient.

Further limitations of natural ventilation occur when outside air is warmer than the air inside of the barn, a situation that occurs for a period of several hours almost every day as the sun warms the air outside of the barn more quickly than inside. During these periods of time, air entering the cooler interior of the barn through eaves will rise and leave the barn without good mixing near the floor.

Because of these occasional limitations with natural ventilation, we have advocated the use of positive-pressure tube ventilation systems to supplement naturally ventilated calf barns to provide the minimum ventilation rate of 4 air changes per hour. Our preference is based on the widespread success in improving calf health,[10,14]

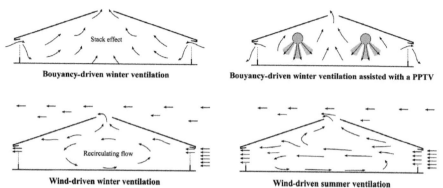

Bouyancy-driven winter ventilation

Bouyancy-driven winter ventilation assisted with a PPTV

Wind-driven winter ventilation

Wind-driven summer ventilation

Fig. 1. On still, winter days, cold air enters a naturally ventilated barn through the eaves and exits out of the ridge as it heats up. Positive-pressure tube ventilation (PPTV) systems ensure the appropriate winter ventilation rate and direct fresh air to calves year-round, especially on still days. When wind is present, wind enters through the sidewalls and mixes with the air inside of the barn before exiting through the ridge. The sidewalls should be open as much as possible to capture prevailing winds during warm weather.

and the modest installation and operating costs compared with full mechanical approaches.

Barn Requirements for Natural Ventilation

Traditional recommendations for naturally ventilated barns focus on ridge openings, eave openings, and interior roof slope for winter conditions, along with a method to open the sidewalls and having sufficient distance from obstructions to wind for warm and hot weather.

The recommended ridge opening provides a net opening of 2 in per 10 ft of building width (5 cm/3 m),[15] and it is critical for ventilation by wind and thermal buoyancy to work. Because calves are commonly housed directly beneath the ridge, the ridge openings are commonly covered. Our experience suggests that the elevated ridge cap with upstands on each side is the preferred covering to limit the amount of moisture coming into the barn. A series of cupolas on the ridge can serve the same purpose; however, they need to provide an equivalent cumulative open area to the traditional ridge opening.

The eave openings running above the long walls on both sides of the barn match the net area of the ridge opening, each providing a 1-in opening per 10 ft of building width (2.5 cm/3 m).[15] Sometimes eave openings are constructed into the building structure above the walls, whereas other times there may be a space above or between retractable curtains. If so, the curtains should be fitted with blocks to keep them open to provide the minimal opening.

The interior slope of the roof should rise toward the ridge at a minimum ratio of 1 height to 4 width.[15] With sufficient slope, warmed air will rise toward the ridge opening much like water moves downward toward a drain.

As weather warms, it is important to open sidewalls and allow winds to move directly into and through the naturally ventilated barn. To allow this, the sidewalls should be able to be opened a minimum of 50% of the sidewall area.[15] In modern barns, opening 80% of the sidewall area is preferable. The recommended total sidewall height is relative to the building width. In general, 12 ft (3.7 m) should be viewed as the minimal sidewall height for buildings less than 40 ft (12.2 m) in width, and reaching

14 ft (4.3 m) in buildings of 60 ft (18.3 m) in width or greater. The permanent foundation wall or footings beneath the curtains should be very short, limited to approximately 2 ft (61 cm) above the floor of the barn. During warm weather when the sidewall curtains are fully open, the low sidewall allows wind to move directly into the calf pens and maximize ventilation. The sidewall should be fitted with retractable curtains, preferably split so that all air does not have to enter above the top of a single curtain.

The naturally ventilated building must be spaced so that winds can enter the open sidewalls in warm weather. Barriers that block winds are called wind shadows and can include adjacent buildings, earthen banks, woodlots, and even seasonal cornfields approaching full height. (See Mario R. Mondaca's article, "Ventilation Systems for Adult Dairy Cattle," in this issue.)

Narrow Barns

The overall rule is: the narrower the barn, the better. Narrow barns are easier to ventilate by wind forces in warm weather. To maximize wind forces across the width of the barn, our preference is to limit the overall barn width to approximately 40 ft (12.2 m) or less. For barns with single or paired calf pens, optimal barns have a single row of pens. Very good performance can be achieved with 2 rows of pens. When barns get wider than 40 ft (12.2 m), natural ventilation is frequently perceived to be insufficient in warm weather.

In addition, it is easier to limit the spread of disease from calf to calf in a long, narrow barn. In single-row calf barns, new calves are placed in freshly cleaned pens, and there is usually a space between them and the oldest calves in the barn. In barns with 2 rows of pens, both rows are filled simultaneously and parallel, similar to a single-row calf barn, leaving the new arrivals in freshly cleaned pens with a few empties between them and the oldest calves about to be weaned. In barns with 3 or more rows, the situation is almost always present in which vulnerable young calves are directly across a service alley from older calves that are potentially shedding pathogens.

Supplemental Positive-Pressure Tube Systems in Naturally Ventilated Barns

Supplemental positive-pressure tubes systems are usually sized to provide the minimum of 4 changes of interior air per hour year-round (**Fig. 2**). This ventilation rate

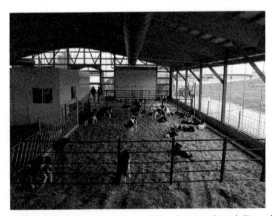

Fig. 2. A supplemental positive-pressure tube system designed to deliver the minimum year-round ventilation rate of 4 air changes per hour in a naturally ventilated calf barn.

assumes a normal stocking density and was recommended as the minimal winter ventilation rate by Bates and Anderson.[16] The tube fan runs 24 hours a day for 365 days per year. If designed properly, the tube systems will deliver fresh air without a draft into the calf's microenvironment.[17] The air introduced through the tubes is distributed around the barn and then exits passively through the typical ridge and eave openings found in naturally ventilated barns.

Typical systems are relatively inexpensive and require modest electricity for operation. For example, a tube system in a 100-ft by 35-ft (30.5-m × 10.7-m) calf nursery might require a single 20-in (51 cm) fan. Depending on what materials are chosen, the fan and tube might cost $1000 plus the design of the system, installation, and wiring bringing the total cost to approximately $2000. The 20-in (51-cm) fan may consume 500 W or 0.5 kWh of electricity, which would yield 12 kWh per day or 4380 kWh per year. If electrical costs are $0.10 per kWh, the annual electrical costs would total approximately $438 per year. These systems can operate as expected for 5 years if properly maintained.

The tubes can be made out of a variety of materials that range from very inexpensive clear polyethylene to moderate-cost woven polyethylene or vinyl, or relatively expensive polyvinyl chloride (PVC) or drainage pipe. Each material has advantages and disadvantages related to cost, durability, and flexibility in options for discharge hole sizing and location. We find the best overall value in the moderately priced woven polyethylene tubes that are supported with double-cable supports on each side of the tube. The linear cost of these tubes is between $5 and $12 per foot ($16–$40/m), depending mainly on the diameter of the tube.

Fresh, clean air is brought into the barn by a fan mounted on an exterior wall. There is typically 1 fan and tube for approximately every 40 ft (12.2 m) of building width, with the tubes running parallel to the length of the barn. Using proper tube design methods, tube systems can be installed up to approximately 250 ft (∼76.2 m) in length with uniform air distribution.[18]

The diameter of the tube relative to the capacity of the fan is critical. The tube should be sized so that the calculated velocity of air in the inlet portion of the tube is less than 1200 ft per minute (6.1 m/s),[17] and is usually larger than the diameter of the fan. When the proximal air speed is greater than this, air discharge becomes less uniform, which results in greater noise and, in more severe cases, fluttering and flapping of the tube nearest the fan, prematurely wearing out the tube.

The diameter and spacing of the holes are custom designed for each installation. The fundamental requirement is that the tube delivers fresh air to the calves without creating a draft. The technical terms are throw distance to still air. Still air is defined as air moving at a speed of less than 60 ft per minute (0.3 m/s) or less than 1 ft per second.[13] The throw distance of air from a tube is determined by the static pressure inside of the tube and by the diameter of the holes or perforations in the tube.[17] At a given static pressure, air exiting a larger diameter hole will travel further than air exiting from a smaller diameter hole.

The desired throw distance will be determined by how high the tube is located above the floor and how far to the side the air needs to travel. Our guidelines are to achieve still air at a point approximately 4 ft (1.2 m) above the floor. The location of the discharge holes is specified by clock positions such as 5:00 and 7:00, which depend on the height to the bottom of the tube from the floor, and the desired width of the throw pattern. The throw distances to desired points of still air are calculated using trigonometry, and the diameters of the discharge holes are sized based on these distances and the estimated static pressure within the tube.

These calculations require the use of fluid mechanics principles that are beyond the scope of this article. Training programs on how to design positive-pressure tube systems using the Positive-Pressure Tube Calculator spreadsheet are offered through The Dairyland Initiative.

Fully Mechanically Ventilated Nursery Calf Barns

There are situations in which natural ventilation with supplemental tubes is not feasible. Common situations include limited land area that precludes adequate spacing between barns and geographic areas with significant hours of still air during warm seasons.

A full discussion of mechanically ventilated barns is beyond the scope of this article. However, a brief summary of the authors' experiences is as follows. Usually, these barns are best designed using negative pressure ventilation calculated to provide approximately 4 air changes per hour in cold weather, 15 air changes per hour in mild spring and fall conditions, and approximately 40 air changes per hour in warm weather. Although this suggests 3 levels of ventilation, it is preferable to stage exhaust fans so that there are 5 or more incremental stages of exhaust rates.

Exhaust rates must be matched with inlets of an appropriate net area. In cold weather, it is important that the inlets are sized so that incoming air enters the space at speeds of about 400 ft/min (2 m/s).[19] This ensures sufficient mixing with the interior air. When inlet speeds are insufficient, cold air does not mix well and may fall to the floor and create severe chilling of calves below the inlets. The matching of inlet area to exhaust rates is not as critical in warm weather; however, the inlets do need to be adjusted for the increased air exchange rates.

Issues that arise in mechanically ventilated nursing calf barns include uneven air distribution throughout the barn, inlet openings and fan maintenance, and inlet location. During cold weather, inlets typically become very small to match the required exhaust fan rate and clog up with debris, limiting air distribution, whereas during warm weather, inlets may not be properly regulated, thus chilling calves during cool nights. Placing the inlets on the nursing calf side of the barn subjects the youngest calves to the freshest but coldest air. Exhausting the air out of the nursing calf side of the barn exposes the youngest calves to the oldest calves' pathogens and contaminants. Automatic controllers should be used to regulate the system based on the inside temperature of the barn.

Tempering Incoming Cold Air

In southern Wisconsin, temperatures rarely drop below −15°F (−26°C). Calf caregivers can prevent hypothermia in calves with excellent bedding management, calf jackets, and good nutrition; therefore, we have generally discouraged the use of supplemental heating because our experience has been that the power costs of heating air usually drives efforts to reduce the winter ventilation rates, which in turn results in increased respiratory disease in calves. However, our experience also suggests that Jersey calves need to be housed in more protected spaces, and there are extreme climates in which it is almost essential to add heat to support most newborn calves during the winter.

Calf barns can be heated in several ways. Although it is relatively easy to install a heating unit within a barn, we discourage their use because of the wide variation in temperature depending on proximity to the heater. Rather, we suggest adding heat to incoming air and distributing it through positive-pressure tubes.

Heat can be added using geothermal or earth tube heat exchangers in which air is warmed by drawing it through long tubes buried 7 to 10 ft (2–3 m) below the surface of the ground. The exact tempering effect is approximate and varies with soil type, depth, moisture content, soil temperature, and other factors.[20] A more common approach is the use of propane or natural gas heaters that warm the air entering a supply plenum or a warming room before entering the positive-pressure tube systems. These heating units are sized to be able to increase a specific airflow a known number of degrees.[20]

Fast-Moving Air in Summer

Very few studies have looked at the effects of heat stress on calves. Hill and colleagues[21] conducted a trial comparing cooling methods for dairy calves and found that calves cooled with fans had a lower respiration rate, improved average daily gain, and increased feed efficiency than those not cooled with fans. Although fans can work well in group housing situations, fans placed perpendicular to individual pens with solid sides will only affect a couple of calves because the solid sides act as baffles, pushing the air up and over the pens.

Although fans provide fast-moving air, they do not ventilate the barn. High, open sidewalls are meant to capture as much of the prevailing winds as possible to achieve an appropriate summer ventilation rate of 40 air changes per hour while providing fast-moving air. However, as previously mentioned, still days occur and there may be impediments to natural ventilation such as nearby buildings. The general target for air speeds to provide a cooling effect is a minimum of 200 ft per minute (1 m/s). These speeds can be achieved with positive-pressure tube systems designed to be used in warm weather, or with either cross-ventilated or tunnel-ventilated mechanical systems designed to move air at those speeds across the entire barn.

PROVIDING AN APPROPRIATE RESTING SURFACE

Deeply bedded resting surfaces are critical for very young calves in cold weather. The thermoneutral zone of newborn calves is 50° to 78°F (10°–26°C), and drops to 32° to 73°F (0°–23°C) by 1 month of age.[13] A newborn calf lying on top of a bare floor at 45°F (7°C) will lose core body temperature without some thermal support. Deep straw bedding allows the calf to build up a layer of heat within the bed and minimize heat loss. The University of Wisconsin School of Veterinary Medicine developed a scoring system called Nesting Score to evaluate the sufficiency of bedding.[1] It is a simple visual evaluation of the visibility of the rear leg of a calf lying down in the bedding. If the entire leg is visible, it is scored as Nesting Score 1 (**Fig. 3**). If the leg is partially

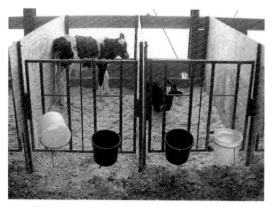

Fig. 3. Nesting Score 1: the entire leg is visible.

obscured by loose bedding, it is Nesting Score 2 (**Fig. 4**). If the rear leg is completely obscured by bedding, it is Nesting Score 3, the desired Nesting Score for cold weather (**Fig. 5**). Calf jackets, which are equivalent to 1 unit of Nesting Score, are often used to provide additional warmth. So, the provision of deep bedding or moderate bedding plus calf blankets are important factors in preventing respiratory disease in calves during cold weather.

Straw bedding is the preferred bedding material for calves; however, it is expensive in some locations. Some dairy operators have successfully used copious quantities of bedding in calf nurseries and find the bedding to be relatively clean after use in the nursery, and subsequently reuse the bedding in growing or yearling heifer barns.

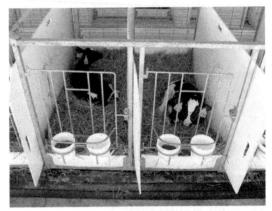

Fig. 4. Nesting Score 2: the rear leg is partially obscured by loose bedding.

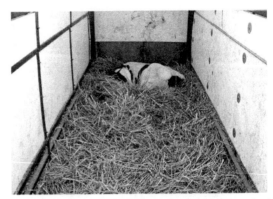

Fig. 5. Nesting Score 3: the rear leg is completely obscured by deep bedding.

Drainage Below the Bedding

To maintain a deeply bedded surface, it is critical that the pen has good drainage so that urine, spilled milk, and water can move out of the pen rather than soak the bedding. Excellent drainage has been achieved using a tiled gravel bed approximately 1.5-ft (0.5-m) deep below the bedded area. The area should be fitted with drainage tiles leading to a collection area outside of the calf barn. With this base, operators typically report that the straw usage to maintain an equivalent bed is half that used to maintain beds over a concrete surface. The tile is covered with gravel and bedding

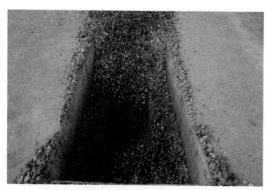

Fig. 6. The drain tile is covered with pea-size gravel and drains to a collection area outside of the calf barn.

is applied on top of the gravel (**Fig. 6**). Sand should not be used in place of gravel because straw bedding becomes churned into the sand as calves walk on the surface. To avoid skid loaders getting stuck, a larger rock gravel can be laid down. Otherwise, a gently sloped concrete floor with a slope of at least 2% that leads to 1 or more drainage channels of 1 to 3 ft (31–91 cm) in width allows skid loaders to ride over the strips of concrete.

Concerns are sometimes raised about the difficulties or impossibility of disinfecting gravel drain areas, particularly with enteric disease such as salmonella. Our experience has been mixed in that several dairies have operated gravel drains for more than a decade without clinical problems, whereas others have had enteric disease problems. To the authors' knowledge, none of the enteric disease problems have been definitively linked to the gravel.

If the surface below the bedding must be solid concrete, 3 issues need to be addressed through floor slopes. First, the floor needs to be sloped to move liquids out of the pen as efficiently as possible with a minimum of a 2% slope, equivalent to 2.4 in (6 cm) per 10 ft (3 m). Second, liquids moved from the pen should not move into an area exposed to the foot traffic of the calf caregiver. Third, the slope needs to prevent water used in service alleys from draining into the pen and bedding. This can be accomplished with a crowned central work alley and a gutter at the immediate front of the calf pen. The pen itself can be sloped toward the front of the pen or, preferably, sloped to the back of the pen with a second drainage gutter at the rear (**Fig. 7**). Drainage gutters should be designed to carry liquids to collection points outside of the building.

In-Floor Heat

In-floor heat is sometimes provided by pumping warmed water through pipes buried in concrete beneath bedded areas or through pipes that form a grid on which the calves lie. Although these techniques can provide some relief in cold weather, both approaches bring some negative attributes. Heating the floor beneath bedding increases the ammonia concentrations in the air around the calf. Ammonia volatility is very temperature-dependent with almost no release from manure at 32°F (0°C), but substantial volatility by 55°F (13°C) and higher.[22] Second, in-floor heat is usually installed in solid floors, which excludes the possibility of drainage immediately beneath the bedding, resulting in higher-moisture beds. For these reasons, we have generally

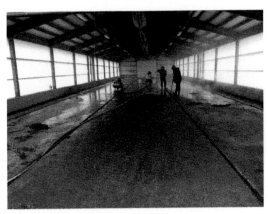

Fig. 7. A 2-row calf barn with a crowned central alley and concrete sloped to a drainage gutter in the back of the pen.

discouraged installation of in-floor heat beneath the calf bedding. However, it is a useful technique in the service alleys and immediately around water fountains to prevent ice accumulation in freezing conditions.

FEED AND WATER ACCESS

Newborn calves should have easy access to fresh, clean, warm water starting at day 1 with access to a palatable starter grain within a couple of days of birth. In group pens, all calves should be able to eat at the same time to ensure that the smallest, most timid calves have the same access to feed as the larger, more high-ranking calves in the group.

The feeding area must be of an appropriate throat and table height for the size of the calves using it. For calves less than approximately 2 months of age, provide 12 in (31 cm) of feeding space per calf, limit the feed manger floor height above the feed alley floor to 4 in (10 cm), and set the throat height to 13 in (33 cm) above the feed alley floor.[23–25] Dividers along the feed area deter socially dominant calves from pushing subordinate calves away from the feed, whereas slat-bar feed fences allow for the use of a taller neck rail to avoid potential injuries from calves reaching for feed. The neck rail height in a slat-bar feed system should be placed 30 in (76 cm) above the feed alley floor.[25] Post-and-rail feed barriers should not be used in nursing calf pens but rather reserved for older heifers greater than 8 months of age.

A minimum of 1 waterer per pen that provides 2 in (5 cm) of accessible water trough per calf is a necessity. Each waterer should not be too tall or placed in the feed table because small calves may have difficulty reaching them. Waterers placed in the bedded pack area should allow access from only 1 side to reduce the spoilage of bedding (**Fig. 8**).

FEATURES SPECIFIC TO CALF BARNS WITH INDIVIDUAL OR PAIR PENS

Calf barns with individual calf pens have some special characteristics for optimal calf health and comfort. These features include an east-west orientation, barns with 1 or 2 rows of pens, solid panels between every other calf, and a walkway between the pens and the outside wall.

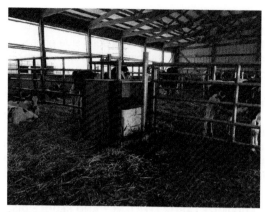

Fig. 8. A concrete barrier limits access to the waterer from the feed alley only, reducing spoilage of bedding.

East-West Orientation

In large group pens, the calves can move to shaded areas during midafternoon to late afternoon. In contrast, a calf confined to a pen near an outside wall may be unable to find shade when the sun is relatively low in the afternoon sky. Therefore, it is important to orient barns with individual calf pens in an east-west orientation.

Separation of Individual Calf Pens from Outside Walls

Individual calf pens should be separated 3 ft (0.9 m) from the outside wall. When the temperature inside of the barn is warmer than the outside temperature, outside air entering through the eaves will fall at relatively high draft speeds into calf pens adjacent to the outside walls. Because of this phenomenon, it has been a common practice in cold climates to place a cover over individual calf pens during the winter. However, a field study showed that a pen cover was associated with tremendous increases in total airborne bacteria counts, which was a risk factor for respiratory disease.[1] Although a cover can eliminate the draft, it also ensures that the air quality in the pen will become very poor. Neither the draft nor the cover is desirable.

The optimal solution is to separate the pen from the outside wall with a 3-ft (0.9-m) wide walkway. There should be a solid vertical rear panel about 20 to 24 in (51–61 cm) high between the calf and the outside walkway. Cold air can fall over the curtain and into the walkway without chilling the calf. If the outside walkway is impossible to install, an acceptable solution is to close the eave on the windward side of the barn and install a well-designed positive-pressure tube system that delivers 4 air changes per hour on a nonstop basis. The pens will be ventilated sufficiently by the tube system, and the curtain sidewall can be opened slightly for natural ventilation when the extreme conditions have passed.

Solid Side Panels with Front and Rear Mesh Panels

In the field trial conducted by Lago and colleagues,[1] the prevalence of respiratory disease was reduced with lower airborne bacterial counts in the pens by greater depth of loose bedding and the presence of a solid panel between each calf. However, the solid panels between each calf tended to increase the airborne bacterial counts; a confounding finding. Because of this finding, we have recommended solid panels between each calf or every other calf, and the use of positive-pressure tube systems to deliver fresh air between the solid panels.

The optimal individual or paired calf pen has solid side panels with relatively open mesh to the front and rear. The rear panel can have an open mesh on the upper portion with a solid base panel to a height of 2 ft (61 cm) because it provides a solid barrier that the calf may nest against during cold weather.

With the open front and rear panel, there is greater opportunity for breezes to move through the pens in warm weather when the sidewall curtains are open (**Fig. 9**). Solid panels on all sides of a calf pen create extreme impediments to natural ventilation. We have done investigative work in open-sided calf barns with positive-pressure tube systems during the summer in which solid panels on all sides of the calf pen prevented prevailing winds from ventilating the pen.

BARN LAYOUT TO MAXIMIZE LABOR EFFICIENCY AND REDUCE DISEASE TRANSMISSION

Comfort considerations for calf caregivers are among the primary reasons to construct barns for calves. Barns can be designed to make work more convenient while minimizing the risk of workers transmitting disease between calves or groups of calves. Rooms for milk preparation, equipment cleaning, record keeping, and other tasks should be temperature controlled to provide comfort for the caregivers. Work rooms and the calf area need to be well-lit so that caregivers can clearly see their tasks. Using general guidelines for milking centers,[26] the milk preparation and bottle cleaning room should have an illumination level of 100-ft candles (1076 lumen/m^2) and the calf housing area should be at least 20-ft candles (215 lumen/m^2).

To avoid the potential of footwear becoming fomites for disease transmission, it is important that solid floors do not drain into areas trafficked by the caregivers. If separate rooms or barns are used for "all-in, all-out" systems, entrance sites can be limited and fitted with disinfectant footbaths (**Fig. 10**).

The nursery should also be designed so that caregivers can easily restrain calves for examination and potential treatment. Although easily done in single or paired calf pens, a swing-gate that allows 1 person to catch and restrain a calf in a large group makes the restraining process easier. Having a scale to weigh calves allows calf performance to be monitored accurately.

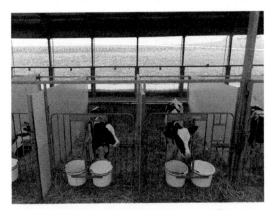

Fig. 9. Solid barriers between individual calf pens limit contact between calves, and an open front and back allow air to flow through the pen.

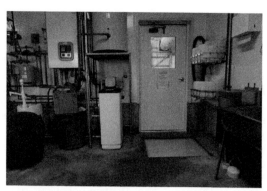

Fig. 10. Caregivers pass through a footbath before entering an "all-in, all-out" pen to reduce disease transmission between pens.

SUMMARY

Over the past decade, our experiences have shown us that calf barns designed and constructed using the techniques described in this article can produce calves as healthy as those raised outside in hutches, while improving the working conditions of calf caregivers. Although there are multiple other management factors that contribute to calf health, the authors believe that a well-designed calf barn sets management up for success and provides calves with an optimal start to life.

REFERENCES

1. Lago A, McGuirk SM, Bennett TB, et al. Calf respiratory disease and pen micro-environments in naturally ventilated calf barns in winter. J Dairy Sci 2006. https://doi.org/10.3168/jds.S0022-0302(06)72445-6.

2. Natural Resource A. dairy housing and equipment systems: managing and planning for profitability: proceedings from the dairy housing and equipment systems: managing and planning for profitability Conference. Camp Hill, PA. Ithaca, NY, February 1–3, 2000. Natural Resource, Agriculture, and Engineering Service, Cooperative Extension; 2000. Available at: http://www.worldcat.org/title/dairy-housing-and-equipment-systems-managing-and-planning-for-profitability-proceedings-from-the-dairy-housing-and-equipment-systems-managing-and-planning-for-profitability-conference-february-1-3-2000-camp-hill-pennsylvania/oclc/42968058. Accessed August 27, 2018.

3. Pedersen RE, Sørensen JT, Skjøth F, et al. How milk-fed dairy calves perform in stable versus dynamic groups. Livest Sci 2009;121(2–3):215–8.

4. Chua B, Coenen E, van Delen J, et al. Effects of pair versus individual housing on the behavior and performance of dairy calves. J Dairy Sci 2002. https://doi.org/10.3168/jds.S0022-0302(02)74082-4.

5. Costa JHC, von Keyserlingk MAG, Weary DM. Invited review: effects of group housing of dairy calves on behavior, cognition, performance, and health. J Dairy Sci 2016. https://doi.org/10.3168/jds.2015-10144.

6. De Paula Vieira A, von Keyserlingk MAG, Weary DM. Effects of pair versus single housing on performance and behavior of dairy calves before and after weaning from milk. J Dairy Sci 2010. https://doi.org/10.3168/jds.2009-2516.

7. Costa JHC, Meagher RK, von Keyserlingk MAG, et al. Early pair housing increases solid feed intake and weight gains in dairy calves. J Dairy Sci 2015. https://doi.org/10.3168/jds.2015-9395.

8. Jensen MB, Duve LR, Weary DM. Pair housing and enhanced milk allowance increase play behavior and improve performance in dairy calves. J Dairy Sci 2015. https://doi.org/10.3168/jds.2014-8272.

9. Svensson C, Liberg P. The effect of group size on health and growth rate of Swedish dairy calves housed in pens with automatic milk-feeders. Prev Vet Med 2006. https://doi.org/10.1016/j.prevetmed.2005.08.021.

10. Jorgensen MW, Adams-Progar A, de Passillé AM, et al. Factors associated with dairy calf health in automated feeding systems in the Upper Midwest United States. J Dairy Sci 2017. https://doi.org/10.3168/jds.2016-12501.

11. Hänninen L, Hepola H, Rushen J, et al. Resting behaviour, growth and diarrhoea incidence rate of young dairy calves housed individually or in groups in warm or cold buildings. Acta Agric Scand Sect A — Anim Sci 2003;53(1):21–8.

12. Babu LK, Pandey H, Patra RC, et al. Hemato-biochemical changes, disease incidence and live weight gain in individual versus group reared calves fed on different levels of milk and skim milk. Anim Sci J 2009;80(2):149–56. https://doi.org/10.1111/j.1740-0929.2008.00620.x.

13. Wathes CM, Jones CD, Webster AJ. Ventilation, air hygiene and animal health. Vet Rec 1983;113(24):554–9. Available at: http://www.ncbi.nlm.nih.gov/pubmed/6670178. Accessed August 27, 2018.

14. Endres MI. 74 automated milk feeders for preweaned dairy calves in the Upper Midwest United States. J Anim Sci 2018;96(suppl_2):38–9.

15. Midwest Plan Service, Ventilation Subcommittee. Natural ventilating systems for livestock housing. Ames (IA): Midwest Plan Service; 1989. Available at: https://www-mwps.sws.iastate.edu/catalog/ventilation-livestock-housing/natural-ventilating-systems-livestock-housing. Accessed August 24, 2018.

16. Bates DW, Anderson JF. Calculation of ventilation needs for confined cattle. J Am Vet Med Assoc 1979;174(6):581–9. Available at: http://www.ncbi.nlm.nih.gov/pubmed/422460. Accessed August 27, 2018.

17. Nordlund KV. Practical considerations for ventilating calf barns in winter. Vet Clin North Am Food Anim Pract 2008. https://doi.org/10.1016/j.cvfa.2007.10.006.

18. Wells CM, Amos ND. Design of air distribution systems for closed greenhouses. Acta Hortic 1994;(361):93–104.

19. Midwest Plan Service, Ventilation Subcommittee. Mechanical ventilating systems for livestock housing. Ames (IA): The Service; 1990. Available at: https://www-mwps.sws.iastate.edu/catalog/ventilation-livestock/mechanical-ventilating-systems-livestock-housing. Accessed August 24, 2018.

20. Midwest Plan Service, Ventilation Subcommittee. Heating, cooling, and tempering air for livestock housing. Ames (IA): Midwest Plan Service; 1990. Available at: https://www-mwps.sws.iastate.edu/catalog/ventilation-livestock-housing/heating-cooling-and-tempering-air-livestock-housing. Accessed August 24, 2018.

21. Hill TM, Bateman HG, Aldrich JM, et al. Comparisons of housing, bedding, and cooling options for dairy calves. J Dairy Sci 2011;94(4):2138–46.

22. Sommer SG, Olesen JE, Christensen BT. Effects of temperature, wind speed and air humidity on ammonia volatilization from surface applied cattle slurry. J Agric Sci 1991;117(01):91.

23. Holmes BJ, Midwest Plan Service. Dairy freestall housing and equipment. Ames (IA): Midwest Plan Service; 2013. Available at: https://www-mwps.

sws.iastate.edu/catalog/livestock/dairy/dairy-freestall-housing-and-equipment. Accessed August 24, 2018.

24. OmslagEXTRAp. The Danish agricultural advisory center Danish recommendations housing design for cattle. 2002. Available at: www.lr.dk. Accessed August 22, 2018.

25. Pennsylvania State University, Agricultural Extension Service. Special circular - Pennsylvania state university, college of agriculture, agricultural extension service. State College (PA): Pennsylvania State University, College of Agriculture Extension Service; 1948. Available at: https://books.google.com/books?id=hFouWd31dN4C.

26. Chastain JP. Lighting requirements for the milking center. Milking Centre Design, Proceedings from the National Milking Centre Design Conference (NRAES-66). Harrisburg, PA, November 17–19, 1992.

Lying Time and Its Importance to the Dairy Cow
Impact of Stocking Density and Time Budget Stresses

Peter D. Krawczel, PhD[a],*, Amanda R. Lee, MS[b]

KEYWORDS

- Stocking density • Behavior • Lying time • Aggression • Time budget

KEY POINTS

- Lying time, regardless of lactation stage, is the behavior that is most consistently reduced by increased stocking density.
- Increased stocking density leads to increased social stress, which is most evident from the increases in aggression commonly observed.
- Understanding how stocking density interacts with other stressors and the role of sleep within a cow's time budget represent the next key areas to evaluation to establish the full effects of overstocking dairy cows' housing facilities.

INTRODUCTION

Increasing stocking density is a common management practice implemented to produce more milk and increase farm profitability. Overstocking of freestall barns can be defined as housing more cows within a pen than the available number of stalls and (or) providing less than the recommended 0.6 m of linear feeding space per cow.[1] Ideal stocking density in freestalls can be defined as 1 cow per freestall and 1 feed bunk spot, with the extent that overstocking is possibly driven by a variety of factors,

Disclosure Statement: The authors have no commercial or financial conflicts of interest with the presented materials. Authors have received funding support from the USDA-ARS-NIFA (United States Department of Agriculture-Agricultural Research Service-National Institute of Food and Agriculture), USDA-ARS-OREI (United States Department of Agriculture-Agricultural Research Service-Organic Agriculture Research and Extension Initiative), and USDA (United States Department of Agriculture) Hatch funds.

a Department of Animal Science, The University of Tennessee, 258 Brehm Animal Science, Knoxville, TN 37996, USA; b Department of Animal Science, The University of Tennessee, 363 Brehm Animal Science, Knoxville, TN 37996, USA
* Corresponding author.
E-mail address: krawczel@utk.edu

including the design and management of the resting space, stage of lactation, formulation of the diet, and environmental factors. In open systems, including compost bedded pack barns, bedded packs, and pastures, the total lying space and feeding space per cow must be factored in. Overstocking, in either system, can inhibit a cow's ability to spend sufficient time doing necessary tasks for maintenance, milk production, and reproductive success.[2]

Implementing elevated stocking density, greater than 100%, has become common to promote increased milk promotion and meet profitability demands. Data collected through the US Department of Agriculture National Animal Health Monitoring System effort reported that 30.4% of US dairy producers overstock their cows at greater than or equal to 110%, with more than 57% of cows overstocked at feeding locations.[3] Maximum stocking density greater than or equal to 110% was reported among 48.5% of herds, suggesting an increasing prevalence, despite potential cow comfort and welfare concerns.[3] Additionally, in a 2012 study, overstocking had an impact on more than 60% of cows within the Northeast United States and Canada.[4] Charlton and colleagues,[5] however, observed that 60% of herds within Canada are housed at less than or equal to 100%, with only 7% stocked at greater than 120%. This variation suggests that stocking density may vary greatly with season, housing environment, and region.

Overstocking decreases cows' ability to spend sufficient time lying, eating, and socializing. Cows allocated more relative time to lying down, suggesting cows place greater priority on meeting lying needs, especially when provided a comfortable environment.[6–8] Furthermore, inability to meet needed lying time has been associated with a greater risk of lameness,[9] reduced growth hormone,[10] and behavioral and physiologic stress responses,[8,11,12] indicating poor biological function. Cows under lying deprivation stomped their legs, repositioned, weight shifted, displayed more restless behaviors, and exhibited more oral stimulation time and frequency than nonlying deprived cows,[8,11] suggesting negative affective state welfare concerns. Therefore, managing stocking density effectively is critical for maintaining milk production, health, and welfare.

DEFINING THE TIME BUDGET

The behavior of dairy cows is dependent on the interaction between the cows and their physical environment. In the big picture, the physical factors of the facility (stall design, flooring type, feed bunk design, and environmental quality) impose baseline limitations on how the cows interact with the housing conditions. Within these limitations, the ability of cows to engage in natural behaviors is further dictated by management routines, such as grouping strategy and stocking density. In general, cows need 12 hours to 14 hours of resting time and 3 hours to 5 hours of feeding time per day (**Table 1**). These time budget requirements constitute 60% to 80% of a 24-hour period, which leaves a limited number of hours for milking and other management procedures. Although there is variation among herds, cows that spend approximately 49% of their time lying and 18% of their time eating may have a greater capacity to maximize individual milk production.[13]

RATIONALE FOR OVERSTOCKING HOUSING FACILITIES

Producer profitability is likely the primary driving force for many management decisions, and stocking density is one of these decisions heavily driven by economic considerations.[14] De Vries and colleagues,[15] reported stocking densities between 110% and 150% can be more profitable when milk sales, after feed cost per cow, results in net gains. When milk loss exceeded 1.0 kg per cow per day and milk price per kg was $0.40 to $0.50, however, there was decreased profit of $8 to $439 per stall per year.[15]

Table 1	
Typical behavioral time budget for lactating dairy cow	
Behavior	**Range of Hours Commonly Devoted Daily to Each Behavior**
Feeding	3–5 (split among 9–14 meals per d)
Lying	10–14
Social interactions	2–3
Ruminating	7–10
Drinking	0.5

General time budget only provides a few hours for management practices to be conducted before they become limiting of key behaviors.

From Grant R. Taking advantage of natural behavior improves dairy cow performance. Proc. Western Dairy Management Conf. Reno, NV. March 7–9, 2007. p. 225; with permission.

Milk price variability can be unpredictable,[14] suggesting that overstocking may be profitable at high milk prices but not at lower milk prices. Other considerations, including feed, labor, replacement, culling, and land, are critical for accurately assessing overstocking costs. Therefore, economic gains associated with varying stocking density may be more attributed to additional and combined management decisions, rather than overstocking alone. Furthermore, overstocking might not produce the economic gain that is often attributed to it, because the milk loss associated with stall availability can exceed 1.0 kg/d.[2]

WHAT ARE THE CURRENT RECOMMENDATIONS FOR STOCKING DENSITY?

Neither the Canadian Code of Practice for the Care and Handling of Dairy Cattle[16,17] nor the Farmers Assuring Responsible Management program manual (www.nationaldairyfarm.com) provides clear recommendations for space requirements of lactating dairy cows. The most specific best practice can be found for postfresh cows, which recommends the provision of 76 cm of feeding space and at least 1 free-stall per cow (100% stocking density as the maximum). Within maternity pens, the Code of Practice recommends providing 15 m^2 of resting space. The main recommendations in the Canadian Code of Practice[16] for space allowances, across all stages of the lactation cycle, are

Stocking density must not exceed 1.2 cows per stall in a freestall system.

Resting areas must provide 120 ft^2 (11 m^2) per mature cow in bedded pack pens.

Adequate linear feed bunk space must be provided to meet the animals' nutritional needs.

For lactating cows outside the immediate postpartum period, the targeted stocking density should be

- One stall per cow in freestall housing is recommended; a maximum of 120% can likely be imposed depending on freestall design, maintenance, and cattle flow through the milking parlor.
- Ten m^2 within loose housing systems; more space may be required if housed on a compost bedded pack to ensure proper function of the bedding system

- One headlock or 60 cm of linear bunk space; headlocks provide a level of protection and are recommended.

The extent that housing systems can be overstocked relies on maintaining cows' ability to meet their time budget requirements. The effects of overstocking on health and productivity are discussed later as they pertain to the resting behavior of the cow. The impact of overstocking at the feed bunk is further discussed in Trevor J. DeVries' article, "Feeding Behavior, Feed Space, and Bunk Design and Management for Adult Dairy Cattle," in this issue.

STOCKING DENSITY ALTERS LYING BEHAVIOR IN FREESTALL SYSTEMS

More than 50% of dairy operations within the United States house their cows entirely indoors, with approximately 20% housed exclusively in freestalls.[18,3] Across multiple studies analyzing short-term overstocking, greater than 113% to 130% overstocking was implemented before behavioral changes occurred.[19-21] Cows stocked at more than 100%, however, were less likely to average at least 12 h/d of lying.[5] Stocking densities of 142% to 150% can reduce lying times by an hour or more, relative to housing the same cows under the same conditions at 100% (or 1 cow per freestall[20,22]). Cows' latency to lay was 13 minutes per opportunity postmilking less when at 150% stocking density,[23] suggesting that the cows might be shifting their behavior away from feeding after milking to lying as a means to guard a key resource. This shift likely increases their risk of mastitis by lying down before teat canals have time to completely close after milking. Cows were initially lying less than 30 minutes after returning to the pen from milking,[23] and overstocked cows spent less time standing within the stall than cows stocked at less than or equal to 100% stocking density.[13,19,23] This suggests that, due to the priority giving to lying by dairy cows, overstocking drives this behavioral drive to maintain use of a key resource by occupying a stall sooner after milking than those in noncompetitive environments and lie down more readily within a stall. Collectively, this may lead to increased risk for environmental mastitis, if the teat end has not had sufficient time to reseal after milking.

The provision of pasture can be an effective means to minimize the negative effects on lying behaviors of increased stocking density within freestall systems. Falk and colleagues[24] reported cow lying time did not change with decreased stall number as long as pasture access was allowed. When given access to both pasture and indoor housing, cows spent a mean of 13.0 h/d on pasture, with 69.4% of lying time on pasture, compared with indoor facilities.[25] When allowed choice, cows spent a majority of their time lying outside rather than in confinement and 54% to 58% of their total time on pasture.[25,26] Legrand and colleagues[25] reported that cows limited to indoor housing spent 1.6 hours per day more lying than when confined to pasture housing, without variation in lying bouts.

Overstocking freestall pens may also alter the diurnal patterns of lying. Increased stocking density increased the overall percentage of cows standing idly waiting for access to freestalls.[19] This effect was most evident between midnight and 4:00 AM; the time period when cows were motivated to lie down. There is a potential for cows to spend more time waiting for a stall to become available than engaging in feeding over the course of a day. Finally, depriving cows of lying for a limited period (2–4 hours), which are similar to those reported in trials evaluating stocking density, resulted in cows attempting to recoup the lost resting time for the next 40 hours.[11] Routine management practices, such as herd health checks or freestall maintenance, could be sufficient to deprive cows of lying for this duration of time.

EFFECT OF STOCKING DENSITY ON FEEDING BEHAVIOR

The impact of stocking density on feeding behavior has been variable across studies. For example, Huzzey and colleagues[27] observed curvilinear decrease in feeding time as feeding space decreased from 81 cm to 21 cm per cow, whereas among cows provided 100 cm per cow at the feed bunk, daily mealtime and feeding activity were 10% and 14% greater, respectively, than when the cows were provided only 50 cm per cow at the feed bunk.[28] Additionally, cows at 50 cm per cow stocking density decreased feeding activity by 24% during the 90 minutes after feed delivery compared with 100 cm per cow stocking density.[28] With a feed bunk fitted with headlocks (which were 60 cm wide), cows at 142% stocking density, denied access to freestalls and headlocks concurrently, decreased feeding time by 0.4 h/d.[21] In other headlock-based feed bunk studies, however, mean feeding time was between 3.7 h/d and 4.4 h/d and was unaffected by stocking density.[20,29] An important distinction to make between these studies is that trials observing a negative effect of overstocking on feeding behavior did not reduce lying space within the pen,[27,28] whereas those that did not report a negative effect on feeding behavior decreased lying space at the same rate that feeding space was reduced.[20,29] This suggests that there is likely a dynamic relationship between the stocking densities of these 2 resources that requires further examination.

EFFECT OF STOCKING DENSITY ON AGGRESSION

In addition to altering lying behavior and, potentially, feeding behaviors, overstocking can cause social stress as evident in aggression at the feed bunk and displacements. Social dominance refers to a dominant animal forcibly removing a subordinate animal from a feeding, lying, drinking, or standing location.[30] This removal occurs predominantly through displacement, in which a cow uses her head or body, via physical contact against a subsequent cow's body, to remove the secondary cow's head or body from a freestall or feed space.[31,32]

Aggressive behaviors related to feed bunk usage increase among overstocked cows.[27] Cows stocked at 120%, 133%, and 150% had more aggressive behaviors per hour than cows stocked at 100% and 109%.[23] Aggression at the feed bunk during 2 hours postfeeding linearly increased with increasing stocking density[20] whereas stocking the feed bunk at 100 cm per cow versus 50 cm per cow reduced displacements by 0.9 per 90-minute observation period.[28] Further decreasing stocking density to 25% did not alter feed bunk aggression or displacements compared with 100%.[22] When housed within freestalls with high stocking density (113%) and low stocking density (67%), cows at the higher stocking density had 0.4 more agonistic interactions per hour than cows at lower stocking densities,[33] whereas in another study, freestall displacements per 24 hours increased numerically by 2.3 as stocking density increased from 75% to 150%.[22]

STOCKING DENSITY IN BEDDED PACKS

Despite the recent interest in compost bedded systems, this was the primary housing system for lactating cows (4.3% of operations) or dry cows (3.6% of operations) on a relatively small number of overall farms.[18] Bewley and colleagues[34,35] reported that the correct amount of space within a compost bedded pack barn is 10 m² per cow for cows producing less than or equal to 50 lb (23 kg) per day. For each 25-lb (11 kg) per day milk production increase, cows should be given an additional 0.9 m².[34] When dealing with ill or lame cows, 12 m² per cow should be provided.[34]

Observed mean stocking rates across multiple studies ranged between 7.4 m² and 9.0 m² ± 2.2 m²,[36–38] somewhat less than the space recommended. A clear recommendation is difficult to make for compost bedded systems, because the space required per cow beyond the minimum needed for comfortably lying is highly dependent on the amount of moisture coming into the system, frequency of bedding, and other associated factors. For noncomposted bedded packs, there is a general recommendation for 11 m² per cow. Fregonesi and Leaver[33] showed that among 6 cows stocked in 2 straw yard housing areas at 27 m² (4.5 m² of lying space per cow; high stocking density) and 54 m² (9 m² of lying space per cow; low stocking density), there were no differences in rumination, feeding, lying, and standing on bed time. As compost bedded pack barns increase in prevalence, more research must be conducted to evaluate the effects of stocking density within this housing system.

EFFECT OF STOCKING DENSITY ON AUTOMATIC MILKING SYSTEMS

As automatic milking systems (AMSs) become more popular, determining proper stocking density will be critical. Deming and colleagues[39] observed mean stocking density among 13 herds in Ontario, Canada, was 55 cows per AMS, with a freestall stocking density of 90%. Unlike traditional systems, in which all cows are milked twice or thrice daily, AMSs may reduce the number of milkings per cow by providing an alternative source for competition.[40] Cows stocked at 150% were displaced more at the freestalls and feed bunk than those housed at 100% and 120%.[41] Similar trends were observed in lying and standing behavior among cows housed at 150% compared with those milked in a traditional parlor.[21,41] Rumination time among cows at 150% was significantly lower, however, than in those housed at 100% and 120%.[41] Establishing a recommendation for overall stocking density within AMS needs to consider the target number of milkings per day per cow, efficiency of cows moving through the milking unit, and traffic flow to ensure that cows can achieve their time budgeting needs while maintaining their productivity.

POTENTIAL EFFECTS OF STOCKING DENSITY ON PRODUCTION AND HEALTH

The reduction of resting time by overcrowding is the most likely explanation of the reduction in performance associated with decreasing stall availability,[2] because cows prioritize rest over other behaviors when resources are limited.[7] This was evident from the behavioral response of cows when housed with diminishing access to resources. The portion of time spent lying increased in an effort to maintain a consistent number of hours of rest whereas feeding and socialization were decreased. In conjunction with reduced productivity, cows may be more at risk for reduced milk quality. Udder hygiene was not affected by increasing stocking density from 100% to 142%.[20,21] At day 14, however, cows stocked at 131% and 142% had increased leg hygiene scores, suggesting overstocking can have negative effects.[20] Additionally, Fregonesi and Leaver[33] reported cows housed with low space allowance had a poorer cleanliness score than those housed with high space allowance on a bedded pack.

Beyond the effects on production, there are several important health-related factors that are detrimentally altered by reduced lying time. First, the predominance of concrete flooring results in a greater strain on the hoof when cows are forced to stand for extended periods of time.[42] The negative impact of the standing time is further worsened from the softening of the hoof by the manure slurry covering the alleyways, which leads to an increased probability of infectious hoof disease.[43] Increased stocking density has also been associated with increased risk of lameness,[44] possibly attributed to decreased lying time.[20] Second, a stress response was evident in the concentration of cortisol in cows subjected to deprivation of lying[12] relative to control cows with unrestricted ability to lie down. Third, increased lying time also has a potential benefit for fetal growth, because significantly more blood flowed to the gravid uterine horn when cows were lying relative to when they were standing during several stages throughout the gestation period.[45]

CONSIDERATIONS REGARDING STOCKING DENSITY OF TRANSITION COWS

Stocking density during the transition period can be a critical factor determining whether or not a cow obtains sufficient intake and an adequate space at calving, which can affect production, behavior, stress response, and health.[46,47] During the late dry period, adequate space has been associated with increased milk production and lower somatic cell count.[48,49] As prefresh stocking density in a freestall pen increased by 10%, above 80%, milk production decreased by 0.7 kg/d.[49] Overstocking may have different impacts, however, based on environment and feeding system. For example, Proudfoot and colleagues[50] observed cows stocked at 100% on an individual feeder versus those stocked at 150% did not differ in milk production. Although ensuring sufficient lying and eating space may decrease the likelihood of postpartum metabolic disease and milk production losses, environmental and housing factors may play a substantial role in understanding the effects of overstocking.

EFFECT OF STOCKING DENSITY ON THE LYING BEHAVIOR OF TRANSITION COWS

Lying time varies as cows approach calving day,[51] regardless of stocking density. Cows at 80% stocking density in freestalls spent more time lying on days 0, 5, and 7 before calving compared with cows stocked at 100%.[52] Proudfoot and colleagues[50] observed that multiparous cows in a competitive feeding environment spent 150 min/d less lying than cows feeding in a noncompetitive manner. These investigators noted that multiparous cows in competition for feeding space spent more time standing during the week before calving, 1 week prepartum, and 2.8 hours more during week 1 postpartum.[50]

EFFECT OF STOCKING DENSITY ON THE FEEDING BEHAVIOR OF TRANSITION COWS

Understanding stocking density's relationship with feed bunk usage is important for providing adequate feed bunk space for sufficient dry matter intake and reduced aggression, particularly during the transition period. Prepartum mean meal time was 10 minutes per meal longer than postpartum,[27] suggesting prepartum cows may need longer to break down a typical dry cow ration targeted at promoting rumen fill. Yet, among dry multiparous cows fed fresh feed once daily, only 65% to 69% visited the feed bunk at the time feed was delivered.[53] Additionally, Huzzey and colleagues,[54,55] observed cows stocked at 150% in the freestalls and at the feed bunk took 30 minutes longer to approach the feed bunk after fresh feed delivery compared with those stocked at 100%. Cows not able to eat freshly delivered feed ate 14% less, leading to decreased dry matter intake and increased disease incidence postpartum.[1,47] Providing sufficient feed bunk space is necessary for allowing cows to eat longer and receive fresh feed immediately after delivery.

Across multiple studies, there is a strange dynamic with dry matter intake and stocking density. Prepartum cows in overstocked pens consistently consumed more feed per head than those at 100% stocking density. Dry matter intake was 1 kg/cow/d more among cows stocked at 150% than those at 100% stocking density,[54,55] suggesting a greater feeding rate and potential for slug feeding and ruminal digestion problems.[56] Feed consumption per cow stocked at 4 cows per individual feeder was 25% more than calculated requirements.[57,58] These cows also spent 4% less time eating.[57]

EFFECT OF STOCKING DENSITY ON THE SOCIAL AGGRESSION OF TRANSITION COWS

Stocking density should be evaluated as a means of reducing negative social interactions between cows,[1] because displacements can decrease a cow's ability to meet dietary needs. Feeding behavior may be more affected by stocking density in primiparous cows, because limited resources are a greater challenge to this group.[55,59] Multiparous cows had a greater social dominance score than primiparous cows when housed together.[59] Among cows that shared an Insentec feeder (Marknesse, the Netherlands), primiparous cows were replaced 25 times/d in a competition situation compared with 7 times/d in a noncompetitive situation.[50] In mixed housing, without individually assigned feeding space, as seen among traditionally housed cows, primiparous cows may be displaced with a greater frequency when overstocked than when stocked at 100%. Lobeck-Luchterhand and colleagues[52] observed that despite multiparous cows spending 47 min/d more feeding than nulliparous cows, no variation in social ranking was observed. Additionally, Proudfoot and colleagues[50] reported no difference in feeding time, frequency of visits to a feeder, dry matter intake per visit, or total daily feeding time among cows stocked at 100% or 150%. Further work must be proposed to explore the development of social hierarchy and the role of feeding behavior among dry cows, considering parity as a confounding factor.

Varying stocking density can have an impact on number of displacements from the feed bunk or feeding space, regardless of parity. Huzzey and colleagues[55] observed 22 more displacements from the feed bunk per day among cows housed at 150% versus those housed at 100%. When 4 cows shared a single automatic feeder, displacements were 38% greater than when an individual cow was assigned an individual automatic feeder.[57] Dry cows stocked at 80% had 6 less displacements from the feed bunk per day than cows stocked at 100% stocking density.[52] This suggests that regardless of stocking density, some low level of displacements occur within any given system.

EFFECT OF STOCKING DENSITY ON THE STRESS RESPONSE AND HEALTH OF TRANSITION COWS

Use of corticotropin has become a common way to assess dry cow stress associated with increased stocking density. Results can vary greatly, however, due to confounding variables within studies. Elevated fecal cortisol metabolite, plasma nonesterified fatty acids, and glucose concentration were greater among cows stocked at 150% versus cows housed at 100%.[55] Furthermore, low ranked cows administered a glucose tolerance test, had a greater insulin response and tended to have greater nonesterified fatty acid response than the high ranked cows.[54] Determining the effects of stocking density on dry cows must be further explored, considering a range of stocking densities from 80% to 200%, to provide a more representative sample of management practices. Although stocking density and management style can vary greatly within a single dry cow group, providing better guidelines for how to manage dry cows in all systems is necessary to promote dairy cow health and decrease stress postpartum.

FUTURE DIRECTIONS FOR UNDERSTANDING THE EFFECTS OF STOCKING DENSITY

To further the current understanding of the role of stocking density on the behavior of dairy cows, there are a few areas that need to be more fully addressed. First, the interaction of stocking density with other stressors needs to be fully understood. Second, the increased understanding of sleep in dairy cows provides the means to start to evaluate the quality of lying time and, therefore, the evaluation of stocking density on lying behavior beyond changes in total daily time may become possible.

Often the effect of increasing or decreasing stocking density is reported to be much greater on commercial farms than in controlled studies. This is likely due to the effort in controlled studies to control stressors beyond stocking density compared with commercial operations where multiple stressors might challenge those cows. This dynamic was evident in the combination of feed restriction and stocking density evaluated by Collings and colleagues.[60] The concept of stressors having an additive effect is much better understood, however, in other species. The combination of stocking density and mixing altered the feeding behaviors of swine in an additive manner.[61,62] The combination of restraint and lipopolysaccharide-challenge reduced growth and increased concentrations of corticosterone in mice to a greater extent than either stressor alone.[63]

The most likely stressors that worsen the effects of stocking density are dietary fiber, feed availability, and heat stress. Physically effective fiber is the fraction of dietary fiber with sufficient particle length to stimulate chewing (ruminative and eating) and create a well-formed rumen digesta mat.[64,65] Feeding diets deficient in physically effective neutral detergent fiber and/or excessive fermentable carbohydrates (primarily starch) may induce subacute rumen acidosis. Associated with subacute rumen acidosis, changes in feeding behaviors caused by increased stocking density may be sufficient to alter rumen biohydrogenation of fatty acids, reduce milk fat synthesis, and alter milk fatty acid composition.[66]

There will also continue to be growing pressure to avoid managing the feed bunk for feed refusals; a survey of western US dairy farms suggests a growing number of producers are targeting 0% feed refusals.[67,68] This is likely due to feed costs accounting for 55% of the total expenses of a dairy operation.[69] A 12-hour restriction of feed decreased total feeding time and increased feeding rate.[7]

Heat stress is another major factor that likely interacts with increased stocking density to exacerbate the detrimental effects of overstocking. A main behavioral response to heat stress from dairy cows was a reduction of lying time,[70] which is consistent with the effects of increased stocking density. Increasing ambient temperature from $25.5°C$ to $40.0°C$ was sufficient to have a negative effect on all aspects of the time budget; with lying time decreased by 34%, feeding time by 46%, and rumination by 22%.[71] The similarity of the detrimental effects of both heat stress and stocking density makes it likely that the combination of the 2 has a greater cumulative effect than either individually.

Understanding sleep in the dairy cow provides critical insight in to how cows use the 12 hours of lying time they are expected to engage in. There is evidence that cows spend 3 hours to 4 hours per day sleeping[72,73]; however, their sleep is fragmented and spread out in short 3-minute to 5-minute bouts throughout the day.[72,73] More specifically, this can be segmented into different vigilance states, with 3 hours per day spent in non–rapid eye movement (REM) sleep, 30 min/d to 45 min/d in REM sleep, and 8 hours per day drowsing.[72,74] To engage in REM sleep, a cow must be in a recumbent posture,[75] which she may have limited access to in an overstocked pen. Consequently, when overall lying time is decreased, a detrimental effect on sleep also is likely.

TAKE-HOME MESSAGES

- Increasing the stocking density of the freestalls above 100% consistently reduces lying time of lactating dairy cows. Overstocking the housing of transition cows worsens the decreases in lying time that are inherent with this portion of the lactation cycle.
- The extent that cows can be housed above a stocking density of 100% is likely driven by the design and maintenance of the lying space. Freestall stocking densities above 120% consistently have negative behavioral and production effects.
- The most consistently observed behavioral response to overstocking at the feed bunk is increased aggression.
- Stocking densities of more novel management systems (compost bedded packs and AMSs) currently lack specific recommendations because the ideal stocking density is dependent on both the behavioral needs of the cows within them and the overall functioning of the system.
- When evaluating the impacts of stocking density on feeding behaviors, the stocking density at the freestalls should also be considered. Cows place a greater priority on resting compared with feeding. Therefore, it is hypothesized that a relationship among freestall stocking density, feed bunk stocking density, and feeding behaviors exists.
- Currently, there is limited research on the impacts of stocking density on the feeding behavior of dairy cows during the dry and transition periods. There is also a lack of information on the feed bunk and freestall management practices during the transition period in North America. Assessment of these transition cow management practices will improve the conduct of applied research on the spatial needs of dairy cows and heifers by providing the means to apply treatments that reflect on-farm practices.
- Understanding the interaction of stocking density with other potential stressors is the next phase to establishing critical stocking densities for dairy cows throughout lactation and ensuring cows are able to meet their time budget needs.

REFERENCES

1. Grant RJ, Albright JL. Effect of animal grouping on feeding behavior and intake of dairy cattle. J Dairy Sci 2001;84:E156–63.
2. Bach A, Valls N, Solans A, et al. Associations between nondietary factors and dairy herd performance. J Dairy Sci 2008;91(8):3259–67.
3. USDA. Facility characteristics and cow comfort on U.S. dairy operations, 2007. Fort Collins (CO): USDA–APHIS–VS, CEAH; 2010.
4. von Keyserlingk MAG, Barrientos A, Ito K, et al. Benchmarking cow comfort on north american freestall dairies: lameness, leg injuries, lying time, facility design, and management for high-producing holstein dairy cows. J Dairy Sci 2012; 95(12):7399–408.
5. Charlton GL, Haley DB, Rushen J, et al. Stocking density, milking duration, and lying times of lactating cows on canadian freestall dairy farms. J Dairy Sci 2014;97(5):2694–700.
6. Haley DB, Rushen J, Passillé A M d. Behavioural indicators of cow comfort: activity and resting behaviour of dairy cows in two types of housing. Can J Anim Sci 2000;80(2):257–63.
7. Munksgaard L, Jensen MB, Pedersen LJ, et al. Quantifying behavioural priorities—effects of time constraints on behaviour of dairy cows, bos taurus. Appl Anim Behav Sci 2005;92(1–2):3–14.

8. Munksgaard L, Ingvartsen KL, Pedersen LJ, et al. Deprivation of lying down affects behaviour and pituitary-adrenal axis responses in young bulls. Acta Agric Scand A Anim Sci 1999;49(3):172–8.
9. Cook NB, Nordlund KV. The influence of the environment on dairy cow behavior, claw health and herd lameness dynamics. Vet J 2009;179(3):360–9.
10. Munksgaard L, Løvendahl P. Effects of social and physical stressors on growth hormone levels in dairy cows. Can J Anim Sci 1993;73(4):847–53.
11. Cooper MD, Arney DR, Phillips CJ. Two- or four-hour lying deprivation on the behavior of lactating dairy cows. J Dairy Sci 2007;90(3):1149–58.
12. Munksgaard L, Simonsen HB. Behavioral and pituitary adrenal-axis responses of dairy cows to social isolation and deprivation of lying down. J Anim Sci 1996; 74(4):769–78.
13. Gomez A, Cook NB. Time budgets of lactating dairy cattle in commercial freestall herds. J Dairy Sci 2010;93(12):5772–81.
14. Wilson P. Decomposing variation in dairy profitability: the impact of output, inputs, prices, labour and management. J Agric Sci 2011;149(4):507–17.
15. De Vries A, Dechassa H, Hogeveen H. Economic evaluation of stall stocking density of lactating dairy cows. J Dairy Sci 2016;99(5):3848–57.
16. National Farm Animal Care Council (NFACC). Code of practice for the care and handling of dairy cattle. 2009. Available at: http://www.nfacc.ca/codes-of-practice/dairy-cattle. Accessed August 15, 2018.
17. National Milk Producers Federation (NMPF). National dairy FARM animal care manual. 2013. Available at: http://www.nationaldairyfarm.com/animal-care-resources.html. Accessed August 15, 2018.
18. USDA. Dairy cattle management practices in the United States, 2014. Fort Collins (CO): USDA–APHIS–VS–CEAH–NAHMS; 2016.
19. Hill CT, Krawczel PD, Dann HM, et al. Effect of stocking density on the short-term behavioural responses of dairy cows. Appl Anim Behav Sci 2009;117(3):144–9.
20. Krawczel PD, Klaiber LB, Butzler RE, et al. Short-term increases in stocking density affect the lying and social behavior, but not the productivity, of lactating holstein dairy cows. J Dairy Sci 2012;95(8):4298–308.
21. Krawczel PD, Mooney CS, Dann HM, et al. Effect of alternative models for increasing stocking density on the short-term behavior and hygiene of holstein dairy cows. J Dairy Sci 2012;95(5):2467–75.
22. Winckler C, Tucker CB, Weary DM. Effects of under- and overstocking freestalls on dairy cattle behaviour. Appl Anim Behav Sci 2015;170:14–9.
23. Fregonesi JA, Tucker CB, Weary DM. Overstocking reduces lying time in dairy cows. J Dairy Sci 2007;90(7):3349–54.
24. Falk AC, Weary DM, Winckler C, et al. Preference for pasture versus freestall housing by dairy cattle when stall availability indoors is reduced. J Dairy Sci 2012;95(11):6409–15.
25. Legrand AL, von Keyserlingk MAG, Weary DM. Preference and usage of pasture versus free-stall housing by lactating dairy cattle. J Dairy Sci 2009;92(8):3651–8.
26. Charlton GL, Rutter SM, East M, et al. The motivation of dairy cows for access to pasture. J Dairy Sci 2013;96(7):4387–96.
27. Huzzey JM, DeVries TJ, Valois P, et al. Stocking density and feed barrier design affect the feeding and social behavior of dairy cattle. J Dairy Sci 2006;89(1): 126–33.
28. DeVries TJ, von Keyserlingk MAG, Weary DM. Effect of feeding space on the inter-cow distance, aggression, and feeding behavior of free-stall housed lactating dairy cows. J Dairy Sci 2004;87(5):1432–8.

29. Campbell MA, Dann HM, Krawczel PD, et al. Effects of stocking density and feed availability on short-term lying, feeding, and rumination responses of holstein dairy cows. Proc. American Dairy Science Association Annual Meeting. Pittsburgh, PA, June 25–28, 2017. p. 367–8.

30. Chebel RC, Silva PRB, Endres MI, et al. Social stressors and their effects on immunity and health of periparturient dairy cows1. J Dairy Sci 2016;99(4):3217–28.

31. Jensen MB, Proudfoot KL. Effect of group size and health status on behavior and feed intake of multiparous dairy cows in early lactation. J Dairy Sci 2017;100(12): 9759–68.

32. Krause KM, Oetzel GR. Understanding and preventing subacute ruminal acidosis in dairy herds: a review. Anim Feed Sci Technol 2006;126(3):215–36.

33. Fregonesi JA, Leaver JD. Influence of space allowance and milk yield level on behaviour, performance and health of dairy cows housed in strawyard and cubicle systems. Livest Prod Sci 2002;78(3):245–57.

34. Bewley JM, Taraba J, Day G, et al. Compost bedded pack barn design: features and management considerations. 2012. Available at: http://www2.ca.uky.edu/agcomm/pubs/id/id206/id206.pdf.

35. Black RA, Krawczel PD. A case study of behaviour and performance of confined or pastured cows during the dry period. Animals 2016;6(7) [pii:E41].

36. Barberg AE, Endres M, Janni KA. Compost dairy barns in minnesota: a descriptive study. Appl Eng Agric 2007;23:231–8.

37. Black RA, Taraba JL, Day GB, et al. Compost bedded pack dairy barn management, performance, and producer satisfaction. J Dairy Sci 2013;96(12):8060–74.

38. Janni KA, Endres MI, Reneau JK, et al. Compost dairy barn layout and management recommendations. Appl Eng Agric 2007;23(1):97–102.

39. Deming JA, Bergeron R, Leslie KE, et al. Associations of housing, management, milking activity, and standing and lying behavior of dairy cows milked in automatic systems. J Dairy Sci 2013;96(1):344–51.

40. Rodenburg J. Robotic milking: technology, farm design, and effects on work flow. J Dairy Sci 2017;100(9):7729–38.

41. Witaifi AA, Ali ABA, Siegford JM. Stall and feed bunk stocking rates impact cows' diurnal behavior and activity in automatic milking system farms. J Vet Behav 2018;24:48–55.

42. Cook NB. The influence of barn design on dairy cow hygiene, lameness and udder health. Proc. 35th Annu. Conf. Am. Assoc. Bovine. Pract. Stillwater, OK, September 26–28, 2002. p. 97–103.

43. Guard C. The importance of locomotion. Midwest DairyBusiness 2002;32–4.

44. Westin R, Vaughan A, de Passillé AM, et al. Cow- and farm-level risk factors for lameness on dairy farms with automated milking systems. J Dairy Sci 2016; 99(5):3732–43.

45. Nishida T, Hosoda K, Matsuyama H, et al. Effect of lying behavior on uterine blood flow in cows during the third trimester of gestation. J Dairy Sci 2004; 87(8):2388–92.

46. Fustini M, Galeati G, Gabai G, et al. Overstocking dairy cows during the dry period affects dehydroepiandrosterone and cortisol secretion. J Dairy Sci 2017; 100(1):620–8.

47. Luchterhand KM, Silva PRB, Chebel RC, et al. Association between prepartum feeding behavior and periparturient health disorders in dairy cows. Front Vet Sci 2016;3:65.

48. Green MJ, Bradley AJ, Medley GF, et al. Cow, farm, and herd management factors in the dry period associated with raised somatic cell counts in early lactation. J Dairy Sci 2008;91(4):1403–15.

49. Oetzel GR, Emery KM, Kautz WP, et al. Direct-fed microbial supplementation and health and performance of pre- and postpartum dairy cattle: a field trial. J Dairy Sci 2007;90(4):2058–68.

50. Proudfoot KL, Veira DM, Weary DM, et al. Competition at the feed bunk changes the feeding, standing, and social behavior of transition dairy cows. J Dairy Sci 2009;92(7):3116–23.

51. Rice CA, Eberhart NL, Krawczel PD. Prepartum lying behavior of holstein dairy cows housed on pasture through parturition. Animals 2017;7(4):32.

52. Lobeck-Luchterhand KM, Silva PR, Chebel RC, et al. Effect of stocking density on social, feeding, and lying behavior of prepartum dairy animals. J Dairy Sci 2015; 98(1):240–9.

53. Lobeck-Luchterhand KM, Silva PRB, Chebel RC, et al. Effect of prepartum grouping strategy on displacements from the feed bunk and feeding behavior of dairy cows. J Dairy Sci 2014;97(5):2800–7.

54. Huzzey JM, Grant RJ, Overton TR. Short communication: relationship between competitive success during displacements at an overstocked feed bunk and measures of physiology and behavior in holstein dairy cattle. J Dairy Sci 2012; 95(8):4434–41.

55. Huzzey JM, Nydam DV, Grant RJ, et al. The effects of overstocking holstein dairy cattle during the dry period on cortisol secretion and energy metabolism. J Dairy Sci 2012;95(8):4421–33.

56. Bargo F, Muller LD, Delahoy JE, et al. Performance of high producing dairy cows with three different feeding systems combining pasture and total mixed rations. J Dairy Sci 2002;85(11):2948–63.

57. Olofsson J. Competition for total mixed diets fed for ad libitum intake using one or four cows per feeding station. J Dairy Sci 1999;82(1):69–79.

58. Pahl C, Hartung E, Mahlkow-Nerge K, et al. Feeding characteristics and rumination time of dairy cows around estrus. J Dairy Sci 2015;98(1):148–54.

59. González M, Yabuta AK, Galindo F. Behaviour and adrenal activity of first parturition and multiparous cows under a competitive situation. Appl Anim Behav Sci 2003;83(4):259–66.

60. Collings LK, Weary DM, Chapinal N, et al. Temporal feed restriction and overstocking increase competition for feed by dairy cattle. J Dairy Sci 2011;94(11): 5480–6.

61. Hyun Y, Ellis M, Johnson RW. Effects of feeder type, space allowance, and mixing on the growth performance and feed intake pattern of growing pigs. J Anim Sci 1998;76:2771–8.

62. Hyun Y, Ellis M, Riskowski G, et al. Growth performance of pigs subjected to multiple concurrent environmental stressors. J Anim Sci 1998;76:721–7.

63. Laugero KD, Moberg GP. Effects of acute behavioral stress and LPS-induced cytokine release on growth and energetics in mice. Physiol Behav 2000;68: 415–22.

64. Mertens DR. Creating a system for meeting the fiber requirements of dairy cows. J Dairy Sci 1997;80(7):1463–81.

65. Weidner SJ, Grant RJ. Soyhulls as a replacement for forage fiber in diets for lactating dairy cows1. J Dairy Sci 1994;77(2):513–21.

66. Bauman DE, Lock AL. Animal products and human health: perceptions, opportunities, and challenges. Proc. Cornell Nutrition Conference. East Syracuse, NY, October 24–26, 2006. p. 45–77.

67. Silva-del-Río N, Heguy JM, Lago A. Feed management practices on California dairies. J Dairy Sci 2010;93(E-Suppl):773 [abstract].

68. Soriani N, Trevisi E, Calamari L. Relationships between rumination time, metabolic conditions, and health status in dairy cows during the transition period. J Anim Sci 2012;90(12):4544–54.

69. USDA-ERS. Monthly cost of production estimates. Washington, DC: USDA–Economic Research Service; 2014. Available at: http://www.ers.usda.gov/data-products/milk-cost-of-productionestimates.aspx. Accessed April 14, 2014.

70. Cook NB, Mentink RL, Bennett TB, et al. The effect of heat stress and lameness on time budgets of lactating dairy cows. J Dairy Sci 2007;90(4):1674–82.

71. Tapkı İ, Şahin A. Comparison of the thermoregulatory behaviours of low and high producing dairy cows in a hot environment. Appl Anim Behav Sci 2006;99(1–2):1–11.

72. Ruckebusch Y. The relevance of drowsiness in the circadian cycle of farm animals. Anim Behav 1972;20(4):637–43.

73. Ternman E, Hänninen L, Pastell M, et al. Sleep in dairy cows recorded with a non-invasive eeg technique. Appl Anim Behav Sci 2012;140(1):25–32.

74. Nilsson E. Quantification of sleep in dairy cows in three different stages of lactation. MS thesis. Uppsala (Sweden): Department of Animal Nutrition and Management. Swedish University of Agricultural Science; 2011. Available at: https://stud.epsilon.slu.se/3108/1/nilsson_e_110809.pdf.

75. Ruckebusch Y. Sleep deprivation in cattle. Brain Res 1974;78(3):495–9.

Feeding Behavior, Feed Space, and Bunk Design and Management for Adult Dairy Cattle

Trevor J. DeVries, BSc (Agr), PhD

KEYWORDS

- Dairy cattle • Feeding behavior • Sorting • Feed space • Bunk design
- Feeding management • Feeding frequency • Feed push-up

KEY POINTS

- The feeding behavior of dairy cows, including how, when, and what cows eat of the feed provided to them, has a significant impact on cow health and productivity.
- Dairy cows need sufficient space to eat simultaneously, and a bunk design that minimizes competition, ensures good feed access, and minimizes risk of injury.
- Continuous feed access throughout the day, through adequate feeding levels, and frequent feed delivery and push-ups, also contribute to ensuring good eating behavior.

INTRODUCTION

Successful management of the nutrition of dairy cows not only ensures the proper formulation and preparation of a diet designed to meet production targets, but also involves ensuring cows consume the diet provided to them in a manner that is going to optimize health, production, and efficiency. In particular, how dairy cows eat, when they eat, and what they actually consume from the feed provided to them are all critical.

Grazing cattle have a natural diurnal feeding pattern, dependent primarily on daylength, whereby cows consume their largest meals each day around the times of sunrise and sunset.[1,2] Despite this natural behavior, in modern, intensive dairy operations, it is management practices that are the major stimuli for lactating dairy cows to consume their total mixed ration (TMR). For example, the delivery of fresh feed, and to a lesser extent, the return from milking, elicit the greatest motivation for feeding activity.[3–5] The traditional recommendation for adequate linear feed bunk space is 0.6 m

The author has nothing to disclose.
Department of Animal Biosciences, University of Guelph, 50 Stone Road East, Guelph, Ontario N1G 2W1, Canada
E-mail address: tdevries@uoguelph.ca

Vet Clin Food Anim 35 (2019) 61–76
https://doi.org/10.1016/j.cvfa.2018.10.003

per cow.[6,7] However, this may be insufficient during peak periods of feeding activity when bunk attendance is highest[3] and for transition cows. If cows are unable to gain access to feed when desired, as in the case of spatial (eg, the physical feed area design or stocking rate) or temporal feed restriction (eg, how long feed is available throughout the day), competition between individuals increases. This in turn, has negative impacts on meal patterning and the composition of diet consumed, having negative consequences on health and production.

There is field evidence to suggest that the full nutritive value of the rations provided are not always realized on farm. In addition, field observations also suggest that housing and management may play as large of a role as the dietary composition itself in the performance and health of dairy cows. This review outlines how many of these observations may be explained by the role that dairy cow feeding behavior patterns have on ensuring cow health, efficiency, and productivity. In particular, it is discussed how that knowledge is used to design feeding areas that allow dairy cows to express that behavior, allowing for optimal dry matter intake (DMI) of the intended diet, while minimizing competition and risk of injury. Finally, the role of feeding management, in terms of providing cows continuous access to feed throughout the day, and stimulation of good eating behavior are discussed.

FEEDING BEHAVIOR OF DAIRY COWS

To understand recommendations for feed area design and TMR management, an explanation of the impact that feeding behavior has on intake, health, and digestive efficiency is needed. Those areas of feeding behavior that need to be considered include how cows eat their ration, when they consume their ration, and what they actually consume from the TMR provided to them.

How Cows Eat Their Ration

Milk production of dairy cows is inherently linked to the amount of nutrients consumed; that consumption is essentially the function of a cow's eating behavior. That is, the total DMI (kilogram per day) of a cow is the result of the frequency of meals consumed daily (number per day) and their size (kilogram per meal).[8] DMI can also be expressed as a function of the total feeding time of a cow per day (minute per day) multiplied by the rate (kilogram dry matter per minute) at which she consumes that feed. Thus, for a cow to consume greater amounts of dry matter, she needs to adjust some aspect of her feeding behavior. For example, by increasing the frequency of daily meals or the average meal size, or some combination of those two, the cow can increase her daily DMI. The same concept applies to the length of eating time per day and the rate at which that feed is consumed. In recent research we[9] have demonstrated, using data from multiple studies of high production cows, that meal frequency and total feeding time were stronger predictors of daily DMI, and subsequently milk yield, than the size of meals consumed or the speed at which they were consumed. Thus, these data suggest that increases in DMI may be achieved more consistently by getting cows to have more frequent meals, spread over a longer period of time at the feed bunk.

Dairy cattle fed a TMR typically consume their daily DMI in 3 to 5 h/d, spread between 7 to 12 meals per day.[10] The size and distribution of those meals not only may impact DMI, but may also influence rumen function. Following a meal, and initial digestion of highly fermentable carbohydrates, volatile fatty acids accumulate and ruminal pH declines. The rate of pH decline increases as meal size increases.[11] Furthermore, with increased rate of feed consumption, daily salivary secretion is reduced,[12] decreasing the buffering capacity of the rumen and further reducing rumen pH. This results in a much more variable fermentation pattern, resulting in within-day depressions in rumen pH characteristic of subacute ruminal acidosis (SARA). As such, it has been suggested that management practices that cause adult dairy cattle to eat fewer and larger meals more quickly have been associated with a greater incidence of SARA.[13] Therefore, maximizing rumen health, efficiency, and productivity involves providing dairy cows with a feeding environment and management of feed therein to promote the frequent, slow consumption of feed in small meals throughout the day.

When Cows Eat Their Ration

It has been demonstrated that the diurnal feeding patterns of group-housed, TMR-fed dairy cows are mostly influenced by the time of feed delivery, feed push-up, and milking,[3] with the most dramatic peaks in feeding activity occurring around the time of feed delivery and the return from the milking parlor. DeVries and von Keyserlingk[4] corroborated that finding in a study where they separated TMR delivery and milking times by 6 hours, and demonstrated that cows shifted their feeding pattern such that the greatest bunk activity was noted after the feed delivery and not after milking. King and colleagues[5] shifted the timing of TMR delivery (two times per day) ahead of milking by 3.5 hours, and found that the initial meal size following feed delivery was similar in that study whether or not cows were milked at that time. Those authors also found that the size of the meal following milking was reduced when cows no longer received fresh TMR on return from milking. Collectively, the results from these studies indicate that TMR delivery acts as the primary influence on cow daily feeding activity patterns, more than that of feed push-up, milking activity, or the time of day.

What Cows Actually Consume from Their Ration

Despite the intended purpose of TMR to provide cows with a homogenous mixture of feed ingredients that are to be consumed as formulated, dairy cattle have been shown to preferentially select (sort) for certain components of TMR, and avoid other components.[14] As a result, the diet consumed is different from that delivered to the cow. Cows typically select against the longer, forage components of the TMR, and select for the smaller, grain components.[15,16] The sorting of TMR by dairy cows can result in the ration actually consumed by cows being lesser in effective fiber and greater in fermentable carbohydrates than intended, thereby increasing the risk of depressed rumen pH.[17] Associated with this, in two studies it was reported that such sorting of a TMR is associated with producing milk with lower fat percentage (milk fat decreases by 0.15% points for every 10% refusal of long forage particles in the ration[18,19]). Miller-Cushon and DeVries[20] also demonstrated that same association, finding that milk fat decreased by 0.10% points for every 10% refusal of long particles.

Miller-Cushon and DeVries[20] also found that milk protein content decreased by 0.04% points for every 10% refusal of long particles. This suggests that sorting also disrupts the balance of nutrients required to optimize microbial protein production. Imbalanced nutrient intake, as a result of sorting, also has the potential to impact the efficiency of digestion and production. In support of this, Sova and colleagues[21] found that efficiency of milk production decreased by 3% for every 1% of group-level selective overconsumption (sorting) of fine ration particles. Finally, sorting may lead to reductions in milk production. Coon and colleagues[22] recently demonstrated that greater sorting, as result of feeding a diet with greater straw particle size, was associated with greater variability in reticulorumen pH, rumination, and DMI over the first 4 weeks of lactation, and a trend for reduced cumulative milk production over that time period.

Sorting of a TMR can also reduce the nutritive quality of the TMR remaining in the feed bunk, particularly in the later hours past the time of feed delivery, after cows have had much time to sort out those desirable components of the TMR.[23,24] In a group feeding situation this may be disadvantageous for those animals that do not have access to feed, particularly at the time when it is delivered. For example, when there is high competition at the feed bunk, some cows may not be able to maintain adequate nutrient intake to maintain high levels of production and growth.[13] Again, there is evidence to suggest that this sorting behavior may impact production at a herd-level; Sova and colleagues[21] showed that every 2% point increase in sorting against the longest TMR particles, at a group level, was associated with a per cow reduction of 0.9 kg/d of 4% fat-corrected milk.

In summary, there is much empirical evidence indicating that the feeding behavior patterns of dairy cows play an important role beyond proper diet formulation, in ensuring good rumen digestion, rumen health, and efficiency of production. Using that knowledge, there is the opportunity to improve the environment within which feed is provided, and how that feed is managed, to promote good eating behavior patterns.

FEED BUNK COMPETITION, SPACE, AND DESIGN
Feed Bunk Competition

When resources are limited, competition between individuals for access to those resources is greater. As herd animals, dairy cows are highly motivated to feed simultaneously with other members of their social group.[8] If there is insufficient space for all animals to feed together, there may be competition for access to the feed. This poses a problem if the competition reaches a level whereby the health and welfare of individual cows are compromised.

Competitive behavior is characterized in the literature in two ways: indirect or direct competition.[25] Indirect competition for feed access is displayed when individuals modify their behavior to obtain access to the feed bunk, such as shifting feeding times to less busy periods of the day,[26] or increasing the rate of feed consumption.[27] Direct competition is displayed through acts or threats of physical aggression between individuals; for example, one cow displacing or replacing another from their position at the feed bunk.[28,29] Alteration of natural behaviors because of competition between cows, either direct or indirect, may have widespread consequences for their physiological health, such as instability in the rumen environment,[13] and psychological health, such as reduced motivation to feed within a certain distance of more dominant individuals.[30]

Social position within the herd has a great influence on the success of dairy cows in competitive interactions.[31] Not all individuals are of equal rank within the social hierarchy of the herd,[32] therefore, dominance is expressed whenever the behavior of one individual deters the behavior of another.[31] In research by Rioja-Lang and colleagues,[33] preference testing was used to examine the importance of avoiding social stress imposed by more dominant cows over feed quality. Subordinate cows were given a choice between consuming low-quality feed alone, or consuming high-quality feed next to a more dominant individual; results indicated that the subordinate cow preferred to feed away from the dominant individual, despite having to sacrifice feed quality. In a follow-up study, the same research group allowed subordinate cows to choose between consuming a low-palatability feed alone versus a high-palatability feed next to a dominant cow, at different intercow distances.[30] When provided with smaller distances of 0.3 or 0.45 m between cows, the subordinate individual chose to feed alone; at greater distances of 0.6 or 0.75 m, the subordinate cow was willing to eat next to the dominant cow. These studies suggest that the social stress imposed by dominant cows may result in a disproportionate impact of increased competition on subordinate cows.

When feed bunk competition increases, cows demonstrate reduced feeding time[34–36]; increased feeding rate[24,27,37]; and consume fewer, larger, and longer meals each day.[24,37] Greater feed bunk competition may also be associated with reduced rumination activity.[38,39]

Modification of the rate of intake and the length of feeding activity allows cows to maintain their daily DMI[37]; individuals may also maintain intakes by shifting their feeding activity to times of the day when fewer cows are present at the bunk.[26] Subordinate cows, in particular, forgo peak feeding times in favor of a later time when there is less competition for feed access.[27,33] Crossley and colleagues[37] recently demonstrated greater variability in feeding time, feeding rate, meal patterns, and milk production between individuals within a group at a high level of feeding competition, suggesting that as competition for feed increases, all cows are not able to compensate equally for the greater competitive pressure.

Shifting the timing of feed access throughout the day also means that, because of feed sorting, cows within a group, end up consuming rations of differential composition. Because the individuals that are typically forced to access feed outside of peak periods are subordinate cows,[23,27] they are more likely to consume a sorted ration. Conversely, dominant cows that access feed during peak times may have increased consumption of the highly fermentable carbohydrate components of the ration, and thus may be at increased risk of developing metabolic disorders, such as SARA.[17]

Competition caused by increased feed bunk stocking density can lead to increased idle standing time, as cows wait to gain access to an occupied feed bunk.[27,35,36] As seen in displacement behavior, inactive standing time is greatest during the peak periods of bunk attendance following the delivery of fresh feed,[35,36] and may also have long-term health impacts. Those cows who spend more time standing inactively, and thus more time in total standing outside the stall on hard, wet floors, may be at higher risk of developing foot problems.[40,41]

Krawczel and colleagues[39] reported an association of blood corticoid response to an corticotropin challenge in competitively fed cows, suggesting the cows experienced a stress response to the alteration of their feeding behavior. Huzzey and colleagues[42] compared dry cows fed at two different stocking densities, and found higher plasma non-esterified fatty acids (NEFA) and fecal cortisol concentrations in cows with the lowest success at displacing conspecifics from the feed bunk, compared with moderately or highly successful cows. Furthermore, these researchers found a higher peak insulin response in low-success cows than higher-success cows, indicating a reduced tissue response to insulin, similar to insulin resistance. In a related study, primiparous cows had higher fecal metabolites when overstocked, whereas no difference was found in multiparous cows, suggesting that younger animals have more difficulty managing increased competition levels.[43]

In a study of competitively fed dairy cows by Hetti Arachchige and colleagues,[44] heart rate was reduced as feeding space increased, indicating a reduction in stress response. Interestingly, heart rates of subordinate cows remained elevated over those of higher-ranked cows regardless of intercow feeding space, suggesting they consistently experienced a stress response when feeding in proximity to more dominant individuals.[44] This increased stress could influence a subordinate cow's motivation to access feed when a more dominant cow occupies the bunk. Competitive feeding stress may also have an impact on reproductive performance; Caraviello and colleagues[45] identified that the probability of pregnancy at 150 days in milk (DIM) increased linearly as feeding space per cow increased from 30 to 60 cm. Similarly, Schefers and colleagues[46] found, in a study of data from 108 herds, that greater bunk space in the breeding pen was associated with improved service rate.

Feed Bunk Space

Reducing feed bunk competition, by providing adequate feed bunk space (to allow animals to eat simultaneously) improves access to feed, particularly for subordinate dairy cattle.[35,36] For example, DeVries and colleagues[34] found that, in a free-stall system, doubling available linear bunk space from 0.5 to 1 m per cow resulted in 60% more space between cows, and a 57% reduction in aggressive interactions at the feed bunk. These changes allowed cows to increase the time spent feeding, particularly in the peak periods following delivery of fresh feed. Similar findings were reported by Hetti Arachchige and colleagues,[44] who supplemented pastured cows with a partial mixed ration on a feed pad, at three different space allowances. They observed that as feeding space increased, cows spent a greater amount of time feeding and were involved in fewer aggressive interactions. These behavioral changes, in turn, contribute to more consistent DMI patterns within and between animals, and promote healthy feeding behavior patterns. It is not surprising that Sova and colleagues[21] found in a cross-sectional study of parlor-milked, free-stall herds that every 10 cm per cow increase in feed bunk space (mean, 54 cm per cow; range, 36–99 cm per cow) was associated with 0.06% point increase in group average milk fat and a 13% decrease in group-average somatic cell count. These changes in milk composition are explained by the previously described impact that feed bunk stocking density has on the behavioral patterns of cows. With greater feeding space, cows may consume their feed in a manner more conducive to stable rumen fermentation, and thus promote greater milk fat production. Furthermore, with more space at the bunk, cows are less stressed, and also not forced to choose to lie down too quickly after milking rather than compete for a feeding spot, thus their risk of mastitis is reduced. Woolpert and colleagues[47] recently demonstrated that herds with high de novo fatty acid concentration in bulk tank milk, as compared with those with low de novo fatty acid concentration, tended to have greater bunk space per cow, and be 10 times more likely to have greater than or equal to 46 cm per cow of bunk space. This again suggests that greater bunk space facilitates improved eating behavior patterns, conducive to better rumen fermentation patterns.

In much work, focused primarily on mid- to late-lactation cows, researchers have not been able to detect any impact of stocking density (at feed bunk and lying stalls) on DMI or milk production.[39,48] These cows seem resilient in terms of maintaining levels of intake needed to maintain their production. This is achieved by altering their feeding behavior patterns (for the worse). That being said, there are examples in the literature where reduced bunk space has been associated with lesser production. For example, Deming and colleagues[49] observed that lesser availability of feed bunk space in automatic milking system herds was associated with lesser herd-average milk yield. The longer-term impacts of bunk overcrowding are also not well described. However, work such as that done by Sova and colleagues[21] sheds some light on the potential impacts.

Reduced feed bunk space during the transition period is one area where the literature is consistent. Reductions in DMI have been reported when transition cows are overcrowded at the feed bunk.[29] Greater feed bunk competition, as a result of lesser space availability, has also been related to the health status of transition cows. Goldhawk and colleagues[50] reported that cows who developed subclinical ketosis in the early postpartum period initiated fewer displacements at the feed bunk during the week before calving. Similarly, Huzzey and colleagues[51] reported that cows who were diagnosed with metritis 1 week after calving engaged in fewer competitive interactions at the feed bunk during periods of peak feeding activity. As result, those cows experienced lower DMI, particularly during peak feeding times. In more recent work by Kaufman and colleagues,[52] it was reported that increasing stocking density by 5% during the week before calving was found to increase the risk of ketosis by 10% for cows on commercial farms. Collectively, these studies suggest that factors that may limit the desire of cows to go to the feed bunk, and compete for feed access, particularly at the peak feeding times of the day, such as an overcrowded feed bunk, may assist in predisposing cows to health issues, such as subclinical ketosis and metritis, in the early postpartum period.

Based on the available literature, the recommendation to the dairy industry, when it comes to feed bunk space availability, is still to provide sufficient space so that all cows may feed simultaneously. Given the typical size of the modern dairy cow (in particular those large breeds, such as Holstein), a significant amount of space per animal is needed to achieve that goal. Specifically, more than the traditional standard of 61 cm of bunk space per cow is required. That being said, the opportunity to provide more space to cows needs to be justified with the potential returns it may provide. For the most vulnerable cows, that is, those in the late dry period and those in the early postpartum period, sufficient feeding space is necessary to ensure cows can maximize DMI and, thus, make a smooth transition to lactation, with minimal risk of disease. For cows at those stages, provision of enough space to allow simultaneous feeding ($\geq$76 cm per cow) is essential to optimize health and production. For other lactating cows, providing good bunk availability is still critical to maximize DMI, and promote good eating, lying, and rumination patterns. As such, the target requirement for those cows is a minimum of 61 cm per cow. From a practical perspective, this means that the construction of pens with three or more rows of freestalls per feed bunk should be avoided, because these typically limit feed bunk space to 40 to 45 cm per cow or less with 100% stall stocking.

Feed Barrier Design

The design of the feed barrier that separates the cow from her feed is another factor that influences the level of competition at the feed bunk. There are examples of studies comparing open-type feed barriers (post and rail) with headlocks (self-locking stanchions). No data exist, to our knowledge, to suggest there is greater (or lesser) DMI and milk production with one system over the other; however, these designs do cause differences in behavior at the bunk. Early research by Bouissou[53] found that physical separation between the heads of feeding cows provided subordinate individuals with better access to feed, potentially because of a greater feeling of protection afforded by the physical barrier.[54] Endres and colleagues[55] demonstrated that during periods of peak feeding activity (90 minutes after fresh feed delivery) cows that had lower feeding times relative to group mates when using the post-and-rail barrier showed more similar feeding times to group mates when using the headlock barrier. Those researchers also reported 21% fewer displacements at the feed bunk when cows accessed feed by a headlock barrier as compared with a post-and-rail barrier. This work suggests that a headlock barrier can reduce aggression at the feed bunk and improve access to feed for socially subordinate cows during periods of peak feeding activity. Huzzey and colleagues[36] also found that subordinate cows were displaced more often with the post-and-rail barrier design, particularly at higher stocking densities. Huzzey and colleagues[36] also reported that daily feeding times were less and the duration of inactive standing in the feeding area was more, when using a headlock compared with a post-and-rail feed barrier. It is possible that the size of the headlocks used in that study contributed to that finding. Those headlocks were spaced at 61 cm center-to-center, which has traditionally been a common dimension adopted by the dairy industry. A challenge with such spacing is that many of modern, large-breed cows (Holsteins) are physically wider in girth than that spacing. As result, it is nearly impossible to fit cows into every headlock at that traditional spacing. As such, for headlocks, spaced 61 cm center-to-center, one often sees at least 2 out of every 10 headlocks empty because of lack of total space availability at the bunk. Thus, if headlocks are used, it may be better to size them appropriately for the cows using them (eg, 71–76 cm wide, center-to-center for Holstein cattle). This may be particularly important for transition dairy cows. Feeding competition for such vulnerable cows is also potentially reduced by using alternative feed barriers. An example is a feed stall that included body dividers at the cow side of the feed bunk. DeVries and von Keyserlingk[35] reported that these further limit competition at the bunk, and improve feed access over and above that provided with just more space.

The height and position of the feed rail (or top of the headlock) is also important in promoting good feed access. These require to be positioned at a small enough distance from the floor to keep cows standing in the feed alley and prevent them from going underneath and escaping. Conversely, neck rails are required to be positioned high enough so that the cow can stand and eat at the feed bunk without experiencing any pressure on her neck. Offsetting the neck rail (toward the feed) may also allow for easier access to the feed. For a headlock, this involves titling the headlock toward the feed; this then helps the cow be able to feed with minimal pressure put on her shoulders (from the headlock). The height of the neck rail is recommended in a post-and-rail system to vary between 122 and 137 cm (from the standing surface to the rail). At a higher placement no offset is necessarily needed; however, at a lower placement (toward 122 cm), an offset of 15 to 25+ cm from the manger wall may be necessary. For headlocks, the top rail of the headlock should be positioned at a minimum height of 122 cm, and titled forward by 15 to 20 cm from the cow side of the manger wall.

To summarize, the provision of sufficient feed bunk space to allow animals to eat simultaneously, particularly when combined with a well-designed physical partition (headlocks or feed stalls), minimizes feeding competition, reducing variability in feed access across cows within the group. As a result, more consistent DMI patterns, and healthier feeding patterns, are observed within and between animals. This is particularly important for close-up and fresh cows who are at greatest risk of low DMI and postpartum health challenges if they are forced to deal with feed access competition during those stages of their production cycle.

FEEDING MANAGEMENT
Feed Access

To maximize DMI and milk production, lactating dairy cattle are typically fed ad libitum. To reduce labor inputs and limit feed wastage, some producers may control feeding amounts to their cows by feeding for 0% refusals, known as "slick-bunk" feeding,[56] which restricts the amount of time that feed is accessible throughout the day. The challenge with such a practice is to minimize the time per day that the bunk is empty (ie, no >30-to-60-minute maximum per day). The feed intake patterns of dairy cows are cyclical, day-to-day, and thus it is difficult when feeding for low refusals to ensure that the bunk remains empty for such short times periods of the day. Under that type of management, without careful reading of the bunks, there may be situations where bunks are empty for multiple hours per day. Sustained periods of time with empty bunks have been shown to have negative impacts on cow behavior, intake, and production. For example, extensive restriction (8 hours) of feed access time has been shown to limit intake and production.[57] Alternatively, moderate limitations have been shown to negatively affect feeding behavior, causing cows to have shorter meals, less feeding time, and faster eating rates.[58,59] Collings and colleagues[56] found that temporal restriction of feed access (14 vs 23 h/d access) resulted in lower feeding times and greater feed bunk competition. Those researchers also found that, at greater stocking densities (ie, creating competition for feed bunk access), this temporal restriction increased the rate of feed consumption across the day.

Miller-Cushon and DeVries[60] found that at lower feeding amounts, feed sorting was reduced, whereas DMI was also reduced. In a field study by Bach and colleagues,[61] with 47 dairy herds with similar genetics that were fed the exact same TMR, they found that herds that fed for refusals averaged almost 1.6 kg/d more milk. The results of this work, and those described previously, suggest that bunks need to be monitored on a continual basis to ensure that cows have consistent access to their feed throughout every 24-hour period. With good management, and proactive adjustments to feeding amounts, low refusal rates are potentially attainable. However, in situations where such a high level of management is not possible, it is advised to feed at higher refusal rates (minimum 3%) to ensure that cows do not run out of feed at any time point in advance of their next feed delivery.

Feed Delivery Frequency

Because the delivery of TMR plays a large role in stimulating cows to eat, the frequency by which that occurs impacts feeding behavior patterns, and thus also cow health and productivity. Compared with two times per day TMR delivery, with delivery once per day, there is a significantly greater peak in feeding activity in the immediate time period following feed delivery,[23] indicative of slug feeding. This may predispose cows to SARA[23] because of large diurnal fluctuations in ruminal pH.[62] However, for cows fed more often than once per day, they end up consuming their TMR more evenly throughout the day, increasing their total feeding time.[23,63] In addition, it has been reported that subordinate cows are not displaced as frequently when fed more often,[23] indicating that these cows would have greater access to feed, particularly fresh feed, when the frequency of feed delivery is greater than once a day. In a study by Oostra and colleagues,[64] increasing feed delivery from two to six times per day for robot-milked cows was reported to promote greater feeding activity and, in turn, reduced waiting times for the milking unit. Finally, providing feed two times per day or more often per day has also been reported to reduce the degree of feed sorting as compared with feeding once per day,[21,23,65] further contributing to more consistent nutrient intake patterns over the course of the day.

The consistent feeding patterns that result from delivering TMR more than once per day may contribute to more consistent rumen pH, and as a result, improved milk fat,[66] fiber digestibility,[67] and possibly production efficiency.[63] Woolpert and colleagues[47] recently reported that dairy herds with high de novo fatty acid concentration in bulk tank milk, as compared with those with low de novo fatty acid concentration, tended to be five times more likely to feed cows twice versus once per day, confirming the positive impacts of feeding more than once per day on rumen fermentation. Although less consistently reported, frequent delivery of TMR may also impact DMI and milk yield. Hart and colleagues[68] reported that DMI was greatest in three times per day milked cows fed three times per day (27.8 kg/d) compared with when fed twice per day (27.0 kg/d) or once per day (27.4 kg/d). In that study, greater DMI came as a result of larger meals following the return from milking and the delivery of feed. Furthermore, in a Canadian field study of freestall herds, delivery of TMR twice per day compared with once per day was reported to be associated with less feed sorting, greater DMI (+1.4 kg/d), and greater milk yield (+2.0 kg/d).[21]

Providing good access to fresh feed, by delivering more frequently throughout the day, may be particularly important in situations where the feed bunk is overstocked. In a recent study Crossley and colleagues[69] demonstrated that for cows fed under high competitive pressure (2:1 stocking density at the bunk) the first meals after feed delivery were, on average, shorter and smaller in size when cows were fed their TMR at a higher frequency (six times per day) compared with a lower frequency (twice per day). The first meals postfeeding coincide with peak periods when most cows are feeding together and the competition for access to feed is typically at its highest level.[3–5] As a result, such a feeding pattern would allow for a greater turnover of cows at the feed bunk, and thus would provide more opportunities for all individuals to access fresh feed. Crossley and colleagues[69] also reported that increasing the frequency of feed delivery for competitively fed cows resulted in a trend for greater rumination time, and reduced milk production variability between cows.

The frequency of feed delivery may also interact with ration moisture content and environmental temperature. Greater sorting of a TMR, when fed once per day, may be particularly troublesome when feeding low dry matter content TMR during periods of high ambient temperatures and humidity. In such cases, delivering feed once per day may increase the risk of sorting and also limit intake.[70,71] These may be the result of greater feed heating and spoilage in the bunk. Therefore, greater frequency of feed delivery may be critical in hot climates, particularly those regions with high humidity and high ambient temperature.

For dairy producers, the decision to deliver TMR more than once per day has to be made by contrasting the potential benefits against the costs. Mixing and delivering TMR more often increases labor and energy (fuel) costs. Such increases in cost must be offset by the potential benefits, which could vary from farm to farm. The most consistent returns would be greater milk fat content and improved efficiency of milk production. Furthermore, all of these benefits have the potential to be greater in situations of overcrowding and areas with high environmental temperature and humidity.

Feed Delivery Timing

The timing of TMR delivery may also play a large role in ensuring good, consistent eating patterns. A goal of TMR management should be to stimulate feeding activity at as many time points across the day as possible, to increase the distribution of feed intake. In addition to using the delivery of fresh TMR to stimulate feeding activity in cows, it is also known that cows are more likely to eat following milking, and near the time of other management events during the day. Knowing that, it is possible then to stimulate greater meal frequency across the day by staggering these management events. For example, more feeding activity throughout the day may be achieved by moving the time of feed delivery away from the time of milking. King and colleagues[5] shifted feed delivery (twice per day) ahead of milking (three times per day) by 3.5 hours, and reported that greater feed stimulation across the day resulted in cows consuming their feed more slowly in smaller, more frequent meals. Those researchers ascribed that change in feeding pattern to have contributed to an improvement in efficiency of milk production. Therefore, producers are encouraged to find ways of staggering times of milking and feed delivery to encourage a wide distribution of feeding activity throughout the day.

The timing of feed delivery, and availability of feed postmilking, is also important for the udder health of lactating dairy cows. There has been a long-standing belief that dairy cows need to remain standing for some period of time after milking to allow their teat orifice and canals to close. This, in turn, is supposed to help prevent bacterial penetration when the cow eventually lies down, and thus reduce the risk of intramammary infection. Delivery of feed at the time of milking has typically been recommended to encourage cows to remain standing following milking, rather than to immediately lie down. In support of that, in our research we have demonstrated that the presence of fresh feed at the bunk encourages longer postmilking standing times.[4,5,72] The study by DeVries and colleagues[72] was the first to document how postmilking standing time relates to the risk of intramammary infection. It was reported that cows that lay down, on average, for the first time 40 to 60 minutes after milking tended to have lower odds of a new intramammary infection caused by environmental bacteria compared with cows that lay down within 40 minutes after milking. In subsequent work, Watters and colleagues[73] reported that the amount of time spent standing following milking is longer for those cows milked three times per day, and thus cows need to spend even more time standing after milking to reduce the risk of infection. Collectively, the results of these studies indicate that management practices that discourage cows from lying down immediately after milking, such as providing fresh feed near the time of milking, or ensuring there is adequate feed available in the bunk following milking, may help decrease the risk of intramammary infection.

Feed Push-Up

A primary factor influencing feed availability throughout the day is how and when feed is pushed back to cows in the bunk. Dairy cows have a natural tendency to continually sort through their TMR, push it around with their head, and toss it forward where it is no longer within reach. In a flat feeding surface, this is problematic, resulting in producers needing to push the feed closer to the cows in between feed deliveries to ensure continuous TMR access. In our research we have demonstrated that TMR push-up does not have the same stimulatory impact on feeding activity as does the delivery of fresh TMR.[3] There is also no scientific evidence to suggest that pushing up feed more frequently stimulates more DMI. Regardless, TMR push-up is critical to ensure that feed is accessible when cows want to eat; feed push-up needs to occur frequently enough such that any time a cow decides to go to the feed bunk, there is feed available to her at that time. Researchers have shown that greater lying duration is associated with greater frequency of feed push-ups,[5,49] suggesting that frequent push-up minimizes the time cows need to spend waiting for feed access and can devote more time to lying down. Feed push-up also ensures that DMI is not limited, and thus production is optimized. Evidence for this was shown in a cross-sectional study of 47 herds, all with similar genetics and feeding the exact same TMR, by Bach and colleagues,[61] where those herds that did not push up feed (5 out of 47 herds) produced 3.9 kg/d less milk per day per cow (−13% difference). In a more recent observational study of robot herds, Siewert and colleagues[74] reported that farms with automatic feed push-up produced 352 kg more milk/robotic unit and 4.9 kg more milk/cow per day than farms that manually pushed up feed. It is presumable that this effect is not directly attributable to the use of an automated feed pusher, but rather that those farms using such automated equipment had more consistent feed push-up, and thus continual feed access, than those pushing up feed manually. In situations where manual feed push-up is done consistently and frequently, the same results should be achievable.

Feed push-up also helps minimize variation in feed consumed, by mixing up the feed that is no longer in reach with that which is currently available in the bunk. Thus, frequent pushing up of TMR in the bunk is necessary, particularly in the first few hours after feed delivery, when the bulk of the feeding activity has occurred. There are two primary ways to evaluate whether or not feed push-up is occurring frequently enough on farm. The first is to evaluate for the presence (or not) of neck injuries (eg, hair loss, scabbing, lesions, swelling) on the backside of the neck of the cows. Such injuries typically indicate that cows are pushing against the neck rail at the feed bunk, trying to get access to feed that may not be within reach. The position of the neck rail is often blamed for such neck injuries; however, even at low aggressive neck rail placements, these injuries do not necessarily need to be an issue if feed is always available and pushed up. The second indicator of the adequacy of the frequency of the feed push-up is the reaction of cows themselves to that feed push-up. Some may claim that pushing up feed has the same stimulatory effect on eating as does the delivery of fresh TMR; from the scientific literature, that does not seem to be the case. In situations where feed push-up has a large stimulation effect on cows to get up and eat, it would indicate that the cows are hungry, and have gone too long without good access to the TMR that is supposed to be available to them. Therefore, it is recommended in those situations to push-up feed more frequently. In those scenarios the stimulatory effect of pushing up the feed diminishes over time, resulting in cows consuming feed when they want to, and eating a more consistent ration overall.

In summary, greater intake, production, and efficiency may be achieved by ensuring cows have continual access to their TMR across the day, by ensuring adequate feeding amounts, increasing the frequency of feed delivery, altering the timing of feed delivery to create multiple stimulation points for feeding across the day, and pushing up feed frequently. These all not only ensure cows are stimulated to eat across the day, but that there is feed continuously available to them when they want to eat, and that the feed consumed is consistent with that originally formulated for them.

SUMMARY

Despite many advances in the nutritional management of dairy cows, it is known that DMI is not always maximized, nor is the way feed is consumed always ideal for the cow. The feeding behavior of dairy cows, including how, when, and what cows eat of the feed provided to them, has significant impacts on health and productivity. Housing and management strategies may be implemented to optimize access to feed and feeding patterns, thus promoting good health, productivity, and welfare. Reducing competition for feed access, by providing sufficient amounts of space at the feed bunk for all cows to eat simultaneously, along with proper design of the feed bunk barrier, may all have significant impacts on ensuring cows can get to feed when they want to. Ensuring feed is provided in sufficient amounts across the day, so that feed is available at any time of the day when cows go to the bunk, helps prevent inconsistent feed intake patterns from developing. Frequent push-up of feed in the bunk across the day is also critical to maintain that continuous feed access. Finally, the frequent delivery of fresh feed (particularly of TMR) may help in limiting sorting, and thus reducing the variability in composition of feed consumed, and also promote the consumption of frequent, smaller meals across the day. These housing and management strategies are all recommended with the goal of promoting healthy feed consumption patterns that are conducive to high levels of intake, good rumen health, production, and welfare.

ACKNOWLEDGMENTS

Much of the research reviewed in this paper was funded in part by Natural Sciences and Engineering Research Council of Canada (NSERC; Ottawa, ON, Canada) Discovery Grants awarded to T.J. DeVries and Ontario Ministry of Agriculture Food and Rural Affairs (OMAFRA)/University of Guelph Production Systems research grants. Thanks also to the many students and staff at the University of Guelph and University of British Columbia for their contributions to much of this research.

REFERENCES

1. Gonyou HW, Stricklin WR. Diurnal behaviour patters of feedlot bulls during winter and spring in northern latitudes. J Anim Sci 1984;58:1075–83.
2. Ray DE, Roubicek CB. Behaviour of feedlot cattle during two seasons. J Anim Sci 1971;33:72–6.
3. DeVries TJ, von Keyserlingk MAG, Beauchemin KA. Diurnal feeding pattern of lactating dairy cows. J Dairy Sci 2003b;86:4079–82.
4. DeVries TJ, von Keyserlingk MAG. Time of fresh feed delivery affects the feeding and lying patterns of dairy cows. J Dairy Sci 2005;88:625–31.
5. King MTM, Crossley RE, DeVries TJ. Impact of timing of feed delivery on the behavior and productivity of dairy cows. J Dairy Sci 2016;99:1471–82.
6. Grant RJ, Albright JL. Effect of animal grouping on feeding behaviour and intake of dairy cattle. J Dairy Sci 2001;84(E. Suppl.):E156–63.
7. National Farm Animal Care Council. Code of practice for the care and handling of dairy cattle. Ottawa (Canada): Dairy Farmers of Canada; 2009.
8. Nielsen BL. On the interpretation of feeding behaviour measures and the use of feeding rate as an indicator of social constraint. Appl Anim Behav Sci 1999;63:79–91.
9. Johnston C, DeVries TJ. Associations of feeding behavior and milk production in dairy cows. J Dairy Sci 2018;101:3367–73.
10. DeVries TJ, von Keyserlingk MAG, Weary DM, et al. Measuring the feeding behavior of lactating dairy cows in early to peak lactation. J Dairy Sci 2003a; 86:3354–61.
11. Allen MS. Relationship between fermentation acid production in the rumen and the requirement for physically effective fiber. J Dairy Sci 1997;80:1447–62.
12. Beauchemin KA, Eriksen L, Nørgaard P, et al. Salivary secretion during meals in lactating dairy cattle. J Dairy Sci 2008;91:2077–81.
13. Krause KM, Oetzel G. Understanding and preventing subacute ruminal acidosis in dairy herds: a review. Anim Feed Sci Tech 2006;126:215–36.
14. Miller-Cushon EK, DeVries TJ. Feed sorting in dairy cattle: causes, consequences, and management. J Dairy Sci 2017b;100:4172–83.
15. DeVries TJ, Beauchemin KA, von Keyserlingk MAG. Dietary forage concentration affects the feed sorting behavior of lactating dairy cows. J Dairy Sci 2007;90:5572–9.
16. Leonardi C, Armentano LE. Effect of quantity, quality, and length of alfalfa hay on selective consumption by dairy cows. J Dairy Sci 2003;86:557–64.
17. DeVries TJ, Dohme F, Beauchemin KA. Repeated ruminal acidosis challenges in lactating dairy cows at high and low risk for developing acidosis: feed sorting. J Dairy Sci 2008;91:3958–67.
18. DeVries TJ, Holsthausen L, Oba M, et al. Effect of parity and stage of lactation on feed sorting behavior of lactating dairy cows. J Dairy Sci 2011;94:4039–45.
19. Fish JA, DeVries TJ. Varying dietary dry matter concentration through water addition: effect on nutrient intake and sorting of dairy cows in late lactation. J Dairy Sci 2012;95:850–5.

20. Miller-Cushon EK, DeVries TJ. Associations between feed push-up frequency, feeding and lying behavior, and milk composition of dairy cows. J Dairy Sci 2017a;100:2213–8.

21. Sova AD, LeBlanc SJ, McBride BW, et al. Associations between herd-level feeding management practices, feed sorting, and milk production in freestall dairy farms. J Dairy Sci 2013;96:4759–70.

22. Coon RE, Duffield TF, DeVries TJ. Effect of straw particle size on the behavior, health, and production of early lactation dairy cows. J Dairy Sci 2018;101:6375–87.

23. DeVries TJ, von Keyserlingk MAG, Beauchemin KA. Frequency of feed delivery affects the behavior of lactating dairy cows. J Dairy Sci 2005;88:3553–62.

24. Hosseinkhani A, DeVries TJ, Proudfoot KL, et al. The effects of feed bunk competition on the feed sorting behavior of close-up dry cows. J Dairy Sci 2008;91:1115–21.

25. Giraldeau LA, Caraco T. Social foraging theory. Princeton (NJ): Princeton University Press; 2000.

26. Forbes JM. Voluntary food intake and diet selection in farm animals. Wallingford (United Kingdom): CAB Int.; 1995.

27. Olofsson J. Competition for total mixed diets fed for ad libitum intake using one or four cows per feeding station. J Dairy Sci 1999;82:69–79.

28. Huzzey JM, Weary DM, Tiau BYF, et al. Short communication: automatic detection of social competition using an electronic feeding system. J Dairy Sci 2014;97:2953–8.

29. Proudfoot KL, Veira DM, Weary DM, et al. Competition at the feed bunk changes the feeding, standing, and social behavior of transition dairy cows. J Dairy Sci 2009;92:3116–23.

30. Rioja-Lang FJ, Roberts DJ, Healy SD, et al. Dairy cow feeding space requirements assessed in a Y-maze choice test. J Dairy Sci 2012;95:3954–60.

31. Bielharz RG, Zeeb K. Social dominance in dairy cattle. Appl Anim Ethol 1982;8: 79–97.

32. Bouissou MF. Behaviour of domestic cattle under modern management techniques. In: Hood DE, Tarrant PV, editors. The problem of dark-cutting in beef. The Hague (The Netherlands): Martinus Nijhoff; 1981. p. 141–69.

33. Rioja-Lang FC, Roberts DJ, Healy SD, et al. Dairy cows trade-off feed quality with proximity to a dominant individual in Y-maze choice tests. Appl Anim Behav Sci 2009;117:159–64.

34. DeVries TJ, von Keyserlingk MAG, Weary DM. Effect of feeding space on the inter-cow distance, aggression and feeding behavior of free-stall housed lactating dairy cows. J Dairy Sci 2004;87:1432–8.

35. DeVries TJ, von Keyserlingk MAG. Feed stalls affect the social and feeding behavior of lactating dairy cows. J Dairy Sci 2006;89:3522–31.

36. Huzzey JM, DeVries TJ, Valois P, et al. Stocking density and feed barrier design affect the feeding and social behavior of dairy cattle. J Dairy Sci 2006;89:126–33.

37. Crossley RE, Harlander-Matauschek A, DeVries TJ. Variability in behavior and production between dairy cows fed under differing levels of competition. J Dairy Sci 2017;100:3825–38.

38. Batchelder TL. The impact of head gates and over-crowding on production and behaviour patterns of lactating dairy cows. In: Dairy housing and equipment systems. Camp Hill (PA): Managing and Planning for Profitability, Natural Resource, Agriculture, and Engineering Service Publ #129; 2000. p. 325–30.

39. Krawczel PD, Klaiber LB, Butzler RE, et al. Short-term increases in stocking density affect the lying and social behavior, but not the productivity, of lactating Holstein dairy cows. J Dairy Sci 2012a;95:4298–308.

40. Galindo F, Broom DM. The relationships between social behaviour of dairy cows and the occurrence of lameness in three herds. Res Vet Sci 2000;69:75–9.
41. Greenough PR, Vermunt JJ. Evaluation of subclinical laminitis in a dairy herd and observations on associated nutritional and management factors. Vet Rec 1991; 128:11–7.
42. Huzzey JM, Grant RJ, Overton TR. Short communication: relationship between competitive success during displacements at an overstocked feed bunk and measures of physiology and behaviour in Holstein dairy cattle. J Dairy Sci 2012a;95:4434–41.
43. Huzzey JM, Nydam DV, Grant RJ, et al. The effects of overstocking Holstein dairy cattle during the dry period on cortisol secretion and energy metabolism. J Dairy Sci 2012b;95:4421–33.
44. Hetti Arachchige AD, Fisher AD, Wales WJ, et al. Space allowance and barriers influence cow competition for mixed rations fed on a feed-pad between bouts of grazing. J Dairy Sci 2014;97:3578–88.
45. Caraviello DZ, Weigel KA, Craven M, et al. Analysis of reproductive performance of lactating cows on large dairy farms using machine learning algorithms. J Dairy Sci 2006;89:4703–22.
46. Schefers JM, Weigel KA, Rawson CL, et al. Management practices associated with conception rate and service rate of lactating Holstein cows in large, commercial dairy herds. J Dairy Sci 2010;93:1459–67.
47. Woolpert ME, Dann HM, Cotanch KW, et al. Management practices, physically effective fiber, and ether extract are related to bulk tank milk de novo fatty acid concentrations on Holstein dairy farms. J Dairy Sci 2017;100:5097–106.
48. Krawczel PD, Mooney CS, Dann HM, et al. Effect of alternative models for increasing stocking density on the short-term behavior and hygiene of Holstein dairy cows. J Dairy Sci 2012b;95:2467–75.
49. Deming JA, Bergeron R, Leslie KE, et al. Associations of housing, management, milking activity, and standing and lying behavior of dairy cows milked in automatic systems. J Dairy Sci 2013;96:344–51.
50. Goldhawk C, Chapinal N, Veira DM, et al. Prepartum feeding behavior is an early indicator of subclinical ketosis. J Dairy Sci 2009;92:4971–7.
51. Huzzey JM, Veira DM, Weary DM, et al. Behavior and intake measures can identify cows at risk for metritis. J Dairy Sci 2007;90:3220–33.
52. Kaufman EI, Leblanc SJ, McBride BW, et al. Association of rumination time with subclinical ketosis in transition dairy cows. J Dairy Sci 2016;99:5604–18.
53. Bouissou MF. Role du contact physique dans la manifestation des relations hiérarchiques chez les bovines. Consequences pra- tiques. Ann Zootech 1970;19: 279–85.
54. Konggaard SP. Feeding conditions in relation to welfare for dairy cows in loose-housing systems. In: Baxter SH, Baxter MR, MacCormack JAD, editors. Farm animal housing and welfare. Dordrecht (The Netherlands): Martinus Nijhoff; 1983. p. 272–80.
55. Endres MI, DeVries TJ, von Keyserlingk MAG, et al. Effect of feed barrier design on the behavior of loose-housed lactating dairy cows. J Dairy Sci 2005;88:2377–80.
56. Collings LKM, Weary DM, Chapinal N, et al. Temporal feed restriction and overstocking increase competition for feed by dairy cattle. J Dairy Sci 2011;94:5480–6.
57. Martinsson K, Burstedt E. Effect of length of access time to feed and allotment of hay on grass silage intake and production in lactating dairy cows. Swed J Agric Res 1990;20:169–76.
58. French P, Chamberlain J, Warntjes J. Effect of feed refusal amount on feeding behavior and production in Holstein cows. J Dairy Sci 2005;88(E. Suppl. 1):175.

59. Munksgaard L, Jensen MB, Pedersen LJ, et al. Quantifying behavioural priorities - Effects of time constraints on behaviour of dairy cows, Bos taurus. Appl Anim Behav Sci 2005;92:3–14.

60. Miller-Cushon EK, DeVries TJ. Feeding amount affects the sorting behavior of lactating dairy cows. Can J Anim Sci 2010;90:1–7.

61. Bach A, Valls N, Solans A, et al. Associations between nondietary factors and dairy herd performance. J Dairy Sci 2008;91:3259–67.

62. Shabi Z, Bruckental I, Zamwell S, et al. Effects of extrusion of grain and feeding frequency on rumen fermentation, nutrient digestibility, and milk yield and composition in dairy cows. J Dairy Sci 1999;82:1252–60.

63. Mantysaari P, Khalili H, Sariola J. Effect of feeding frequency of a total mixed ration on the performance of high-yielding dairy cows. J Dairy Sci 2006;89: 4312–20.

64. Oostra HH, Stefanowska J, Sällvik K. The effects of feeding frequency on waiting time, milking frequency, cubicle and feeding fence utilization for cows in an automatic milking system. Acta Agr Scand A-An 2005;55:158–65.

65. Endres MI, Espejo LA. Feeding management and characteristics of rations for high-producing dairy cows in freestall herds. J Dairy Sci 2010;93:822–9.

66. Rottman LW, Ying Y, Zhou K, et al. The daily rhythm of milk synthesis is dependent on the timing of feed intake in dairy cows. Physiol Rep 2014;2:1–12.

67. Dhiman TR, Zaman MS, MacQueen IS, et al. Influence of corn processing and frequency of feeding on cow performance. J Dairy Sci 2002;85:217–26.

68. Hart KD, McBride BW, Duffield TF, et al. Effect of frequency of feed delivery on the behavior and productivity of lactating dairy cows. J Dairy Sci 2014;97:1713–24.

69. Crossley RE, Harlander-Matauschek A, DeVries TJ. Mitigation of variability between competitively-fed dairy cows through increased feed delivery frequency. J Dairy Sci 2018;101:518–29.

70. Felton C, DeVries TJ. Effect of water addition to a total mixed ration on feed temperature, feed intake, sorting behavior, and milk production of dairy cows. J Dairy Sci 2010;93:2651–60.

71. Miller-Cushon EK, DeVries TJ. Effect of dietary dry matter concentration on the sorting behavior of lactating dairy cows fed a total mixed ration. J Dairy Sci 2009;92:3292–8.

72. DeVries TJ, Dufour S, Scholl DT. Relationship between feeding strategy, lying behavior patterns, and incidence of intramammary infection in dairy cows. J Dairy Sci 2010;93:1987–97.

73. Watters MEA, Barkema HW, Leslie KE, et al. Relationship between post-milking standing duration and risk of intramammary infection in free-stall housed dairy cows milked three times per day. J Dairy Sci 2014;97:3456–71.

74. Siewert JM, Salfer JA, Endres MI. Factors associated with productivity on automatic milking system dairy farms in the Upper Midwest United States. J Dairy Sci 2018;101:8327–34.

Maximizing Comfort in Tiestall Housing

Harold K. House, MSc, PEng[a],*, Neil G. Anderson, DVM, MSc[b]

KEYWORDS

- Tiestall • Cow comfort • Tie rail • Stall partition • Electric trainer

KEY POINTS

- Stall size must be designed for the size of cow to accommodate lunging space and lying space.
- Base and bedding must provide comfort and traction while minimizing hock lesions.
- Feed and water must be easily accessible.
- Electric trainers can be used to promote stall cleanliness if managed properly.
- Proper ventilation is necessary for fresh air and heat stress relief.

INTRODUCTION

It is important in all forms of dairy cow housing to maximize comfort by designing and building for the cow, and tiestall housing is no exception. This article focuses on key areas that have an overall effect on the comfort of the dairy cow in tiestall housing and lead to improved comfort and producer satisfaction.

Tiestall housing is the name given to dairy cattle housing where the cows are individually tethered in distinct stalls (**Fig. 1**). This option is often considered with herd sizes up to 100 cows but can be used with larger herds as well. Cows are milked in place and fed individually. Producers with smaller herds believe that it is a lower cost option to milk with a pipeline in the stall compared with a milking parlor capable of milking many more cows. Producers also like the concept of treating cows as individuals.

TIESTALL LAYOUTS

Traditionally, the tiestall barn was a 2-story barn with a loft area above and a stable area below (**Fig. 2**). This allowed for convenient storage of hay and straw that could be transferred to the cows in the stable below. Tiestalls were arranged in a double

The authors have nothing to disclose.
[a] DairyLogix, 34049 Saltford Road, RR#4, Goderich, Ontario N7A 3Y1, Canada; [b] 14789 Creditview Road, Cheltenham, Ontario L7C 3G6, Canada
* Corresponding author.
E-mail address: harold@dairylogix.com

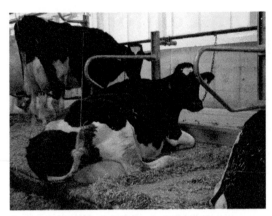

Fig. 1. Cows are tethered in individual stalls in tiestall housing.

row running the length of the barn with possible maternity pens and young stock pens along 1 side or at 1 end.

The modern tiestall barn is a single-story barn with feed stored in an adjacent building or silos (**Fig. 3**). Tiestalls are still arranged in a double row running the length of the barn, and the most common arrangement is a tail-to-tail configuration, because approximately two-thirds of the time is spent behind the cows for milking and bedding maintenance. Some producers prefer a head-to-head arrangement because this allows for feeding options that may include some form of automation. Long narrow tiestall barns allow for tunnel ventilation options that are not as economical in wider barns. Some larger tiestall operations have been constructed with 4-row configurations, but 2 rows of tiestalls are the most common arrangement.

Another layout option that has gained some popularity is a row of 2 stalls with an adjacent row of bedded pack pens along 1 side (**Fig. 4**). This allows for the housing of mature cows and replacements under 1 roof.

STALL AREA

Cow measurements and their space requirements are needed to design stalls. Stall dimensions must be appropriate for standing, lying, rising, and resting without injury,

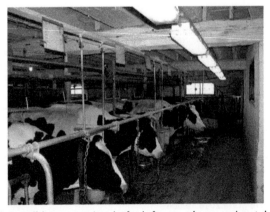

Fig. 2. Traditional tiestall barns consisted of a loft area above and a stable area below.

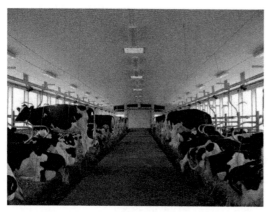

Fig. 3. Modern tiestall barns consist of single story barns with adjacent feed storage.

pain, or fear. Stalls must meet the needs of the cow for comfort and of the caregiver for cleanliness and ease of milking. This article describes cow dimensions, space requirements, and tiestall dimensions for Holstein cows typically seen in North America. The concepts shown in **Tables 1** and **2** may be used to design stalls for Holstein heifers or other dairy breeds.

Cow Dimensions

Cows vary in size between and within herds. The first step in planning stall size is the measurement of primiparous and multiparous cows in a herd (**Fig. 5**). Rump heights and hook-bone widths are useful measures to estimate several other body dimensions. Because several body dimensions are proportional, ratios provide reasonable estimates of dimensions for calves, heifers, or other dairy breeds. Stalls may be built in 3 sizes (sized for primiparous cows, multiparous milking cows, and dry or special-needs cows) in recognition of the variation in cow size and their needs within a herd. Anderson[1] proposed measuring a sample of small, medium, and large cows. A barn with 1 stall size poses several challenges to both management and cows. Stall and cow cleanliness, labor, mastitis, lameness, and cow comfort are issues to consider in choosing tiestall sizes.

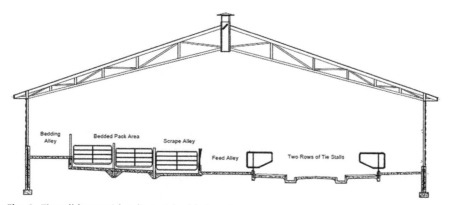

Fig. 4. Tiestall barn with adjacent bedded pack area.

Table 1
Body dimensions, example measurements for mature Holsteins, and estimated ratios to rump height and hook-bone width

Body Dimension	Inches	Proportions
Nose-to-tail length	102 (range 96–110)	1.6 × rump height
Imprint length—resting	72 (68–76)	1.2 × rump height
Imprint width	52 (48–54)	2.0 × hook-bone width
Forward lunge space	24 (23–26)	0.4 × rump height
Stride length when rising	18	0.3 × rump height
Rump height—mature	Median 60 (range 58–64)	
Rump height—lactation 1	Median 58, top 25% - 59	
Stance—front-to-rear feet	60 (range 58–64)	1.0 × rump height
Withers (shoulder) height	60 (range 58–64)	1.0 × rump height
Hook-bone width	26 (range 24–27)	

Table 1 shows measurements of multiparous Canadian Holsteins at a dairy herd and some calculated proportions. For example, multiparous cows had a rump height of 60 in, a nose-to-tail length of 8.5 ft, and a hook-bone width of 25 in. Their weight exceeded 1550 lb.

Space Requirements

Research by the University of British Columbia determined that a 1350-lb cow uses 118 in longitudinal space and 43 in lateral space when lying.[2] Observations of cows freely lying and rising reveal that a multiparous Holstein cow uses 102 in × 52 in of living space and another 20 (16–24) in of forward space for lunging motions.

Nose-to-tail length describes the measurement from the tail to the nose of a cow standing with her head forward. A cow has a normal crook in her neck when lying and her nose-to-tail length is less than while standing.

Imprint length describes the length from folded foreknee to tail while lying in the narrow position. It defines the bed length needed for resting with all body parts on the stall. Imprint length is greater when the cow extends her front legs forward in a normal (long) resting position.

When resting in the narrow position, the point of the hock on the upper hind leg and the extension of the abdomen on the opposite side define the imprint width. This width is the minimum stall width for a resting cow. For improved comfort, however, most new tiestall barns are built with stalls wider than the imprint width of a cow in the

Table 2
Stall dimensions, estimated relationships to body dimensions, and example calculations for mature Holsteins in a study herd

Stall Dimension	Ratio and Reference Body Dimension	An Example a Median Cow
Bed length = imprint length	1.2 × rump height	1.2 × 60 = 72 in
Tie rail height above cow's feet	0.80 × rump height	0.80 × 60 = 48 in
Stall width[a] = imprint width	2.0 × hook-bone width	2 × 26 = 52 in

[a] Producers are building most new tiestalls wider than this minimum width. They mount loops on 54-in centers to provide 50 in of width.

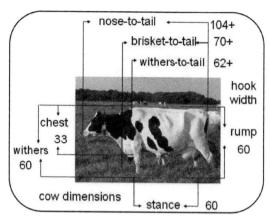

Fig. 5. Cow measurements (in inches) useful for designing stalls.

narrow resting position. This increased space also allows easy access to the cow at milking time for the milker.

Lunging space is the room needed for lying and rising motions and it extends forward, downward, and upward for head lunge and bob, vertically and forward for standing, and laterally for hindquarter movements. Knowledge of lunging space is needed to properly size the opening at the front of tiestalls, position tie rails, choose the shape and dimensions of stall dividers, and avoid hazards when turning out of stalls. A cow's nose uses the space 4 in to 12 in above the surface when lying or rising.

Stall Dimensions as Ratios of Body Dimensions

Although nose-to-tail length is essential, it is a difficult dimension to gather. Hookbone width and rump height are easy to measure and because many body dimensions are proportional; these 2 cow dimensions are useful references for sizing stalls. **Table 2** shows stall dimensions, estimated relationships to body dimensions, and example calculations for mature Holsteins in a study herd.

Fig. 6 shows a tie-rail stall and example dimensions. Cows should be measured before choosing stall sizes.

Tie Rail (Head Rail) Location

A tie rail (sometimes called a head rail) is the pipe used as the attachment for the tie chain and often serves a dual purpose, acting as the water line supply to the water bowls. The tie rail controls the forward location of a cow while she stands in the stall. The standing surface (eg, mat or mattress) is the reference for vertical placement of the tie rail. The vertical location above the bed may be approximately 0.8 × rump height. In practice, the tie rail may be mounted 44 in to 48 in higher than the top surface of the bed. Higher tie rails improve udder cleanliness,[3,4] but they may have an adverse effect on neck lesions, lying time, and lameness,[5] so some debate exists regarding the appropriate height.

There is greater confidence regarding the horizontal location of the head rail relative to the feed manger. The tie rail forward location is a horizontal measurement from the gutter curb. The tie rail mounts 8 in to 12 in forward of the center of the manger curb and over the manger. A tie rail placed 86 in horizontally forward of the gutter curb allows cows with approximately 58-in to 60-in rump height to stand straight in the stall. Providing greater space behind the rail decreases the risk for neck and knee injuries

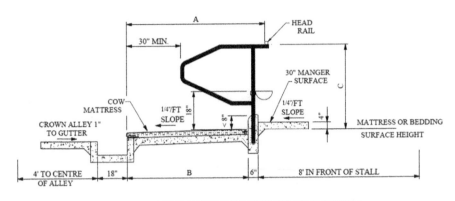

Fig. 6. Tiestall partition showing dimensions for cows of various stages of lactation.

	DIMENSIONS (IN)				
Holstein Cows	A	B	C	WIDTH	CHAIN LENGTH
Primiparous	84	70	44	50	C - 8
Multiparous	86	72	48	54	C - 8
Dry Cow	86	72	48	60	C - 8

and increases both the frequency and duration of lying bouts but also slightly increases the risk for dirty udders.[5]

Proper location of the tie rail lets a cow stand parallel to the dividers with all 4 feet in the stall and rise or lie with minimal or no contact with it. Measure vertical placement from the concrete platform during construction and allow for the bed. Standing in the gutter, diagonal standing or neck injuries are obvious signs of incorrect placement or obstructions at the front of the stall.

Injuries to the sensitive supraspinous processes of the neck may occur with tie rails located higher than 48 in to 50 in and when cows reach for feed. Injuries to supraspinous processes may be avoided by mounting the tie rail lower and keeping feed within reach. The distance between the manger curb and the tie rail may be ample enough to allow a cow to pass through without entrapment.

Tie Chain—Length and Safety

A tie chain confines a cow to her stall space and allows for ease of lunging, resting in the head back position, or grooming. Longer neck chains have been shown to reduce the risk for hock lesions[3–6] and neck and knee injuries.[5] A tie chain with snap should extend only to the height of the manger curb (**Fig. 7**). Prevention of entrapment of a leg is assured by installing the proper length of chain. The "tails" of the bracket should be oriented to extend fore and aft rather than downward and upward. Longer chains give cows freedom to show strong signs of estrus, but they may be shortened (eg, wrap the chain around the tie rail) temporarily (12–24 h) when a cow is in heat or when a cow must be handled to facilitate the administration of treatment, for example.

Wide Opening—Forward or Diagonal Lunge

When rising or lying normally, a multiparous Holstein cow uses approximately 10 ft of space measured from her tail to her most forward lunge distance. Therefore, unobstructed forward space for frontward lunging and bobbing of the head should be provided by designing a wide front opening and paying attention to feed curb height. Obstructions in the lunging space lead to diagonal (corner-to-corner) standing, lying,

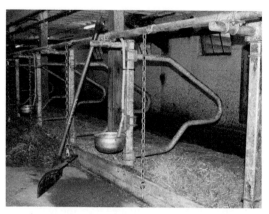

Fig. 7. The tie chain with snap should extend to the height of the manger curb.

and rising. Cows still lunge forward relative to their body direction but diagonal or side-wise to the stall. For side lunging, choose a divider with an opening wide enough to permit easy lunging for rising or lying.

Manger Curb

A manger or feed curb defines the forward limit of the bed length measured from the gutter curb. Manger curbs keep bedding out of feed and feed in the manger. Tradition-ally, the curb height has been built at 10 in to 12 in measured from the concrete plat-form for mattress stalls, making the final curb height 8 in higher than the cow's feet (eg, top of mattress or mat with bedding). The height of the manger curb (and the manger surface) must not interfere with forward lunging motions and a disadvantage of this traditional design has been that the feed curb does interfere with the normal stride taken during rising. Even then, however, some cows stride into the manger and a slip-pery surface poses a secondary hazard. Concrete and wood are the most common materials used to build manger curbs and concrete is typically poured 6 in wide to sup-port divider mounting posts. Cows extend their legs forward into the manger and rest with their necks on the curb (**Fig. 8**). Curb edges should be beveled, smooth, or rounded on the cow and manger sides. A flat manger surface and a wooden curb may save the cost of forming and pouring a concrete curb and this approach has emerged more recently to replace the traditional approach. With this technique, pro-ducers attach a board (eg, 2 × 4) to the posts that support the stall dividers, and, by minimizing height, this design allows more freedom for front leg movement.

Manger Height and Surface

The height of the manger surface (feed table) is designed relative to the cow's feet on the bed.

Manger height is chosen to minimize pressure on the front claws, optimize foot health, and make eating more comfortable for cows. Manger height should allow for nearly normal lunging motions with minor compromises for bobbing the head. Cows may choose to kneel to eat when the manger is level with or lower than their feet or when the tie rail is too low. Traditionally, the manger surface is built 4 in higher than the level of the cow's feet (top of the mattress or bedding). This is approximately 6 in to 7 in measured from the concrete platform, but, in alternative designs without a large concrete feed curb, they are level with the standing surface. The eating surface

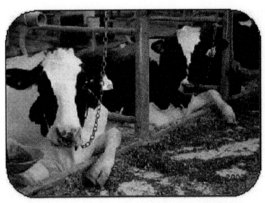

Fig. 8. The manger curb separates the bedding area from the feed area and should be beveled to allow the cow to extend her legs comfortably over the curb.

is built approximately 24-in wide and made with an acid-resistant, relatively smooth finish. Ceramic tile, plastic, and special concrete are common surfaces for mangers. Each provides benefits, challenges, or hazards for consideration because slippery surfaces are a hazard for workers. Feed should be kept within 24 in of the manger curb. An elevated feed alley keeps feed closer to cows, reduces reaching for feed and stepping forward, minimizes injuries to necks or manure contamination of beds, and reduces labor for pushing up feed. The disadvantage is that this design requires a higher manger curb, which may obstruct the forward movement of the forelimb while rising.

Water Bowls

Nose-to-poll length establishes the space required for access to a water bowl. This length is approximately 24 in for multiparous Holstein cows. 24 in of space should be provided from the top of the water bowl to any obstruction above it. An obstruction may be a tie rail, manger divide, or stall divider, depending on location of the water bowl (**Fig. 9**). Tie rails mounted 44 in, 46 in, or 48 in above the bed allow water bowls to be mounted over the manger and to provide greater than or equal to 24 in above the bowl for drinking and adequate space below the bowl for cleaning mangers.

The bowl may be placed within a manger divide over the manger when there is 24 in of unobstructed space above the bowl. Dominant cows may keep submissive cows away from the water bowl and a hinged panel within a manger divide is one solution to the problem. Other solutions include a bowl on each side or moving the cow to another stall. Do not mount the water bowl above the tie rail. The risk of wet bedding, mastitis, or slippery beds is greater with bowls over the stall platform. Size the water line for peak flow—often a 2-in to 3-in line is large enough in most facilities.

Platform—Length and Slope

The length of the stall platform is the distance from the gutter curb to the manger curb.

The imprint length of the resting cow should be used as a guide for determining the correct platform length. Platform length should allow cows to rest parallel to the dividers in the short position with tail and legs on the bed. Consider a 70-in platform for primiparous cows that have a rump height of 58 in to 59 in. Consider a 72-in platform for multiparous Holstein cows measuring 60 in at the rump. Increased stall platform length is associated with decreased risk for hind claw rotation—an indication of

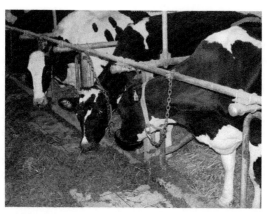

Fig. 9. The cow should have 24 in of clearance to comfortably drink from the water bowl.

poor claw health[3,4]—and knee lesions[5] but a slight increase in the risk of dirtier udders.[3–5]

In practice, bed or platform length ranges from 68 in to 72 in. Some producers have built longer beds for cows standing greater than 60 in at the rump. For stalls with mattresses or mats, bed length should be measured from the gutter curb to the manger curb. With stalls using a bedding retainer, it is important to use sufficient bedding so that the bedding retainer is never exposed. Measure bed length from the gutter side of the bedding keeper when the bedding keeper is kept covered with bedding. The minimum platform length described previously does not permit cows to lie straight with their forelegs extended. They lie diagonally or lie with their rumps over the gutter to attain this normal resting posture. Stalls are seldom built with longer beds, however, because they pose challenges with stall and cow cleanliness and the risk of mastitis.

A slope of 2% to 3% should be built into the concrete platform (higher at the front) (eg, approximately 1.5–2.0 in, in a 72-in stall) and the interior of the barn should slope from 1 end to the other to keep the milk line the same height above the platform.

Stall Bed or Cushion

Concrete platforms require a cushion for a resting surface. Ample bedding is a best management practice installed in most animal welfare audit programs, and cows need a cushioning surface with good traction to avoid injuries. Obstructions to normal resting positions and choices in beds or bedding contribute to restlessness and hock blemishes or injuries. Rubber-filled, foam mats with rubber top covers; mats of various compositions; and organic (straw, sawdust, or peat moss) or inorganic (sand) bedding provide varying degrees of cushioning for the stall platform. Mattresses or mats have a limited life expectancy for softness and require replacement after a few years in service. They should be bedded with chopped straw, sawdust, kiln-dried softwood shavings, or peat moss. Hardwood shavings or wood chips are unacceptable bedding materials because they are not very absorbent, and their hardness and sharpness may lead to hock damage. Solid mats provide varying amounts of cushioning and they require a generous (eg, >3 in) cover with bedding. Nash and colleagues[7] found, when comparing bedding depth, that farms using as little as 1 in or more of bedding on a mattress base had an increased average herd lying time of 72 minutes per day compared with herds with less than 1 in of bedding on rubber mats. The herds bedded with 1 in or more of bedding on mattresses also had 24% fewer hock injuries and 25% fewer knee injuries.

Some mattresses or mats allow a basin to form that collects urine and milk. This results in wet teats, udders, and flanks and a hazard for mastitis. Some mats or top covers are slippery and become slipperier with straw and moisture. Water bowls mounted over the bed can contribute to wetness and slipperiness in the stall and are not recommended. Poor traction with 1 foot on a slippery bed and the other on ceramic tile in a manger may contribute to a falling-forward hazard while rising or reaching feed.

Sand bedding, although not common in tiestall applications, is a material that significantly reduces lameness in free stalls and can be used in tiestalls as well. Concrete platforms can be converted to sand by fixing a 6-in × 6-in post cut at a 45° angle or a 3-in dia Polyvinyl chloride or fiberglass pipe to the rear of the stall (**Fig. 10**). Manure removal is a challenge, and some reinforcement of the manure gutter is required to deal with the extra wear caused by the sand, particularly at right-angle turns. Usually an organic substrate, such as paper or hay, is added to the manure channel to facilitate movement of the sand laden manure along the gutter. Some producers have filled in gutter cleaner channels with concrete and then bedded with straw at the curb and removed the manure straw sand mix with a skid steer loader.

Loops or Dividers and Stall Width

Loops or dividers define the width of the stall space for each cow, and imprint width should be used to determine minimum stall width (approximately 2 times hook-bone width). Because minimum width prevents cows from resting in wider positions, producers frequently build stalls wider than the minimum and tiestalls are often installed wider than in freestall barns. Dividers are often mounted on 54-in centers for average-sized multiparous Holstein cows (gives 52 in of space). In practice, loops are being mounted on 50-in to 60-in centers to provide 48 in to 58 in of space, depending on cow size or special needs. Wider stalls have been shown to promote longer lying times, reduce lameness, and decrease the risk for neck lesions but also carry a low risk for dirtier legs and flanks.[5,6]

A loop mounted on each side defines the stall space and prevents cows from swinging widely, contaminating beds with manure or urine, or tramping on teats. A loop design for ease of use by the cow when exiting the stall or the worker when moving milkers between adjacent stalls is preferred. Generally, this is a loop with the rear part of the top pipe lower than the forward part of the top pipe, and provides 30 in of space at the back of the stall (eg, a 42-in loop for 72-in platforms). Cows need

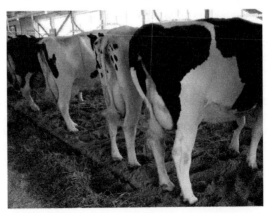

Fig. 10. Tiestall cows bedded with sand using a 3 in. dia. PVC pipe for retaining the bedding.

this space to back into while turning to exit a stall safely; 12 in of space between the top of the bed and the bottom pipe of the divider should be provided to avoid entrapment of a cow's head (**Fig. 11**). The supports should be mounted for milking equipment to the posts. This allows a cow to swing her head easily over the loop without obstructions. Many companies manufacture support posts that allow adjustment of the height of the tie rail, loop, or water bowl.

There has been interest in flexible dividers for tiestall partitions similar to the interest shown in freestall barns. Flexible dividers allow the cow more freedom of movement, but at the same time the cow can take advantage of the flexibility to crowd into the adjacent stalls.

End Stalls

An end stall must provide space for backing around with the rump, swinging the head for turning out of the stall, and resting postures. A stall divider (loop) should be used for the end partition.

A section of brisket locator or plastic pipe should be used as an end curb. Use the post for mounting milk and vacuum lines. Vertical and horizontal pipes in end stalls obstruct normal backing or head swinging motions and they may contribute to slips or falls while attempting to cross the gutter when cows exit the stall. Concrete curbs in end stalls are hazards for injuries to hook bones when resting, and they restrict normal leg postures for resting cows, making these end stalls less desirable locations in the barn. Cows may avoid end stalls with obstructions when re-entering the barn after being out for exercise.

Stall Height

Stall height is the difference in elevation between the walkway and the stall platform. Stall height affects cow and worker safety or comfort and the stall platform level is typically built 2 in higher than the walkway to facilitate ease of entry or exit for cows and avoidance of cows jumping across gutters. Ease of entry or exit for workers (eg, ergonomics, fatigue, or longevity) and ease of doing reproductive examinations and artificial insemination—ergonomics for technicians and veterinarians—should also weigh on the choice of platform level. The depth of the gutter and frequency of gutter cleaning to avoid overflow of slurry onto walkways or beds are also factors that have an impact on the height chosen.

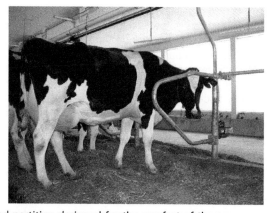

Fig. 11. Suspended partition designed for the comfort of the cow.

Gutter and Walk Alley

The width of the gutter must be less than the step length of a cow. Step length of a cow varies with traction (slipperiness of the floor), lameness, and cow size. The walk alley and bed must provide good traction and the gutters should be made wide enough to accommodate 18-in flites on a gutter cleaner. Gutter grates provide a visual clue to cows crossing a gutter and help keep tails out of slurry. Tail ties help keep tails out of slurry as well. The walk alley can be crowned 1 in from center to gutter, and some producers install rubber with excellent elasticity and traction for the walk alley to facilitate cow flow.

Electric Cow Trainers

Electric trainers train cows to step back when arching their backs for defecation or urination.

The purpose is to position cows so they defecate or urinate in the gutter rather than the stall bed. Electric trainers must not restrict the normal eating, standing, or lying behavior of cows and they must not restrict access to feed or water. Cow trainers are banned in some European countries but continue to be used in North America. Zurbrigg and colleagues[3,4] noted 76% of 317 Ontario tiestall farms used trainers, and, in large spacious stalls, with long neck chains, some producers view cow trainers as essential for positioning the cow to keep the stalls clean. The scientific evidence to support their use is, however, weak. Several studies[3,4] have associated cow trainer use with dirtier udders and hind limbs and a greater risk for hock lesions, but perhaps this reflects poor positioning and use rather than an inherent risk of their use per se, because in many herds they clearly keep stalls and cows cleaner when properly adjusted to the cows using the stalls.

Certainly, if cow trainers are used they should be correctly positioned 48 in (eg, range 47–49 in, horizontal measurement) forward of the gutter curb for Holsteins in stalls with 68-in to 72-in platforms. The trainer should be positioned 42 in (eg, range 41–43 in) forward of the gutter curb for Jerseys in stalls with 62-in to 66-in platforms. The trainer should be located approximately 2 in above the chine for training purposes (approximately 24 h) and raised to approximately 4 in above the chine after the training period. The trainer may be lowered to 2 in for remedial training (24 h) and then raised again to 4 in above the chine (**Fig. 12**). Trainers must have a height adjustment and a fore and aft adjustment for each cow, and they must have secure attachment so they do not fall on a cow. The distance between the trainer bow and the cow must be at least 2 in and be raised to a higher position when a cow is expected to be or is in heat. The power supply must be of low voltage (eg, 2500 V) and power output (eg, 0.1–0.2 J). The power supply must be grounded to a dedicated rod outside the barn and not to any stabling within the barn.

Incorrectly positioned trainers prevent a cow from showing strong signs of heat, making heat detection difficult and contributing to poor reproductive performance. Incorrectly positioned trainers force cows to eat while on their knees and make cows urinate or defecate without arching their back. The location of the milk and vacuum lines must not interfere with the correct location for the trainer because the trainer location has the priority. The directions for installation should include the indications for use.

Diet and consistency of manure affect stall cleanliness and usefulness of electric trainers. The posture and the arc in a cow's spine defecating vary with feeds and feeding husbandry.

Generally, a diet of dry hay and some corn silage leads to firm manure—and an arc in the spine during defecation; however, there may be no arc in the spine and very

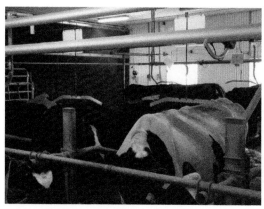

Fig. 12. The cow trainer should be positioned 48 in forward of the gutter curb and 2 in above the chime for training purposes.

slight elevation of the tail with diets that predispose cows to diarrhea. Cow cleanliness concerns and apparent failure of trainers may be corrected by feeding for firmer manure and regaining the arced posture for defecation.

Tethering and Exercise

The most significant difference between tiestall housing and other methods of housing and managing dairy cattle is the restriction of movement imposed by tethering the cow in the stall. In many herds, tiestall cows are allowed outside to an exercise lot for a few hours each day, while the barn is bedded and feed is mixed and delivered. Others producers, however, do not allow daily exercise and cows are tethered 24/7. This is becoming more commonplace in larger facilities with lack of labor.

Proponents of exercise identify 2 main benefits for tiestall housed dairy cows: improved health and improved behavioral freedom. Popescu and colleagues[8] and Regula and colleauges[9] noted a significant reduction in lameness in tiestall herds, and Loberg and colleauges[10] showed an improvement in claw conformation and heel horn erosion with regular access to outside exercise. Keil and colleauges[11] and Gustafson and colleauges[12] found outdoor access improved hock abrasions, with the former study stressing the importance of the duration of access to observe a positive effect, recommending a minimum of 50 hours of outdoor access within a 4-week period, equivalent to 1.5 hours to 2 hours per day.[11] Gustafson and colleauges[12] observed reduced risk for illness with daily exercise.

These are important issues, but it can also be argued that many of these negative effects are a result of poor cow comfort inside the barn—which may be directly addressed through the design improvements discussed thus far in this article. The restriction of movement imposed by tiestalls can be alleviated by daily release for untethered exercise, but ultimately consumers will likely decide whether this is sufficient for tiestall housing to continue into the future.

VENTILATION

Ventilation is another important aspect of comfort in tiestall barns. Tiestall barns can be ventilated naturally or with fans, but the preferred method is naturally with some form of fan ventilation for heat stress relief. Heat stress is an issue in tiestall barns similar to cows in freestall barns and may be an even greater issue because cows

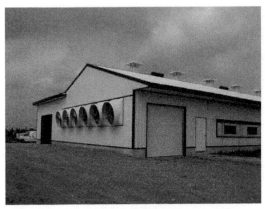

Fig. 13. Two-row tiestall barns are ideally suited for tunnel ventilation.

cannot move to find a place that provides more fresh air. The solutions to provide more convective heat stress relief by increasing the airflow over the cows are similar to free-stall barns, those being the use of panel fans, high-volume low-speed fans, and tunnel ventilation.

The application of panel fans is similar to the application in freestall barns, where the panel fans are placed over the top of the tiestalls to increase the air speed. The use of high-volume low-speed fans is only applicable in wider tiestall barns where the ceiling height is sufficient for the installation and proper functioning of these fans. Tunnel ventilation is a good option in many tiestall barns because a 2-row tiestall barn is long and narrow, and because the air speed is proportional to the cross-sectional area of the barn; higher air speeds can be achieved with less fan power than in wider barns **(Fig. 13)**.

Misting systems can be added to tunnel ventilation to provide evaporative cooling. Another option is to pull the air through a water curtain. This inlet looks like a honey comb or corrugated cardboard type material. Water is distributed at the top of this curtain and allowed to trickle down through the corrugations. The air is pulled through the curtain and the rise in humidity from the water results in a drop in temperature. The curtain needs to be cleaned periodically so that the air flow is not reduced. If misting systems or water curtains are used, care must be taken that they do not increase the moisture content of the bedding, which could lead to mastitis problems.

SUMMARY

Maximizing comfort in tiestall barns is as important as maximizing comfort in other forms of dairy housing. Because the tiestall cow is tethered in 1 place, the stall dimensions, base and bedding, and partition type all play a significant role in providing for the comfort of the cow. Ease of access to feed and water is also a critical factor because mangers and waterers make up part of the tiestall area. Proper ventilation is also important because the cow cannot move to a more comfortable location within the barn.

REFERENCES

1. Anderson NG. Tie-stall dimensions. Guelph (Canada): Ontario Ministry Of Agriculture, Food and rural affairs, Infosheet; 2014. Available at: http://omafra.gov.on.ca/english/livestock/dairy/facts/tiestalldim.htm.

2. Ceballos A, Sanderson D, Rushen J, et al. Improving stall design: use of 3-D kinematics to measure space use by dairy cows when lying down. J Dairy Sci 2004;87(7):2042–50.

3. Zurbrigg K, Kelton D, Anderson N, et al. Tie-stall design and its relationship to lameness, injury, and cleanliness on 317 Ontario dairy farms. J Dairy Sci 2005; 88:3201–10.

4. Zurbrigg K, Kelton D, Anderson N, et al. Stall dimensions and the prevalence of lameness, injury, and cleanliness on 317 tie-stall dairy farms in Ontario. Can Vet J 2005;46:902–9.

5. Bouffard V, de Passillé AM, Rushen J, et al. Effect of following recommendations for tiestall configuration on neck and leg lesions, lameness, cleanliness and lying time in dairy cows. J Dairy Sci 2017;100:2935–43.

6. Nash CGR, Kelton DF, DeVries TJ, et al. Prevalence of and risk factors for hock and knee injuries on dairy cows in tiestall housing in Canada. J Dairy Sci 2016; 99:6494–506.

7. Nash C, Zaffino J, Haley DB, et al. Stall, base, bedding type and depth, lying time and leg injury prevalence on Canadian tie-stall dairy farms. Dairy Cattle Welfare Symposium. Guelph, Ontario, Canada, October 24–26, 2012. p. 200–1.

8. Popescu S, Borda C, Diugan EA, et al. Dairy cows welfare quality in tie-stall housing system with or without access to exercise. Acta Vet Scand 2013;55:1089–91.

9. Regula G, Danuser J, Spycher B, et al. Health and welfare of dairy cows in different husbandry systems in Switzerland. Prev Vet Med 2004;66:247–64.

10. Loberg J, Telezhenko E, Bergsten C, et al. Behaviour and claw health in tied dairy cows with varying access to exercise in an outdoor paddock. Appl Anim Behav Sci 2004;89:1–16.

11. Keil NM, Wiederkehr TU, Friedli K, et al. Effects of frequency and duration of outdoor exercise on the prevalence of hock lesions in tied Swiss dairy cows. Prev Vet Med 2006;74:142–53.

12. Gustafson GM, Luthman J, Burstedt E. Effect of daily exercise on performance, feed efficiency and energy balance of tied dairy cows. Acta Agric Scand A Anim Sci 1993;43:219–27.

Optimizing Resting Behavior in Lactating Dairy Cows Through Freestall Design

Nigel B. Cook, BSc, BVSc, Cert CHP, DBR, MRCVS

KEYWORDS

- Freestall • Time budget • Resting behavior • Lunge and bob

KEY POINTS

- Freestalls should be designed to optimize resting behavior of dairy cattle and provide a safe, comfortable, clean, and dry place to lie down.
- The time available for rest is dependent on stall design, stocking density, time spent away from the pen, heat stress, and cow-related factors, such as lameness.
- Freestall pens should be designed for group sizes that minimize time out of the pen milking, with alleys and crossovers that facilitate flow around the pen and access to feed and water.
- Optimal stall design provides a deep-bedded cushioned surface and a resting area sized correctly to the size of the cow using it and should be delineated by a brisket locator and stall dividers that do not have a negative impact on the ability of the cow to rise and lie down.

INTRODUCTION

The daily time budget of the lactating dairy cow has been a topic of significant research interest over recent years, with greater awareness of the importance of adequate time for rest, feeding, milking, and socialization behavior. It is now known that dairy cattle are highly motivated to gain adequate rest and demonstrate a relatively inelastic demand for 12 hours to 13 hours of lying time per day, which they value over other important activities, such as feeding.[1,2] The cost of inadequate rest is considerable, with cows at risk for health problems, such as lameness,[3] and associated lowered milk production.

A freestall facility for dairy cattle should be designed to optimize resting behavior. This article discusses those elements of design that have a direct impact on cows' ability to lie down for sufficient time each day. Tiestall design to achieve the same goal is discussed elsewhere in this issue and readers will note common themes in the 2 articles (see Harold K. House and Neil G. Anderson's article "Maximizing Comfort in Tiestall Housing" in this issue).

Disclosure Statement: The author has nothing to disclose.
Department of Medical Sciences, University of Wisconsin–Madison, School of Veterinary Medicine, 2015 Linden Drive, Madison, WI 53706, USA
E-mail address: nigel.cook@wisc.edu

vetfood.theclinics.com

FACTORS DETERMINING THE TIME FOR ADEQUATE REST

Several factors interface to determine whether a cow can optimize resting behavior. Design of the resting space is chief among these factors and is discussed as it pertains to freestall facility design, but other factors that must be considered include stocking density, time spent out of the pen and lock-up time, heat stress, and cow-related factors, such as lameness.

Competition and overstocking are significant factors influencing the resting time of cows in the pen. Studies consistently demonstrate reduced lying times at elevated stocking densities,[4] and the impact of overstocking on the cow is discussed (see Peter D. Krawczel and Amanda R. Lee's article "Lying Time and Its Importance to the Dairy Cow–Impact of Stocking Density and Time Budget Stresses" in this issue.)

Gomez and Cook[5] showed a significant relationship between increased time out of the freestall pen milking and reduced lying time, and Espejo and Endres[6] noted that time out of the pen milking was associated with an increased risk for lameness. Milking order is not random,[7] and allowance must be made for the time away from a place to feed and rest for the last cow in the group, not the average cow.[8] Similarly, it is commonplace in freestalls to lock cows up at the feed bunk to perform management tasks, such as reproductive examinations and vaccinations. Prolonged time spent locked up can have an impact on resting behavior; for example, Cooper and colleagues[9] showed that cows recovered only 40% of lost lying time within 40 hours after a 2-hour to 4-hour deprivation of available rest.

Heat stress is another significant factor having an impact on the ability of the cow to rest. Heat-stressed cows lie down for a constant number of lying bouts per day but accumulate heat when lying down at a rate of approximately 0.5°C/h to 0.6°C/h.[10] At some point, determined by core body temperature gain, the cow must stand to cool down, and, at higher ambient temperatures, the duration of each lying bout becomes shorter, thus decreasing lying time. Cook and colleagues[11] showed an impact of heat stress on resting behavior at a temperature humidity index of 68 and a reduction in lying times associated with a tendency to stand up and cool beneath fans and soakers in the feed alley. The addition of heat abatement strategies to freestall design is, therefore, essential to ensuring adequate rest in warmer climates. These challenges are discussed (see Mario R. Mondaca's article "Ventilation Systems for Adult Dairy Cattle"; Jennifer M.C. Van Os's article "Considerations for Cooling Dairy Cows with Water" in this issue.) with regard to ventilation design and the use of water cooling strategies.

Although low resting times may contribute to lameness,[3,8] resting behavior is in turn significantly impacted once cows become lame. The primary change in behavior observed in the lame cow is a difficulty performing rising and lying movements in the stall.[8] This difficulty manifests in altered stall use behavior where lame cows have a hard time rising after lying down and are reluctant to lie back down once they have risen.[12–14] Whether or not lame cows lie down for longer or shorter daily times than nonlame cows depends on other aspects of the cow's time budget and bedding surface. For example, with herds that milked predominantly 3 times per day, lame cows on average lay down for less time,[5] whereas in smaller herds milking 2 times per day, lame cows tend to lie down for longer periods of time than nonlame cows.[15,16] Ito and colleagues[14] noted that severely lame cows lay down longer on deep-bedded stalls but not on rubber mats, similar to the findings from the author's original study with sand beds.[12] There is uniform agreement that lame cows demonstrate abnormal resting behavior, as shown in **Fig. 1**. A central aim of facility design is to normalize rest for both lame and nonlame cows, making a goal of achieving a mean

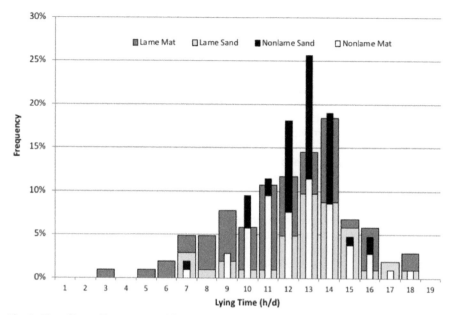

Fig. 1. The effect of lameness and freestall bedded surface (Mat or Sand) on lying time (h/d). Note that the frequency distribution for nonlame cows is relatively normal whereas the distribution is skewed for lame cows with greater numbers of lame cows with very short and very long daily lying times. (*Data from* Gomez A, Cook NB. Time budgets of lactating dairy cattle in commercial freestall herds. J Dairy Sci 2010;93(12):5772–81.)

average lying time of 12 hours per day realistic and significant. It is, therefore, problematic when numerous studies performed on commercial dairy herds demonstrate average lying times less than this goal.[15,17]

Proper freestall design optimizes stall comfort for both lame and nonlame cows; facilitates cow flow around the pen between the resting area, feed bunk, and waterers; and maximizes behavioral freedom by minimizing the potential for competition. Factors important to consider to achieving these goals are pen sizing, layout of the pen, stall layout, and design of the stall.

PEN SIZING

In parlor-milked herds, cows should be penned in groups that can be moved to the parlor and back within a period of time that does not have an impact on the time available for rest. From the commercial herd data collected by Gomez and Cook,[5] the author suggested that time out of the pen should not exceed 3 h/d when lameness and different facility designs are taken into consideration. So, for herds milking 3 times per day, cows should not be out of the pen for longer than 1 hour for milking whereas herds milking 2 times per day should have a maximum time out of the pen of 1.5 hours. Data from commercial herds show that time milking (the time from the first cow leaving the freestall pen to the last cow returning) varies enormously, with a range from 2 h/d to 8 h/d and herd averages in excess of 4 h/d.[18,19] The likely reasoning for this is an overestimate of parlor throughput during the design phase, with oversizing of pen groups and a tendency to add more cows over time without increasing parlor capacity.

A few herds still practice more frequent milkings per day for the entire herd or for subgroups, such as fresh cows. This practice seems rare now in Upper Midwest free-stall herds,[20] however, when implemented, the maximum time out of the pen per day should still not exceed 3 h/d.

Parlor throughput and distance traveled from the pen to the parlor are the key factors driving the time spent milking because cows walk at a relatively constant pace of 3 ft/ min[21] (0.02 m/s). Although traditional parlor turn times may exceed 5 turns per hour (defined as the number of times the whole capacity of the parlor is turned over each hour), the average among typical herringbone and parallel parlors rarely exceeds 4 turns per hour. Rotary parlors can milk cows efficiently, with maximum rotation speeds of approximately 6 seconds per stall, but, even in these facilities, it is often forgotten that the cow needs time for transfer to and from the pen.

Allowing for 10 minutes of transfer time, the maximum group size should be 83% of the maximum cows milked per hour for herds milking 3 times per day (60 min − 10 min = 50 min/1 h milking) whereas the maximum group size for herds milking 2 times per day should be 89% of the maximum cows milked per hour (90 min − 10 min = 80 min/ 1.5 h milking). As a rule of thumb with traditional parlors, the author maintains group sizes of less than 4 times the number of milking units in the parlor. For example, for a double-10 parallel parlor, the group size should be less than 2 × 10 milking units = 20 × 4 turns per hour × 1 h milking = 80 cows for a 3-times-a-day milking herd and 20 × 4 turns per hour × 1.5 h milking = 120 cows for a 2-times-a-day milking herd.

Modern rotary parlors may support group sizes of 400 cows to 500 cows. At some point, however, these pens become so large that parlor throughput stops becoming the limiting factor and other factors come into play, such as social stresses among large groups of cows, the amount of walking the cow must do within the pen to access feed and water and a place to rest, and the amount of time it takes and the disruption it causes when milk pushers enter the pen to get the cows to exit for the parlor. The process of emptying a large pen of cows can take 30 minutes to 45 minutes without factoring in time for milking. Practically, a maximum of approximately 250 cows seems the upper limit for pen capacity before these other issues start to come into play, but currently there are no studies documenting the impact of pen size on cow time budgets and welfare.

For automated milking systems (AMSs), group size is set by the maximum number of cows that can be supported by the robot milking units attached to the pen, and their design is discussed elsewhere in this issue. In a recent large-scale survey of 635 AMS herds in North America, 50 cows per robot was the mean cited.[22] Practically, the author suggests a group size of 50 cows to 55 cows per robot to optimize milk per cow and achieve acceptable fetch rates.

PEN LAYOUT

Pens can be designed with 1 or 2 feed bunks and between 1 row and 6 rows of stalls. Traditionally, the author has designed pens in barns with drive-through feeding down a center feed lane and pens with either 2 rows or 3 rows of stalls on either side. With more AMSs being installed and a greater reliance on mechanical ventilation systems, recent designs have promoted outside feed lanes with back-to-back pens each with 2 rows, 2.5 rows (where 1 row of stalls is shared equally between 2 pens), or 3 rows of stalls.

The cost of adding more rows of stalls per feed bunk potentially reduces feeding space per cow. Design of the feeding area and access to the feed bunk are discussed (see Trevor J. DeVries's article "Feeding Behavior, Feed Space and Bunk Design and

Management for Adult Dairy Cattle" in this issue.). There is evidence, however, to support the concept of allowing all of the cows in a pen to eat at the same time, especially when fresh feed is delivered, because this mimics the natural allelomimetic behavior patterns of the dairy cow.[23] Although feed space is not the only factor driving feed intake, with management of the feed in the bunk equally as important, the author still favors the provision of 24 in to 30 in (60–75 cm) of bunk space per cow, which is possible with pen layouts with up to 3 rows of stalls, depending on the number and width of the crossovers between the feed and stall alleys.

Crossovers between the feed and stall alleys within a pen are essential for cow flow and are used for transfer, water access, and robot access and increasingly as areas for environmental enrichment, such as the use of cow brushes for grooming behavior (**Fig. 2**). A typical crossover with a waterer should be a minimum of 14 ft (4.3 m) wide. This allows 2 ft (0.6 m) for the waterer, 6 ft (1.8 m) for the body of the cow drinking, and 2×3 ft for 2 cows to pass back and forth behind the drinking cow. Crossovers without waterers could be 2 ft (0.6 m) narrower, but those with robot access are frequently a minimum of 20 ft (6 m) in width. The frequency of crossovers has an impact on access to water in the pen and the feed bunk space allowance per cow. Guidance on waterer allowance per cow is weak; however, 2 recent surveys indicate a mean allowance of 3.1 in (8 cm) per cow on a large number of commercial herds,[18,19] but with a wide range from 0.8 in to 9.4 in (2–24 cm) per cow. In the absence of more objective science, it seems reasonable to make sure that pens with more than 10 cows to 15 cows each have more than a single waterer, and the total accessible waterer perimeter should provide 3.1 in to 3.9 in (8–10 cm) per cow in the pen. With this as a goal, crossovers with waterers should be located every 20 stalls to 25 stalls in most lactating cow pen designs, and, where bunk space is prioritized, such as in transition and sick cow pens, more frequent spacing at every 12 stalls to 15 stalls can be justified.

Alleys should be wide enough so as not to impede cow flow around the pen and provide sufficient space for exercise but are limited by cost and by the ability for the area to be scraped clean of manure. Optimal alley dimensions are shown in **Table 1** based on purpose. A stall alley is one which cows use only to enter and leave stalls; a feed alley is one where cows feed along one side; and a feed-stall alley has feed access along one side and stall access along the other.

Whatever the width, the alleys should be sloped along their length to facilitate drainage. The degree of slope depends on the length of the alley, the system used

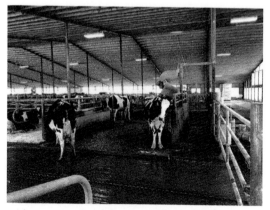

Fig. 2. A crossover with a waterer to allow free access for drinking and cow flow between the feed and stall alleys, fitted with a cow brush and footbath.

Table 1
Suggested alley dimensions for freestall pens based on type

	Recommended Alley Width, m (ft)	
Alley Type	Standard	Optimum
Stall alley	3.0 (10)	3.4–3.7 (11–12)
Feed alley	3.7 (12)	4.0–4.3 (13–14)
Feed and stall alley	4.0 (13)	4.3–4.6 (14–15)

for manure removal (eg, flushing compared with scraping), and the type of bedding. The author recommends 1% to 1.5% slopes for manually scraped alleys and 2% for flush alleys.

STALL LAYOUT

For most pen layouts, a 2-row design is favored over 3 or more rows of stalls. There are 3 potential stall layouts for the 2-row option. Stalls can be laid out head-to-head, where there is a single stall platform and the cows face each other; tail-to-tail, where there are 2 separate platforms for a single cow either side of a stall alley, with the cows facing in opposite directions with their tails toward the stall alley; or head-to-tail. This third option is essentially a tail-to-tail design with both platforms facing away from the feed bunk and is favored by some for prefresh pens operating just in time calving, so that the maternity pen workers can observe the rear of every cow in a stall from the feed lane without having to enter or walk around the pen. There are some minor pros and cons of each of the 3 options that favor moving cows away from the side wall (head-to-head), providing a clean feed alley for working behind cows locked up at the feed bunk (tail-to-tail), more stalls per square foot (tail-to-tail and head-to-tail), or reduced loop anchorage costs (head-to- head). One additional factor is that in the tail-to-tail layout, water access and dominance behavior in the crossovers become more important because cow flow may be limited between the resting and feeding areas. With this design, the author argues the need for more frequent crossovers than with the other designs, with no more than 20 stalls between crossovers.

ASPECTS OF STALL DESIGN

Freestalls should be designed to promote rest for lame and nonlame cows, facilitate rising and lying movements without significant obstruction, and provide sufficient resting area for the size of the cows using them. The design should also ensure that the cows remain clean and dry.
   Design of the freestall should consider

1. Stall surface
2. Resting and lunge space
3. Stall hardware

Stall Surface

Numerous studies support the use of deep, loose-bedded stalls as the ideal bed for a dairy cow. Deep-bedded comfortable stalls reduce the risk for lameness,[19,24–27] reduce the risk for hock injury,[19,28–30] reduce standing time in the stall,[5,12] and enhance lying times.[12,14,15] Deep bedding, especially deep sand, promotes longer lying bouts and easier transitions between standing and lying than mat or mattress surfaces with minimal bedding.[5] Because cows are motivated to rest for approximately 12 h/d, the longer lying bouts mean that the cows need to take fewer bouts per day. The deep bed gives the cow cushion, traction, and support, facilitating rising and lying movements.[8] Mat and mattress surfaces consisting of rubber crumbs, foam, air, or water have yet to provide equivalent performance to well-managed deep beds and increase the risk for lameness.[8] Waterbeds, in particular, have been shown to deliver disappointing lying times.[15] They significantly increase the risk for lameness, especially severe lameness,[31] likely related to the lack of cushion and support as the cow attempts to rise on the platform, leading to abnormal resting behavior and a worsening in the severity of the lameness.

Sand-bedded stalls carry with them an economic benefit. In a Wisconsin study,[32] the rolling herd average milk production for herds bedded with sand was 2401 lb (1089 kg) greater than herds using recycled manure solids and 1859 lb (843 kg) greater than herds using organic bedding, typically over a rubber crumb–filled mattress. Similar differences have been reported elsewhere.[33] Although the cost of handling sand laden manure is likely significant in these herds, the milk response alone likely covers the cost.

Typically, deep beds of sand have 12 in to 18 in (30–46 cm) of sand over an earth or limestone base (**Fig. 3**), with new bedding added twice a week, which amounts to approximately 20 lb to 80 lb (9–36 kg) of sand per stall per day. The bed requires daily maintenance to keep the bedded surface level with the rear curb and to remove the contaminated bedding.

Resting and Lunge Space

Cows should be able to lie down comfortably in a stall without their resting area being compromised by the cows in adjacent stalls. The width and length of the stall platform have been debated continuously over the past decade. There is now ample evidence to demonstrate the benefits of appropriately sized stalls, such as improved lying times[15,34] and a decreased risk of lameness.[35] Specific dimensions are discussed later.

The divider loop delineates the lateral boundaries of the stall. There are considerable variations in design, with the manufacturers of some claiming that they can be paired

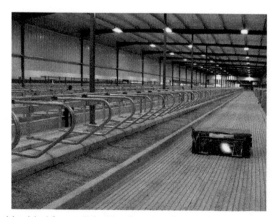

Fig. 3. A new sand-bedded freestall facility showing the earth and limestone base below the curb prior to the addition of sand. These stalls are also designed with a brisket slope to position the cow in the stall.

with smaller dimensions for the resting area. There is no evidence, however, to support this claim, and the area that a resting cow occupies is independent of the type of divider loop.

The boundary of the resting area in the front of the stall is demarcated by the brisket locator. Brisket locators that impede the forward movement of the front limb as the cow rises in the stall reduce stall usage and are not preferred by cows.[36] Cows can raise their forelimbs over obstructions approximately 4 in (10 cm) in height, and use of a brisket locator is associated with a cleaner stall platform. In deep-bedded stalls, the dairy industry has gravitated toward 2 solutions—a pipe attached to an adjustable bracket mounted to the lower divider rail of the divider loop (**Fig. 4**) or a concrete brisket slope formed in front of the stall (see **Fig. 3**). Both are located 68 in to 75 in (1.7–1.9 m) from the rear point of the curb, depending on the size of the cow, and are positioned no higher than 4 in (10 cm) above the rear point of the curb. The gentle brisket slope allows the cow to plant her leg on the slope as she rises, facilitating a step backward in the stall (**Fig. 5**). In mattress stalls, a plastic curb or pipe has been commonly used, secured to the concrete platform.

For cows to lie straight in the stall, it is preferable that they lunge to the front of the platform rather than to the side into the adjacent stall. This typically requires at least 3 ft (0.9 m) of space in front of the resting space to accommodate the shift of the head forward (the lunge), down, and up (the bob) as the cow transfers weight from her rear legs to facilitate rising and lying. In single stalls facing a side wall or alley, there is usually a retaining wall of 18 in to 24 in (45–61 cm) in height that typically compromises the downward movement of the head, so platforms are usually sized at 120 in (305 cm) in length (**Fig. 6**). In head-to-head stalls where cows are face-to-face with each other, the platform is made to be 17 ft to 18 ft (5.2–5.5 m) in length to accommodate some sharing of space (**Fig. 7**). Shorter platforms are not recommended because most Holstein cows at rest measure approximately 8 ft (2.4 m) in length from nose to tail, and a dominant cow in front of a subordinate one acts as a social obstruction to her lunge. Because of the unpredictability of social obstructions to front lunge, the author recommends that all divider loops allow for side lunge as an option. To allow for this, the upper edge of the lower divider rail can be no higher than 10 in to 13 in (25–33 cm) above the stall surface, depending on the size of the cow.

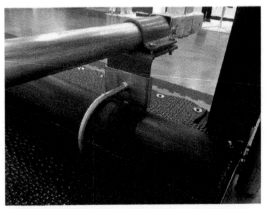

Fig. 4. A cylindrical brisket locator with an adjustable bracket fixed to the lower divider rail of the freestall loop. The adjustment is required to set the height of the brisket locator above the stall surface correctly.

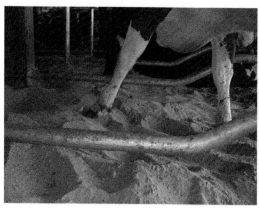

Fig. 5. Note the ability for the cow in this stall to make a forward stride as she rises. Below the sand is a concrete brisket slope facilitating this movement pictured without bedding in **Fig. 3**.

Stall Hardware

Producers building a freestall barn must choose between different types of stall hardware, notably the divider loop, mounting brackets, and neck rail.

The freestall divider loop performs several functions. It defines the lateral limits of the resting space, positions the cow, permits or prevents side lunge, and determines the height of the neck rail. It should perform these functions without injuring the cow. There are numerous designs available without rigorous testing available to critique them, so the comments herein are empirical and based on experiences troubleshooting stall design problems over the past 20 years.

The most important part of the divider loop is the lower rail. This rail's purpose is to suggest to the cow just enough, but not too much, where to lie down, and it must allow her to rise without obstruction or risk of injury. The height of the lower rail is critical. It must allow for at least a 5-in (13 cm) gap between the lower edge of the bar and the top of any brisket locator to prevent any front leg entrapment below the rail and be

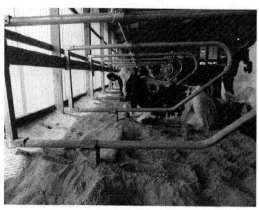

Fig. 6. A side wall stall with ample front lunge space and a divider loop that positions the cow in the stall without impeding side lunge.

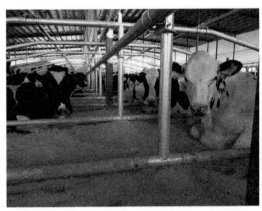

Fig. 7. A head-to-head stall platform designed 17 ft (5.2 m) in length with loop mountings that are adjustable but do not impede the front lunge area of the cow.

positioned at the correct height above the stall surface. Divider rails placed too low allow cows to rise with their front legs over the lower rail, leading to entrapment and a cow caught in the middle of the loop. Divider rails that are too high prevent side lunge into the adjacent stall unless they are so high that the cow lunges below them, commonly seen with Michigan and dog-bone loop designs (**Fig. 8**). Previously, the author made the case that cows should be permitted to lunge both to the front and to the side to prevent social dominance behavior having an impact on the ability for a cow to rise. The target height of the lower rail above the level stall surface (or rear point of the curb in a deep, loose-bedded stall) should be between 10 in and 13 in (25–33 cm), typically 12 in (30 cm) for most mature Holstein cows. The rail should be level and not angled down to the surface. This angled rail promotes side lunge and diagonal lying as the cow takes advantage of the lower rail height at the front of the stall. Loops designed for side lunge, where the cow lunges below the lower rail, also promote diagonal lying, dirty stalls, and medial hock injuries and, therefore, are

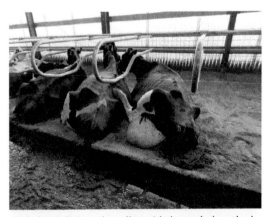

Fig. 8. A dog-bone–style loop designed to allow side lunge below the lower divider rail and access for equipment to level the beds. The issue with this design is obvious—diagonal lying in the stall and manure contamination. Medial hock injuries also may result from the rear leg hanging over the concrete curb.

not recommended. Similarly, loops where the lower rail starts level but bends down to mount onto the top of the stall surface in front should also be avoided because these also invite the cow to lie too far forward and lunge to the side.

The lower rail should extend back toward the rear curb horizontal to the stall surface just enough to suggest where the cow should lie straight in the stall but not so far back that the rail has an impact on the hooks and rump of the cow as she lies down, before it angles upward and out of the way. The author recommends that the angle be 20 in to 22 in (51–56 cm) toward the rear curb back from the brisket locator. Because the location of the brisket locator typically ranges from 68 in to 72 in (173–183 cm) from the rear curb and stall length may vary, different sized loops are needed for different sized stalls. Stall divider designs that use a straight fiberglass pipe struggle to position the cow correctly because they provide a side lunge point in front and too much space in the rear of the stall (**Fig. 9**).

The open diameter of the loop determines the height of the neck rail. A distance of 33 in to 36 in (84–91 cm) from the upper edge of the lower rail to the lower edge of the upper rail should locate the neck rail at the target height of 46 in to 52 in (117–132 cm) depending on the size of the cow. Neck rails determine the standing position of the cow in the stall[37] and are always in the way because cows usually step forward when they rise. In a correctly designed stall, however, provided that there is sufficient height, cows adapt and step backward if it is ensured there are no other obstructions to the normal rising movement of the cow.

Lastly, in relation to the loop, the rear limit of the divider should be 9 in to 12 in (23–30 cm) inside of the rear curb—close enough to prevent cows from walking along the back of the stalls but not so close that it gets hit by passing machinery.

The loop mounting hardware is also an important consideration. The author no longer recommends mounts that require posts mounted onto the stall platform, preferring to retain flexibility for loop positioning and to keep the hardware above the bedding. Over time, wet bedding corrodes the mounting beams, clamps, and wooden posts, leading to a failure of the structure. It is also important, however, for any mounting system to avoid creating an obstruction to the lunge and bob area of the cow. Horizontal rail or beam mounting systems are commonplace and are now preferred (**Fig. 10**). It is critical that the lower edge of the lowest mounting rail is level with the tops of the cows' heads at rest (see **Fig. 7**), typically greater than 36 in (91 cm)

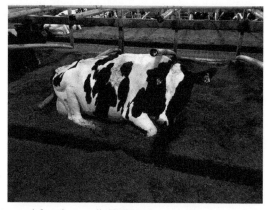

Fig. 9. Originally termed *freedom stall dividers* that consist of 1 or 2 straight pipes struggle to delineate the resting area for the cow leading to aberrant lying behavior.

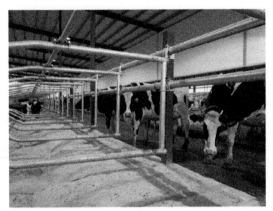

Fig. 10. A twin rail horizontal mounting system that provides flexible divider mounting while ensuring that the rails do not impede front lunge.

above the lying surface. Systems using a lower mounting rail closer to the stall surface present an obstruction to lunge and bob and, therefore, are not recommended.

The final piece of stall hardware is the neck rail. The neck rail provides lateral stability to the stall dividers while positioning the cow in the stall while she is standing.[37] Neck rails have less impact on the lying position of the cow. The correct standing position limits the amount of manure deposited on the stall bed without impeding stall use. In mat or mattress stalls, the neck rail should invite cows to stand up on the stall platform, square in the stall, and the rail is typically mounted directly above a correctly positioned brisket locator using the same horizontal distance from the rear curb for the location. With this location, the risk of the cow perching—standing with the front feet in the stall and the rear feet in the alley, which has been associated with an elevated risk for heel horn erosion—is reduced.[38]

Neck rail position is complicated in deep, loose-bedded stalls because of the raised rear curb, which cows avoid standing on. When the neck rail is located, as described previously for a mattress stall, cows stand inside the curb, diagonally across the resting space, and contaminate the bedding with urine and manure. For that reason, in deep-bedded stalls with raised curbs, the author positions the neck rail approximately 6 in (15 cm) closer to the rear curb, making the cow step back out of the stall and perch. In a well-designed deep-bedded stall facility, approximately 90% of stall

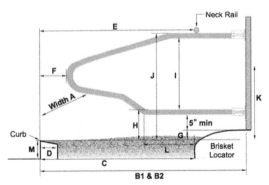

Fig. 11. Stall diagram to identify critical dimensions referred to in **Table 2**.

Table 2
Target freestall dimensions based on an estimate of a cow's body weight

Stall Dimension (in [cm])	Body Weight Estimate (lb [kg])							
	600 (270)	800 (360)	1000 (450)	1200 (550)	1400 (640)	1600 (730)	1800 (820)	2000 (910)
Center-to-center stall divider placement (stall width) (A)	34 (86)	38 (96)	42 (107)	45 (114)	48 (122)	50 (127)	54 (137)	57 (145)
Total stall length facing a wall (B1)	80 (203)	88 (224)	96 (244)	108 (274)	108 (274)	120 (305)	120 (305)	126 (320)
Outside curb to outside curb distance for head-to-head platform (B2)	156 (396)	168 (427)	180 (457)	192 (488)	192 (488)	204 (518)	204 (518)	216 (549)
Distance from rear curb to rear of brisket locator (C)	Not recommended		64 (163)	66 (168)	68 (173)	70 (178)	72 (183)	75 (191)
Width of rear curb (D)	6–8 (15–20)	6–8 (15–20)	6–8 (15–20)	6–8 (15–20)	6–8 (15–20)	6–8 (15–20)	6–8 (15–20)	6–8 (15–20)
Horizontal distance between rear edge of neck rail and rear edge of curb for mattress stalls (E)	46 (117)	55 (140)	64 (163)	66 (168)	68 (173)	70 (178)	72 (183)	75 (191)
Horizontal distance between rear edge of neck rail and rear edge of curb for deep-bedded stalls (E)	40 (102)	49 (125)	58 (147)	60 (152)	62 (157)	64 (163)	66 (168)	69 (175)
Distance from rear edge of divider loop to point of curb (F)	9 (23)	9 (23)	9 (23)	9 (23)	9 (23)	9 (23)	9 (23)	9 (23)
Height of brisket locator above top of curb (loose-bedded stall or mat/mattress surface) (G)	Not recommended	3 (8)	3 (8)	3 (8)	4 (10)	4 (10)	4 (10)	4 (10)

(continued on next page)

Table 2
(continued)

Stall Dimension (in [cm])	Body Weight Estimate (lb [kg])								
	600 (270)	800 (360)	1000 (450)	1200 (550)	1400 (640)	1600 (730)	1800 (820)	2000 (910)
Height of upper edge of bottom stall divider rail above top of curb (loose-bedded stall or mat/mattress surface) (H)	8 (20)	8 (20)	10 (25)	10 (25)	12 (31)	12 (31)	13 (33)	14 (36)
Interior diameter of the stall divider loop (I)	24 (61)	28 (71)	30 (76)	33 (84)	33 (84)	36 (91)	36 (91)	36 (91)
Height of neck rail above top of curb (loose-bedded stall or mat/mattress surface) (J)	34 (86)	38 (97)	42 (107)	45 (114)	48 (122)	50 (127)	52 (132)	54 (137)
Obstruction height (K)	5–35 (13–89)	5–35 (13–89)	5–35 (13–89)	5–35 (13–89)	5–35 (13–89)	5–35 (13–89)	5–35 (13–89)	5–35 (13–89)
Horizontal distance from brisket locator to loop angle (L)	Not recommended	20–22 (51–56)	20–22 (51–56)	20–22 (51–56)	20–22 (51–56)	20–22 (51–56)	20–22 (51–56)	20–22 (51–56)
Rear curb height (M)	6 (15)	8 (20)	8 (20)	8 (20)	8 (20)	8 (20)	8 (20)	8 (20)

The letters in parentheses refer to **Fig. 11**.

standing behavior is perching[39] and lameness prevalence is generally low, so the relationship between perching and lameness found for mattress herds seems not to apply in this situation. Sufficient height is required below the neck rail for the cow to avoid injury as she rises below it when this compromise location is used in deep-bedded stalls.

Recent curved neck rail designs that are attached to dividers whose upper rail is lower than that described in this article aim to force the cow to stand straight in the stall. They are unlikely, however, to influence lying position and are not recommended.

STALL DESIGN RECOMMENDATIONS

Recommendations for stall design and sizing are shown in **Fig. 11** and **Table 2** based on an estimate of the cow's body weight. Stall sizing and use is optimized in pens where there is limited variation in size among the cows using them, making dedicated pens for primiparous and multiparous cows attractive. In groups where there is a wide range in age and size of cow, however, some level of compromise must be reached. The author's preference is to size the stalls to satisfy the needs of the upper quartile of cows in the pen, rather than hamper stall use by larger cows in an attempt to keep the stalls clean for the smallest-sized animals.

SUMMARY

Freestalls can be designed to provide dairy cattle a comfortable place to rest for 12 hours per day. Designs must minimize the time spent out of the pen milking and have layouts that support cow flow between the resting, drinking, and feeding areas. Deep-bedded stalls optimize comfort for the dairy cow, for both nonlame and lame cows, and stalls should be designed to accommodate the size of the cows using them and avoid obstructions to the normal rising and lying movements of the cow.

ACKNOWLEDGMENTS

The author would like to thank the dairy producers who were prepared to take a leap of faith over the years to remodel old freestall facilities and build new barns following the author's recommendations. Without their commitment to improving cow comfort, we would not be where we are today. The author would also like to acknowledge the funding support for the Dairyland Initiative at https://thedairylandinitiative.vetmed. wisc.edu/home/housing-module/supporters/.

REFERENCES

1. Jensen MB, Pedersen LJ, Munksgaard L. The effect of reward duration on demand functions for rest in dairy heifers and lying requirements as measured by demand functions. Appl Anim Behav Sci 2005;90(3–4):207–17.
2. Munksgaard L, Jensen MB, Pedersen LJ, et al. Quantifying behavioural priorities - effects of time constraints on behaviour of dairy cows, Bos taurus. Appl Anim Behav Sci 2005;92(1–2):3–14.
3. Proudfoot KL, Weary DM, von Keyserlingk MAG. Behavior during transition differs for cows diagnosed with claw horn lesions in mid lactation. J Dairy Sci 2010; 93(9):3970–8.
4. Fregonesi JA, Tucker CB, Weary DM. Overstocking reduces lying time in dairy cows. J Dairy Sci 2007;90(7):3349–54.
5. Gomez A, Cook NB. Time budgets of lactating dairy cattle in commercial freestall herds. J Dairy Sci 2010;93(12):5772–81.

6. Espejo LA, Endres MI. Herd-level risk factors for lameness in high-producing hol-stein cows housed in freestall barns. J Dairy Sci 2007;90(1):306–14.

7. Rathore AK. Order of cow entry at milking and its relationships with milk yield and consistency of the order. Appl Anim Ethol 1982;8(1–2):45–52.

8. Cook NB, Nordlund KV. The influence of the environment on dairy cow behavior, claw health and herd lameness dynamics. Vet J 2009;179(3):360–9.

9. Cooper MD, Arney DR, Phillips CJC. Two- or four-hour lying deprivation on the behavior of lactating dairy cows. J Dairy Sci 2007;90(3):1149–58.

10. Hillman PE, Lee CN, Willard ST. Thermoregulatory responses associated with lying and standing in heat-stressed dairy cows. Trans ASAE 2005;48(2):795–801.

11. Cook NB, Mentink RL, Bennett TB, et al. The effect of heat stress and lameness on time budgets of lactating dairy cows. J Dairy Sci 2007;90(4):1674–82.

12. Cook NB, Bennett TB, Nordlund KV. Effect of free stall surface on daily activity patterns in dairy cows with relevance to lameness prevalence. J Dairy Sci 2004;87(9):2912–22.

13. Cook NB, Marin MJ, Mentink RL, et al. Comfort zone-design free stalls: do they influence the stall use behavior of lame cows? J Dairy Sci 2008;91(12):4673–8.

14. Ito K, von Keyserlingk MAG, LeBlanc SJ, et al. Lying behavior as an indicator of lameness in dairy cows. J Dairy Sci 2010;93(8):3553–60.

15. Solano L, Barkema HW, Pajor EA, et al. Associations between lying behavior and lameness in Canadian Holstein-Friesian cows housed in freestall barns. J Dairy Sci 2016;99(3):2086–101.

16. Westin R, Vaughan A, de Passillé AM, et al. Lying times of lactating cows on dairy farms with automatic milking systems and the relation to lameness, leg lesions, and body condition score. J Dairy Sci 2016;99(1):551–61.

17. Ito K, Chapinal N, Weary DM, et al. Associations between herd-level factors and lying behavior of freestall-housed dairy cows. J Dairy Sci 2014;97(4):2081–9.

18. von Keyserlingk MAG, Barrientos A, Ito K, et al. Benchmarking cow comfort on North American freestall dairies: lameness, leg injuries, lying time, facility design, and management for high-producing Holstein dairy cows. J Dairy Sci 2012; 95(12):7399–408.

19. Cook NB, Hess JP, Foy MR, et al. Management characteristics, lameness, and body injuries of dairy cattle housed in high-performance dairy herds in Wiscon-sin. J Dairy Sci 2016;99(7):5879–91.

20. Brotzman RL, Döpfer D, Foy MR, et al. Survey of facility and management char-acteristics of large, Upper Midwest dairy herds clustered by Dairy Herd Improve-ment records. J Dairy Sci 2015;98(11):8245–61.

21. Telezhenko E, Bergsten C. Influence of floor type on the locomotion of dairy cows. Appl Anim Behav Sci 2005;93(3–4):183–97.

22. Tremblay M, Hess JP, Christenson BM, et al. Factors associated with increased milk production for automatic milking systems. J Dairy Sci 2016;99(5):3824–37.

23. Cook NB, Nordlund KV. Behavioral needs of the transition cow and consider-ations for special needs facility design. Vet Clin North Am Food Anim Pract 2004;20(3 SPEC. ISS):495–520.

24. Cook NB. Prevalence of lameness among dairy cattle in Wisconsin as a function of housing type and stall surface. J Am Vet Med Assoc 2003;223(9):1324–8.

25. Espejo LA, Endres MI, Salfer JA. Prevalence of lameness in high-producing hol-stein cows housed in freestall barns in Minnesota. J Dairy Sci 2006;89(8):3052–8.

26. Chapinal N, Barrientos AK, von Keyserlingk MAG, et al. Herd-level risk factors for lameness in freestall farms in the northeastern United States and California. J Dairy Sci 2013;96(1):318–28.

27. Solano L, Barkema H, Pajor E, et al. Prevalence of lameness and associated risk factors in Canadian Holstein-Friesian cows housed in freestall barns. J Dairy Sci 2015;98:6978–91.
28. Weary DM, Taszkun I. Hock lesions and free-stall design. J Dairy Sci 2000;83(4): 697–702.
29. Barrientos AK, Chapinal N, Weary DM, et al. Herd-level risk factors for hock injuries in freestall-housed dairy cows in the northeastern United States and California. J Dairy Sci 2013;96(6):3758–65.
30. Chapinal N, Liang Y, Weary DM, et al. Risk factors for lameness and hock injuries in Holstein herds in China. J Dairy Sci 2014;97(7):4309–16.
31. Salfer JA, Siewert JM, Endres MI. Housing, management characteristics, and factors associated with lameness, hock lesion, and hygiene of lactating dairy cattle on Upper Midwest United States dairy farms using automatic milking systems. J Dairy Sci 2018;0(0):8586–94.
32. Rowbotham RF, Ruegg PL. Association of bedding types with management practices and indicators of milk quality on larger Wisconsin dairy farms. J Dairy Sci 2015;98(11):7865–85.
33. Andreasen SN, Forkman B. The welfare of dairy cows is improved in relation to cleanliness and integument alterations on the hocks and lameness when sand is used as stall surface. J Dairy Sci 2012;95(9):4961–7.
34. Tucker CB, Weary DM, Fraser D. Free-stall dimensions: effects on preference and stall usage. J Dairy Sci 2004;87(5):1208–16.
35. Westin R, Vaughan A, de Passillé AM, et al. Cow- and farm-level risk factors for lameness on dairy farms with automated milking systems. J Dairy Sci 2016; 99(5):3732–43.
36. Tucker CB, Zdanowicz G, Weary DM. Brisket boards reduce freestall use. J Dairy Sci 2006;89(7):2603–7.
37. Tucker CB, Weary DM, Fraser D. Influence of neck-rail placement on free-stall preference, use, and cleanliness. J Dairy Sci 2005;88(8):2730–7.
38. Bernardi F, Fregonesi J, Winckler C, et al. The stall-design paradox: neck rails increase lameness but improve udder and stall hygiene. J Dairy Sci 2009;92(7): 3074–80.
39. Cook NB, Bennett TB, Nordlund KV. Monitoring indices of cow comfort in free-stall-housed dairy herds. J Dairy Sci 2005;88(11):3876–85.

Maternal Behavior and Design of the Maternity Pen

Kathryn L. Proudfoot, MS, PhD

KEYWORDS

- Labor • Transition cow • Pain • Stressor

KEY POINTS

- Labor is a painful and stressful event for most mammals, including dairy cattle.
- Dairy cows with prolonged labor are at high risk of disease after calving.
- Housing for dairy cows during labor is highly variable.
- Understanding maternal behavior in cattle can lead to more appropriate housing designs for cows during labor.
- An ideal maternity pen should be clean and dry, should provide cows the opportunity to hide from barn noise and other cows, and should be free of environmental and social stressors.

INTRODUCTION

A dairy cow will give birth approximately once per year on a modern dairy facility. Like other mammals, labor in cattle is thought to be painful,[1,2] and may result in complications that can put the life of the dam and her calf at risk.[3] It has been estimated that approximately 13.7% to 29% of multiparous cows and 22.6% to 51% of first-calf heifers in the United States experience a difficult birth, resulting in assistance from farm staff or a veterinarian[3,4] (dystocia). Cows with difficult births are at higher risk of morbidity,[5] and their newborn calves are more likely to be stillborn or become ill in early life compared with cows that give birth naturally.[4,6] Thus, ensuring that proper care is provided to cows during labor is critically important for animal welfare, farm productivity, and the overall sustainability of the dairy industry.

Considerable research has focused on improving the nutrition, management, and housing of dairy cows before and after they give birth.[7,8] This research has allowed for major advancements in the understanding of pathologic disease, and the relationship between animal behavior, nutrition, and immunity. Most research has focused on the 3 weeks before to the 3 weeks after calving (the transition period). However, less work has specifically focused on the cow's environment when she is in labor.

Disclosure: The author has nothing to disclose.
Veterinary Preventive Medicine, College of Veterinary Medicine, The Ohio State University, 1920 Coffey Road, Columbus, OH 43210, USA
E-mail address: proudfoot.18@osu.edu

Vet Clin Food Anim 35 (2019) 111–124
https://doi.org/10.1016/j.cvfa.2018.10.007
vetfood.theclinics.com

The housing of dairy cows during labor and calf delivery is highly variable, and depends on the region and farm size. For the purpose of this article, any area where the cow delivers her calf will be referred to as a maternity pen. According to the 2014 US Department of Agriculture (USDA) National Animal Health Survey, 69.4% of farms surveyed reported having a usual place to move cows to deliver their calves.[9] The remaining 30.6% of farms allow cows to give birth in stanchions, tie stalls, or other areas not specifically designated for calving. Use of a separate maternity area was reportedly highest in large farms (95%; 500 lactating cows or more) and lowest in small farms (33%; fewer than 30 lactating cows). Similarly, in a survey of farms in Quebec, Canada, 51.3% of farms reported having a designated maternity pen, the remaining farms calved cows in tie stalls.[10] In the United States, of the farms with designated maternity pens, 64.3% births were reported to occur in pens that hold multiple animals (group maternity pens) and 31.1% of births were reported to occur in pens designated to hold 1 animal at a time (individual maternity pens).[9] Most farms reported keeping cows in a designated maternity pen for a short time (41.9% for 1 day or less and 18.7% for 3 days or less) and some farms house cows in these pens for longer durations (28.1% for 3–14 days, and 11.3% for 14 days or more) before their expected delivery date.

An appropriate environment for the cow during labor and delivery is different from other life stages because the cow undergoes several hormonal and behavioral changes as she approaches birth. An understanding of cows' natural maternal behavior at calving can help caretakers design and manage maternity pens to accommodate the cows' unique needs. The purpose of this article is to describe the current literature on maternal behavior in dairy cattle, as well as best-practices for maternity pen design and management.

MATERNAL BEHAVIOR IN DAIRY CATTLE

For mammals, the survival of offspring depends on the care given by their mothers, especially in early life. Dairy cows, like other ungulates, give birth to offspring that are well-developed at birth (precocial), requiring dams to substantially alter their behavior to help protect their active young.[11,12] These maternal behaviors have been defined as the suite of behaviors expressed by mothers in late gestation, and directed toward the offspring until weaning.[13] The cow may begin altering her behavior before labor begins but the most intensive changes in behavior occur during the few hours before and after giving birth.[14]

Maternal behaviors in dairy cows are thought to be driven in part by changes in hormones involved in the onset and progression of labor (eg, estradiol, progesterone, prolactin, and oxytocin).[12] For cattle, labor occurs in 3 stages that gradually move from 1 to the next. During the first stage of labor (stage I; dilation phase), the cow's cervix begins to dilate, her pelvic ligaments relax, she begins to experience myometrial contractions, and her calf is moved into position for delivery.[15] This stage has been estimated to last between 4 and 24 hours; however, an accurate estimation of this duration is difficult because it requires palpation of the cervix.[16] As cows progress through the first stage of labor, myometrial contractions increase in duration, frequency, and amplitude.[14] Stage I ends when the cervix of the cow is fully dilated and the calf is prepared to move through the birth canal.

During the second stage of labor (stage II; expulsion phase), the calf is propelled through the birth canal through forces in the uterus (myometrial contractions) and the abdomen (abdominal contractions).[15,17] The landmark of this stage is the breaking of the amniotic sac or the sac becoming visible outside of the vulva (water bag), which has been estimated to occur about 10 minutes after the first abdominal contractions.[17] Every 15 minutes thereafter, the cow should show labor progress characterized by the calf's feet, head, shoulders, and eventually hips appearing outside the vulva if the calf's position is forward. Stage II is estimated to last about 45 plus or minus 12 minutes (mean ± SD; time from amniotic sac to birth) in Holstein dairy cows that give birth naturally; however, it can be longer for those experiencing dystocia (87 ± 22 minutes, mean ± SD).[17] Stage II ends when the calf is delivered, and the third stage of labor ends with the expulsion of the placenta.

Cows likely experience variable levels of pain during each stage of labor. Pain is defined by the International Association for the Study of Pain as "an unpleasant sensory and emotional experience associated with actual or potential tissue damage, or described in terms of such damage." In women, pain during labor has been measured using subjective pain scales; most women report moderate, intense, or very intense pain during labor.[18] Although measuring pain in dairy cattle is more difficult, it can be assumed that dairy cows experience labor pain similar to humans and other mammals.[2] During the first stage of labor, the cow likely experiences visceral pain associated with myometrial contractions, distention of the uterus, and dilation of the cervix. During stage II, the cow likely experiences sharper, more localized somatic pain associated with contractions and the movement of the calf through the birth canal.[2]

Research has also documented changes in behavior that coincide with each stage of labor (**Fig. 1**). One of the earliest indications that a cow is in, or is entering, the first stage labor is isolation from the herd to find a suitable place to give birth. Like wild ungulates, dairy cows will distance themselves from other members of the herd to find a secluded area to give birth.[11] In a study of free-ranging beef cattle kept on 86 acres and dairy cattle kept on 50 acres, researchers recorded the characteristics of a calving site and an estimation of the distance between cows on the day of calving.[19] Both beef and dairy cows were found to be more than 15 m from their nearest neighbor on the day of calving compared with the 4 previous days, and both sought high-altitude calving sites with tree cover and branches overhead, or a human-made shelter with water, minerals, and hay. This isolation-seeking behavior is thought to be an antipredator strategy and may help facilitate the bond between the dam and her calf without interference from other cows.[11,20]

Studies using beef and dairy cattle in natural settings provide valuable insights into the innate maternal behavior of dairy cows; however, most dairy cows in North America are kept indoors to give birth. An indoor environment protects dairy cows from predators and inclement weather during parturition but may limit the cow's ability to

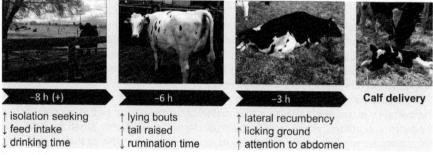

−8 h (+)	−6 h	−3 h	Calf delivery
↑ isolation seeking	↑ lying bouts	↑ lateral recumbency	
↓ feed intake	↑ tail raised	↑ licking ground	
↓ drinking time	↓ rumination time	↑ attention to abdomen	

Fig. 1. Behavioral changes in dairy cows as calving approaches. (*Courtesy of* Gosia Zobel, MSc, PhD, AgResearch New Zealand, Magnus Campler, MSc, PhD, University of Kentucky, and Nigel Cook, BVSc, University of Wisconsin-Madison.)

seek a secluded birthing environment. In a study using Holstein dairy cattle, researchers determined that some cows retain the motivation to hide during labor when housed indoors.[21] Cows were given the choice between a large plywood shelter with 3 walls and a doorway that cows could enter and leave as they chose (2.4 × 6.1 m) and an open bedded pack without walls (2.4 × 7.3 m). When cows were housed alone in the pen, 61% of cows used the shelter to give birth. The use of the shelter for calving was highest during the daytime; 81% of cows that calved during the day used the shelter during labor, suggesting that cows may be more motivated to hide during periods of high activity and noise compared with the relative dark and quiet of night. Cows began using the shelter more often approximately 8 hours before giving birth, which may coincide with the first stage of labor.

In addition to isolation-seeking, several other behaviors change during the first stage of labor, including a reduction in feeding and drinking behavior. Approximately 6 to 8 hours before calving, cows begin to eat less,[22] spend less time eating,[14,23] spend less time ruminating,[22] and spend less time drinking water.[14] Compared with previous days, cows consume approximately 30% less feed on the day of calving.[22] This decline in feeding and drinking behavior is likely driven by a shift in motivational priorities of the cow, as well as pain likely associated with the onset of labor.

Dairy cows kept indoors show restless behavior 4 to 6 hours before giving birth, characterized by an increase in position changes from standing to lying (lying bouts).[14,23,24] Dairy cows kept in an individual maternity pen during labor nearly doubled their lying bouts on the day of calving compared with previous days.[24] This increase in bouts is particularly high for heifers calving for the first time[25] and may also be affected by the cow's environment during labor because cows kept on pasture to give birth showed fewer lying bouts compared with those kept in indoor individual maternity pens.[26] The increase in restless behavior may be driven by pain associated with labor or may reflect the indoor-housed cow's frustration with not being able to find an adequate site to give birth.[11]

Cows show other behaviors as calving approaches, such as raising their tails (4 hours before calving for heifers and 2 hours before calving for cows),[23] sniffing or licking at the ground (3 hours before calving),[23] turning their heads toward their abdomens (2 hours before calving),[14] and increasing the amount of time they spend in lateral recumbency (4 hours before calving).[27] Cows may also become attracted to new odors and pheromones as they approach labor, including amniotic fluids in the 28 and 24 hours before calving compared with earlier periods.[28] Some cows choose to calve near locations where other cows' have given birth, which may be partially driven by odors and pheromones of amniotic fluid left behind by the previous cows because they may indicate a safe place to give birth.[29]

During the second stage of labor, the cow is often in sternal or lateral recumbency to help facilitate calf delivery[17]; cows will spend approximately 50 minutes of the last hour before calving lying down.[30] Researchers monitored the posture of cows before and during calf delivery, and found that 87% of cows and 69% of heifers delivered their calves in a laterally recumbent position.[31]

Immediately after giving birth, the cow directs her attention to her newborn calf.[32] This behavior is thought to be driven by maternal hormones, as well as a combination of olfactory, auditory, visual, and tactile cues from the newborn. When housed with their calves for the first 24 hours after birth, cows spent over 50% of their time licking and sniffing the calf in the first hour after calving.[32] These behaviors are thought to help stimulate calf activity by increasing circulation, urination, and defecation, and may help facilitate the bond between the dam and her calf.[33] After the first hour of birth, cows progressively decreased the time spent directing behaviors toward the calf, and spent more time engaging in lying and feeding behaviors.[32]

The behavior of the dam–calf pair after calving depends on their social environment. When cows give birth alone, they can direct their attention to their own calf in the first few hours after birth without interference from other dams.[32] When cows calve in a group, other preparturient cows may become attracted to the odor and pheromones emitted by the dam and her newborn.[28,34] Cows housed in groups to give birth spent less time licking their own calves compared with cows that calve alone; this reduction in licking time was thought to be due to other cows in the group licking the newborn calf.[34] In addition to licking a newborn, other preparturient cows may attempt to nurse newborn calves that are not their own. A study of group-housed cows found that approximately 30% of calves were nursed by a cow other than their mother.[35] Colostrum quality declines rapidly after calving,[36] so this mismothering behavior may interfere with passive transfer of antibodies to the cow's own newborn.

Research on the maternal behavior of dairy cattle before and after giving birth can provide insights into the design of appropriate housing and management of these animals. The next section focuses on the research to date on maternity pen designs and management of cows during labor that accommodate these behaviors. The section also includes additional research on other important features of the maternity pen, including a reduction of stressors and pathogen exposure to the dam and her newborn calf.

MATERNITY PEN DESIGN AND MANAGEMENT

Although there is probably no perfect maternity pen design, the ideal maternity area should allow the cow to express her innate maternal behaviors before and after labor, including the ability to seek a quiet, comfortable place to give birth. In addition, the pen should be managed to reduce pathogen spread to the cow and her calf, and should minimize environmental and social stressors experienced by the cow during labor.

A maternity pen should allow a cow to find a quiet, secluded area to give birth. Individual maternity pens provide separation from herd mates but are sometimes located in high-traffic areas of the barn (eg, near the office or milking parlor where farm staff can keep close watch on cows in labor). Dairy producers can reduce noise and activity in individual pens by providing a barrier between the cow and her herd mates or noisy parts of the barn (**Fig. 2**). For example, researchers constructed individual maternity pens directly adjacent to the close-up group pen; the maternity pens included a 1.5 by 1.8 m plywood barrier (corner) and a 1.5 m-wide window where cows could see and have nose-to-nose contact with other cows in the group pen.[37] Cows were moved into these pens approximately 8 hours before giving birth and the side of the pen (corner or window) was recorded at calving. Most cows chose to give birth in the corner (79%) and spent most of their time in the corner during the 1 hour before calving. Thus, providing something as simple as a corner to hide from other cows may be beneficial to cows as they give birth.

The size and shape of a hiding space that a cow wants during labor may depend on her experience during labor. For example, researchers constructed maternity pens directly adjacent to a group pen with 3 options for a hiding space: (1) a tall and narrow barrier (1.8 × 1.5 m), (2) a low and wide barrier (1.0 × 2.5 m), and (3) a tall and wide barrier (1.8 × 2.5 m).[38] Cows generally had no preference for barrier shape; however, cows that experienced prolonged labor (an average of 159 minutes for stage II labor, measured as the latency from the first abdominal contractions to calf delivery) were more likely to use the most secluded barrier option (the tall and wide barrier) compared

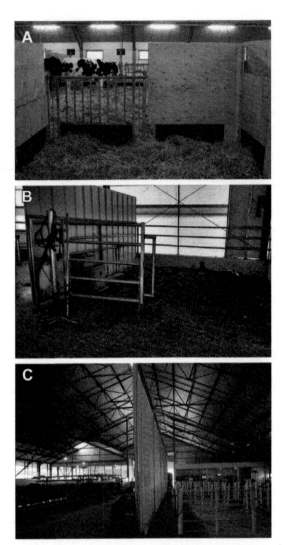

Fig. 2. Practical ways to create seclusion in an individual maternity pen. (*A*) The maternity pen design used in Proudfoot and colleagues[37] (2014b). (*B*) A farm using corrugated metal to divide the maternity pen from the holding pen and milking parlor. (*C*) A farm using a curtain to divide individual maternity pens (*right side* of the curtain) from the feed alley (*left side* of the curtain). (*Courtesy of* [A] the author, Ohio State University; and [B] VanderMade farms, Sherwood, OH; and [C] Ken Nordlund, DVM, University of Wisconsin-Madison.)

with those without prolonged labor (an average of 75.6 minutes for stage II labor). Cows experiencing prolonged labor may also be experiencing additional pain and restless behavior that may have motivated them to seek further seclusion. Thus, cows with prolonged labor may be particularly in need of a quiet, secluded place to give birth without distractions from human caretakers, other cows, or noises in the environment. This finding is, however, at odds with traditional calving management practice because these cows likely need the most care from farm staff because they are at higher risk of experiencing a dystocia and needing assistance during birth.[17] Care should be taken to assist with labor while maintaining a relatively calm environment for the cow (eg, using gentle handling techniques and not moving the cow very far away from her home pen to assist with labor).

Like individual pens, group maternity pens should ideally be in quiet areas of the barn, and be separated from the rest of the herd. However, creating a secluded environment for individual cows within a group maternity pen may be challenging. For example, researchers found that when 2 cows were in a maternity pen with 1 hiding space, the first cow to give birth was more likely to calve outside of the hiding space.[21] This behavior may be driven by competition for the hiding space because the other cow in the pen may have valued that space and guarded it from the cow in labor. Similarly, researchers have found that cows that are more socially dominant over other cows (measured using displacements from the feed bunk) in a group calving pen are the most likely to use the hides to give birth.[39] Thus, an area for individual cows to find seclusion from herd mates at calving should be designed to limit social competition over the space.

Group-housed cows may be motivated to hide to give birth but they may not be willing to work very hard to obtain access to a secluded area. For example, researchers designed a group maternity pen with individual L-shaped hides along the outside of the pen; each hide was protected by a gate that a cow could push through to access the hiding space, not allowing other cows to enter in after her.[39] Investigators recorded the calving location of cows when these gates were closed (and individual cows could push through them) or permanently open. About 50% of cows used 1 of the hides to give birth, regardless of the gate being open or closed. Cows were more likely to use the hide if the gates were permanently open, suggesting that cows were less motivated to push through a gate to access a hidden space. Exhaustion or pain associated with labor may have prevented the cow from accessing the hide when there was an obstacle between her and a secluded space. Together, these findings suggest that many cows are motivated to seek a secluded place to give birth but may be less willing to work very hard to obtain access to this space. Thus, an area for seclusion in a group pen should be designed to reduce competition (eg, avoiding dead-ends such as the L-shape in a group pen) and should not be difficult for cows to access (eg, no gates or other obstacles between the cow and the hiding space).

In addition to being in a quiet area of the barn, the maternity area should also accommodate other normal calving behaviors, such as the restlessness potentially caused by labor pain. Thus, the maternity pen should be well-bedded and comfortable to allow for the cow to get up and lie down with ease. In a study in which cows were given the choice between different flooring surfaces to give birth, researchers found that cows preferred to give birth on a layer of sand with a layer of straw bedding compared with a rubber mat with the same amount of straw bedding.[40] Although less research has been done with cows at calving, the depth of straw bedding in tie stalls has been found to affect lying time in lactating cows; cows increased their lying time by 12 minutes with every addition of 1 kg of straw in the stall.[41] In addition to improving comfort, straw bedding may also decrease disease risk in cows compared with other materials. For example, straw bedding in the maternity pen decreased the herd prevalence of subclinical endometritis by 10% compared with other bedding such as sand, sawdust, paper, or a combination of these materials.[42] Thus, maternity areas should include a thick layer of straw, ideally with a layer of sand underneath (at least 30–46 cm)[43] for extra drainage and comfort.

A wet and dirty maternity environment may increase the risk of illness after calving for cows and calves. Farms that did not clean and disinfect maternity pens after each birth had higher rates of clinical mastitis compared with farms that cleaned between each calving.[44] Calves born on medium-sized herds (100–199 adult cows) that cleaned the maternity pen after each calving also had less risk of diarrhea compared with those born on farms that cleaned less regularly.[45] A dirty environment may be especially problematic in tie stall herds that allow cows to give birth to their calves into the manure gutter (nearly half of farms surveyed in Quebec, Canada).[10] Despite this increased risk of illness, many farms do not clean pens between calving; in a survey of management practices from 153 herds across the United States, researchers found that less than half of respondents reported cleaning their maternity pens after every calving, and many allowed up to 4 births between cleaning.[46]

In addition to affecting disease risk, the hygiene of the maternity pen may also affect the cow's comfort before she gives birth. Although no research has been done with cows during labor, researchers have found that dry cows spent 5 hours less time lying down per day when the sawdust bedding in a freestall was wet (26.5% dry matter) compared with dry (86.4% dry matter).[47] When cows were given the choice between lying down in wet or dry sawdust in a freestall, cows almost completely avoided lying down in wet stalls. Because cows arguably need the most comfortable environment during labor, a dry maternity environment is key. To keep the maternity environment clean and dry, it is recommended that fresh bedding be added daily, the whole pen be cleaned completely every 3 to 4 weeks,[43] and pens be cleaned between calvings to remove the placenta and areas with wet amniotic fluid.

Some epidemiologic research has found associations between maternity pen type (individual or group) and disease risk in calves; however, a cause-and-effect relationship between pen type and disease is still unclear. Calves on farms with individual maternity pens have been found to have a lower risk for diarrhea in medium-sized herds (100–199 adult cows)[45] and reduced risk for respiratory disease,[48] Salmonella shedding,[49] and paratuberculosis infections[50] compared with those with group maternity pens. These associations may be due to the hygiene of the maternity area rather than the pen type because individual pens may be more likely to be cleaned out between births. However, in a clinical trial assessing the effect of individual pens cleaned between calvings compared with group maternity pens, researchers found no differences in the risk of clinical diarrhea, respiratory disease, or any other disease in calves.[51] In addition, researchers found that individual calving areas were a positive predictor of diarrhea in larger herds (>200 adult cows).[45] Thus, the type of maternity pen on its own may not explain disease risk in cows and calves; the management of the pen is also critical.

To further limit disease risk to the cow and calf, the maternity pen should not double as a hospital pen. According to the USDA National Animal Health Monitoring System, 24.9% of farms reported allowing sick cows in maternity pens and 36% reported allowing lame cows in maternity pens.[9] Housing sick or lame cows in the same pen as maternity cows is more common on small to medium farms (<500 head) because there may be fewer designated areas for a hospital. Researchers conducted a survey of hospital pens used on Iowa, USA, dairy farms and found that 36% of hospital pens were also used for calving.[52] Similarly, in a survey of Quebec, Canada, dairy farms, researchers found that 52.8% of farms used the calving pens to house sick animals.[10] Creating 2 smaller, separate areas for sick and maternity cows is recommended to help reduce disease spread from sick animals to the dam and her newborn.

Reducing environmental and social stressors in the maternity pen is also important to consider. For the purposes of this article, a stress response is defined as arising from "real or perceived environmental demands that can be appraised as threatening or benign, depending on the availability of adaptive coping resources to an individual."[53] Environmental stressors in cattle include heat or cold stress, and poor ventilation.[54] Social stressors include competition or agonistic behaviors from other cows,[55] isolation from the herd,[56] and negative human handling.[57]

Although there is little research on the impacts of environmental stressors on labor progress in dairy cows, there is evidence that heat stress can affect cow behavior and health during the final weeks of gestation. Cows that were heat stressed during late gestation had impaired mammary growth before calving and lower milk production in the next lactation compared with cooled cows.[58] Calves from heat-stressed cows have also been found to have lower passive immunity and impaired cell-mediated immune function compared with calves born from cooled cows.[59] Heat stress can also affect cow comfort by increasing standing time[60] and reducing dry matter intake.[58] Thus, the maternity pen, like other pens holding pregnant cows, should be sufficiently cooled to improve cow comfort and avoid problems with the cow and calf after calf delivery.

Reducing social stressors, including agonistic social interactions in a group maternity pen, is also important to consider for the maternity area. During late gestation, agonistic behaviors (eg, head-butting, displacements from feed or lying space) increase when cows are overcrowded[61,62] or when new animals are added to a group pen.[63] Cows, like other social animals, form a social hierarchy in their groups in which dominant animals have first access to valuable resources such as feeding and lying spaces over subordinate animals with lower social status.[64] To determine this hierarchy, cows will engage in agonistic interactions when meeting a newcomer to the pen, and then these interactions will decrease as cows learn their place in the group (approximately 3 days).[65] Cows regrouped into new pens during late gestation ate 9% less and doubled their physical displacements at the feed bunk on the day of regrouping compared with previous days.[63] Thus, a group maternity pen should limit the number of times per week cows enter it (eg, once per week instead of once per day).

An alternative approach to traditional group maternity pens is to create a stable social environment using an all-in-all-out maternity pen.[43] In a stable group maternity pen, a group of cows would enter the pen together and no new cows would be added. As cows calved, they would either leave the pen or be on the other side of a movable fence until all cows in the group calved. Although not all farms are able to use this approach, cows would likely experience less social stress related to regrouping in this stable group environment. Researchers compared moving cows into group pens weekly compared with all-in-all-out stable groups and found no benefits of stable housing on disease risk after calving.[66] However, cows in the stable groups experienced fewer agonistic behaviors compared with those in pens with weekly entries.[67] These types of stable pens may be particularly beneficial to younger and more socially subordinate cows that may experience the most stress with social disturbance in the maternity pen.[43]

Space allowance in the maternity pen may also be important to improve hygiene and allow the cow sufficient movement during labor in any maternity pen type, as well as limit agonistic behaviors and allow cows to find seclusion from other prepartur-ient cows in group maternity pens. High stocking density during the 2 to 3 weeks before calving has been found to be detrimental to dairy cows, particularly those with low social status.[62] For example, researchers housed cows at 100% versus 200% stocking density (at the feed bunk and lying stalls), and found that cows with lower social status at the feed bunk, regardless of age, had the highest fecal cortisol metabolites, a physiologic indicator of stress.[62] However, less research has specifically focused determining the ideal space allowance in the maternity pen, so recommendations for space allowance in the maternity pen are highly variable (eg, 11–19 m^2 per cow).[43,68] Considering a cow's natural restless and isolation-seeking behavior before calving, producers are recommended to create maternity areas that are as large as possible given the farms physical constraints. Maternity areas (individual or group) should include at least 13 m^2 per cow; however, even larger spaces (<16 m^2 per cow) may provide additional benefits to cows as they seek a clean and quiet space to give birth.

Human handling during labor may also be a stressor to dairy cows and may affect labor progress. In a study using indoor-housed dairy cows, farm staff moved cows from a group pen into an individual maternity pen during 3 periods relative to labor: (1) before labor (moved on average 74 hours before calving, showing no obvious signs of labor), (2) during the early part of stage I labor (moved on average 11 hours before calving, showing signs of raised tail, tense and enlarged udder, and/or relaxed pelvic ligaments), or (3) during late stage I labor (moved on average 2 hours before calving, showing signs of abdominal contractions and/or viscous mucus outside of the vulva).[30] Cows moved during late stage I took 30 minutes longer to progress through stage II labor, spent the less time lying down in the hour before calf delivery, and had higher inflammation (measured using haptoglobin) after calving compared with those moved earlier. These results indicate that the potential stress or novelty associated with moving cows from a group to an individual pen during the sensitive period between stage I and II labor may be detrimental to the cow. Thus, for herds that move cows to a maternity area during labor, cows should ideally be handled and moved when early signs of labor are present (eg, relaxed pelvic ligaments, restless behavior, engorged or leaky udders).

Cows should not be kept in individual maternity pens for too long before giving birth because this prolonged separation from herd mates may also be a stressor. Cows are herd animals, and show physiologic and behavior indicators of stress when they are isolated from the protection of their group.[56] Keeping cows in individual maternity pens for longer than 3 days may increase their risk of ketosis and displaced abomasum after calving.[69]

To avoid keeping the cow in the maternity area for too long before calving, cows are sometimes moved just in time, when signs of stage II are clear (eg, the amniotic sac or the calf's feet are present outside of the vulva). It is unclear how this practice affects the cow and her calf because the research to date has only compared cows moved before signs of stage II are present. However, it should be noted that this practice requires almost constant surveillance of cows in late gestation because cows may progress from signs of the amniotic sac present outside the vulva to calf delivery in an average of 45 minutes and as short as 20 minutes.[17] Without proper surveillance, the cow may deliver her calf in an inappropriate area, such as a freestall. A cow that delivers her calf in the freestall is likely not able to maintain a comfortable posture during labor, and her calf is born in an unhygienic and potentially crowded environment that may increase its risk of injury or disease. Thus, this practice is not advisable unless farm employees are monitoring cows constantly throughout the day and night to ensure that the cow is moved to a suitable maternity area to deliver her calf. To reduce potential stress from handling, cows should be moved a short distance and with proper low stress handling techniques from farm employees.

In some cases, dairy cows require human handling during labor to assist with calf delivery. In cases of dystocia, the survival of the calf depends on swift and effective handling from farm staff or the veterinarian.[17] In other cases, human assistance with labor may not be necessary and may cause undue stress to the cow during labor. Researchers who have assessed labor progress for cows and heifers recommend that cows experiencing stage II labor (the time from the amniotic sac becoming present outside of the vulva until calf delivery) longer than 70 minutes and/or those that do not show progress every 15 minutes in labor should be provided obstetric intervention.[17] Cows that have shorter stage II labor and show normal progress every 15 minutes do not need assistance and unnecessary handling from caretakers. Providing training to caretakers can reduce unnecessary assistance during labor and improve the recognition of dystocia.[70] Thus, all employees working with cows in the maternity pens should be trained to recognize signs of dystocia and avoid assisting cows during labor when unnecessary.

SUMMARY

Like other mammals, labor is likely a painful and stressful experience for dairy cows. In a more natural setting, dairy cows will separate from the herd to find a secluded, comfortable, and quiet place to give birth. An indoor maternity pen can mimic this type of natural environment by providing the cow an opportunity to seclude from other cows and from barn activity and noise. The maternity pen should also be well-bedded, dry, and cleaned regularly to provide a comfortable environment for the cow and minimize the spread of pathogens to both the dam and her newborn calf. Managing the maternity pen to reduce environmental stressors, such as heat stress, and social stressors, such as agonistic behaviors from other cows and unnecessary human handling, is also important to help the cow transition smoothly into the lactating herd.

REFERENCES

1. Huxley JN, Whay H. Current attitudes of cattle practitioners to pain and the use of analgesics in cattle. Vet Rec 2006;159:662–8.
2. Mainau E, Manteca X. Pain and discomfort caused by parturition in cows and sows. Appl Anim Behav Sci 2011;135(3):241–51.
3. Mee JF. Prevalence and risk factors for dystocia in dairy cattle: a review. Vet J 2008;176:93–101.
4. Lombard JE, Garry FB, Tomlinson SM, et al. Impacts of dystocia on health and survival of dairy calves. J Dairy Sci 2007;90:1751–60.
5. Peeler E, Otte M. Inter-relationships of periparturient diseases in dairy cows. Vet Rec 1994;134(6):129–32.
6. Chassagne M, Barnouin J, Chacornac J. Risk factors for stillbirth in Holstein heifers under field conditions in France: a prospective survey. Theriogenology 1999;51:1477–88.
7. LeBlanc SJ, Lissemore KD, Kelton DF, et al. Major advances in disease prevention in dairy cattle. J Dairy Sci 2006;89(4):1267–79.
8. Sepúlveda-Varas P, Huzzey JM, Weary DM, et al. Behaviour, illness and management during the periparturient period in dairy cows. Anim Prod Sci 2013;53: 988–99.
9. USDA. Dairy cattle management practices in the United States, 2014. Fort Collins (CO): USDA–APHIS–VS–CEAH–NAHMS; 2016.
10. Vasseur E, Borderas F, Cue RI, et al. A survey of dairy calf management practices in Canada that affect animal welfare. J Dairy Sci 2010;93:1307–15.
11. Rørvang MV, Nielsen BL, Herskin MS, et al. Prepartum maternal behavior of domesticated cattle: a comparison with managed, feral, and wild ungulates. Front Vet Sci 2018;5:1–11.
12. von Keyserlingk MAG, Weary DM. Maternal behavior in cattle. Horm Behav 2007; 52(1):106–13.

13. Dwyer CM. Individual variation in the expression of maternal behaviour: a review of the neuroendocrine mechanisms in the sheep. J Neuroendocrinol 2008;20: 526–34.

14. Jensen MB. Behaviour around the time of calving in dairy cows. Appl Anim Behav Sci 2012;139:195–202.

15. Noakes DE, Parkinson TJ, England GCW, et al. Parturition and the care of parturient animals. In: Noakes DE, Parkinson TJ, England GCW, editors. Arthur's veterinary reproduction and obstetrics. Philadelphia: Saunders; 2001. p. 155–87.

16. Jackson P. Normal birth. In: Jackson P, editor. Handbook of veterinary obstetrics. 2nd edition. Philadelphia: Saunders; 2004. p. 1–12.

17. Schuenemann GM, Nieto I, Bas S, et al. Assessment of calving progress and reference times for obstetric intervention during dystocia in Holstein dairy cows. J Dairy Sci 2011;94:5494–501.

18. Bonica J. Textbook of pain. 5th edition. London: Churchill Livingstone; 1994.

19. Lidfors LM, Moran D, Jung J, et al. Behaviour at calving and choice of calving place in cattle kept in different environments. Appl Anim Behav Sci 1994;42: 11–28.

20. Leuthold W. African ungulates. Berlin: Springer; 1977.

21. Proudfoot KL, Weary DM, Von Keyserlingk MAG. Maternal isolation behavior of Holstein dairy cows kept indoors. J Anim Sci 2014;92:277–81.

22. Schirmann K, Chapinal N, Weary DM, et al. Short communication: rumination and feeding behavior before and after calving in dairy cows. J Dairy Sci 2013;96: 7088–92.

23. Miedema HM, Cockram MS, Dwyer CM, et al. Behavioural predictors of the start of normal and dystocic calving in dairy cows and heifers. Appl Anim Behav Sci 2011;132:14–9.

24. Huzzey JM, von Keyserlingk MAG, Weary DM. Changes in feeding, drinking, and standing behavior of dairy cows during the transition period. J Dairy Sci 2005;88: 2454–61.

25. Neave HW, Lomb J, von Keyserlingk MAG, et al. Parity differences in the behavior of transition dairy cows. J Dairy Sci 2017;100:548–61.

26. Black RA, Krawczel PD. A case study of behaviour and performance of confined or pastured cows during the dry period. Animals (Basel) 2016;6:41–57.

27. Barrier AC, Ruelle E, Haskell MJ, et al. Effect of a difficult calving on the vigour of the calf, the onset of maternal behaviour, and some behavioural indicators of pain in the dam. Prev Vet Med 2012;103(4):248–56.

28. Machado FLCP, Hurnik JF, King GJ. Timing of the attraction towards the placenta and amniotic fluid by the parturient cow. Appl Anim Behav Sci 1997;53:183–92.

29. Rørvang MV, Nielsen BL, Herskin MS, et al. Short communication: calving site selection of multiparous, group-housed dairy cows is influenced by site of a previous calving. J Dairy Sci 2017;100:1467–71.

30. Proudfoot KL, Jensen MB, Heegaard PMH, et al. Effect of moving dairy cows at different stages of labor on behavior during parturition. J Dairy Sci 2013;96: 1638–46.

31. Houwing H, Hurnik JF, Lewis NJ. Behavior of periparturient dairy cows and their calves. Can J Anim Sci 1990;70:355–62.

32. Jensen MB. The early behaviour of cow and calf in an individual calving pen. Appl Anim Behav Sci 2011;134:92–9.

33. Metz J, Metz JHM. Maternal influence on defecation and urination in the newborn calf. Appl Anim Behav Sci 1986;16:325–33.

34. Edwards SA. The behaviour of dairy cows and their newborn calves in individual or group housing. Appl Anim Ethol 1983;10:191–8.
35. Illmann G, Špinka M. Maternal behaviour of dairy heifers and sucking of their newborn calves in group housing. Appl Anim Behav Sci 1993;36:91–8.
36. Moore M, Tyler JW, Chigerwe M, et al. Effect of delayed colostrum collection on colostral IgG concentration in dairy cows. J Am Vet Med Assoc 2005;226:1375–7.
37. Proudfoot KL, Jensen MB, Weary DM, et al. Dairy cows seek isolation at calving and when ill. J Dairy Sci 2014;97:2731–9.
38. Rørvang MV, Herskin MS, Jensen MB. Dairy cows with prolonged calving seek additional isolation. J Dairy Sci 2017;100:2967–75.
39. Rørvang MV, Herskin MS, Jensen MB. The motivation-based calving facility: social and cognitive factors influence isolation seeking behaviour of Holstein dairy cows at calving. PLoS One 2018;13:e0191128.
40. Campler M, Munksgaard L, Jensen MB, et al. Short communication: flooring preferences of dairy cows at calving. J Dairy Sci 2014;97:892–6.
41. Tucker CB, Weary DM, von Keyserlingk MAG, et al. Cow comfort in tie-stalls: increased depth of shavings or straw bedding increases lying time. J Dairy Sci 2009;92:2684–90.
42. Cheong SH, Nydam DV, Galvão KN, et al. Cow-level and herd-level risk factors for subclinical endometritis in lactating Holstein cows. J Dairy Sci 2011;94:762–70.
43. Cook NB, Nordlund KV. Behavioral needs of the transition cow and considerations for special needs facility design. Vet Clin North Am Food Anim Pract 2004;20:495–520.
44. Elbers ARW, Miltenburg JD, De Lange D, et al. Risk factors for clinical mastitis in a random sample of dairy herds from the southern part of The Netherlands. J Dairy Sci 1998;81:420–6.
45. Frank NA, Kaneene JB. Management risk factors associated with calf diarrhea in michigan dairy herds. J Dairy Sci 1993;76:1313–23.
46. Caraviello DZ, Weigel KA, Fricke PM, et al. Survey of management practices on reproductive performance of dairy cattle on large US Commercial Farms. J Dairy Sci 2006;89:4723–35.
47. Fregonesi JA, Veira DM, Von Keyserlingk MAG, et al. Effects of bedding quality on lying behavior of dairy cows. J Dairy Sci 2007;90:5468–72.
48. Svensson C, Lundborg K, Emanuelson U, et al. Morbidity in Swedish dairy calves from birth to 90 days of age and individual calf-level risk factors for infectious diseases. Prev Vet Med 2003;58:179–97.
49. Losinger WC, Wells SJ, Garber LP, et al. Management factors related to *Salmonella* shedding by dairy heifers. J Dairy Sci 1995;78:2464–72.
50. Pithua P, Espejo LA, Godden SM, et al. Is an individual calving pen better than a group calving pen for preventing transmission of *Mycobacterium avium* subsp paratuberculosis in calves? Results from a field trial. Res Vet Sci 2013;95:398–404.
51. Pithua P, Wells SJ, Godden SM, et al. Clinical trial on type of calving pen and the risk of disease in Holstein calves during the first 90 d of life. Prev Vet Med 2009;89:8–15.
52. Fogsgaard KK, Herskin MS, Gorden PJ, et al. Management and design of hospital pens relative to behavior of the compromised dairy cow: a questionnaire survey of Iowa dairy farms. Appl Anim Behav Sci 2016;175:50–5.
53. McEwen BS, Gianaros PJ. Central role of the brain in stress and adaptation: links to socioeconomic status, health, and disease. Ann N Y Acad Sci 2010;1186:190–222.

54. Collier RJ, Dahl GE, VanBaale MJ. Major advances associated with environmental effects on dairy cattle. J Dairy Sci 2006;89:1244–53.
55. Proudfoot K, Habing G. Social stress as a cause of diseases in farm animals: current knowledge and future directions. Vet J 2015;206:15–21.
56. Rushen J, Boissy A, Terlouw EMC, et al. Opioid peptides and behavioral and physiological responses of dairy cows to social isolation in unfamiliar surroundings. J Anim Sci 1999;77(11):2918–24. Available at: http://jas.fass.org/content/77/11/2918. Accessed December 18, 2014.
57. Rushen J, de Passillé AMB, Munksgaard L. Fear of people by cows and effects on milk yield, behavior, and heart rate at milking. J Dairy Sci 1999;82:720–7.
58. Tao S, Bubolz JW, do Amaral BC, et al. Effect of heat stress during the dry period on mammary gland development. J Dairy Sci 2011;94:5976–86.
59. Tao S, Monteiro APA, Thompson IM, et al. Effect of late-gestation maternal heat stress on growth and immune function of dairy calves. J Dairy Sci 2012;95: 7128–36.
60. Cook NB, Mentink RL, Bennett TB, et al. The effect of heat stress and lameness on time budgets of lactating dairy cows. J Dairy Sci 2007;90:1674–82.
61. Proudfoot KLL, Veira DMM, Weary DMM, et al. Competition at the feed bunk changes the feeding, standing, and social behavior of transition dairy cows. J Dairy Sci 2009;92(7):3116–23.
62. Huzzey JM, Grant RJ, Overton TR. Short communication: relationship between competitive success during displacements at an overstocked feed bunk and measures of physiology and behavior in Holstein dairy cattle. J Dairy Sci 2012; 95(8):4434–41.
63. Schirmann K, Chapinal N, Weary DMM, et al. Short-term effects of regrouping on behavior of prepartum dairy cows. J Dairy Sci 2011;94(5):2312–9.
64. Kondo S, Hurnik JF. Stabilization of social hierarchy in dairy cows. Appl Anim Behav Sci 1990;27:287–97.
65. von Keyserlingk MAG, Olenick D, Weary DM. Acute behavioral effects of regrouping dairy cows. J Dairy Sci 2008;91(3):1011–6.
66. Silva PRBP, Moraes JJGN, Mendonça LGD, et al. Effects of weekly regrouping of prepartum dairy cows on innate immune response and antibody concentration. J Dairy Sci 2013;96(2008):7649–57.
67. Lobeck-Luchterhand KM, Silva PRB, Chebel RC, et al. Effect of prepartum grouping strategy on displacements from the feed bunk and feeding behavior of dairy cows. J Dairy Sci 2014;97:2800–7.
68. Graves R. Bedded pack barns for dairy cattle. West Dairy Dig. 2006.
69. Nordlund K, Cook N, Oetzel G. Commingling dairy cows: pen moves, stocking density, and health a changing clinical perspective of fresh cow metabolic disease. In: 39th Proceedings American Association Bovine Practitioners. St. Paul, MN, September 21–23, 2006.
70. Schuenemann GM, Bas S, Gordon E, et al. Dairy calving management: description and assessment of a training program for dairy personnel. J Dairy Sci 2013; 96:2671–80.

Designing Facilities for the Adult Dairy Cow During the Nonlactation and Early Lactation Period

Nigel B. Cook, BSc, BVSc, Cert CHP, DBR, MRCVS

KEYWORDS

- Transition • Facility design • Feed access • Regrouping stress

KEY POINTS

- The blueprint for transition facility design provides for sufficient bunk space for all cows to eat at the same time, access to a comfortable soft bed for rest, and the avoidance of regrouping stress 2 to 7 days before calving.
- Fixed-sized transition cow accommodation must be overbuilt to accommodate a biological process, which results in surges in calving from time to time. This is justified because these facilities affect the lactations of multiple cows, not just a single cow.
- The prefresh area represents a significant bottle neck to cow flow through transition since the cow determines when she will leave the pen, once she calves.
- Fresh cows grouped separately for 21 to 30 days postpartum allow for screening of sick cows and the feeding of specialized rations.

INTRODUCTION

Over the last 2 decades, dairy producers who have expanded their herd size have seized opportunities to improve their adult dairy cow housing and provide accommodation for dry cows, maternity cows, and lactating cows during early lactation. Previously, these cows would often be ignored in herd expansions, with a predominant focus on providing new facilities for the milking cows. Often, cows transitioning from the dry period into early lactation were left to occupy the old facilities that were no longer required for the newly accommodated milking herd. This approach often led to disappointing early lactation performance with associated poor postpartum health.

Even when a decision was made to build a new facility for transition cows, there were few guidelines available and dairy producers were left to make numerous errors.

Disclosure Statement: The author has nothing to disclose.
Department of Medical Sciences, University of Wisconsin-Madison, School of Veterinary Medicine, 2015 Linden Drive, Madison, WI 53706, USA
E-mail address: nigel.cook@wisc.edu

Vet Clin Food Anim 35 (2019) 125–138
https://doi.org/10.1016/j.cvfa.2018.10.008
0749-0720/19/© 2018 Elsevier Inc. All rights reserved.

Fortunately, the early 2000s was a time of elevated interest in transition cow performance metrics, moving from traditional measures of peak milk yield and a reliance on poorly defined health records to metrics that incorporated measures of early lactation milk performance (eg, the Transition Cow Index,[1] daily and weekly milk averages over the first few weeks of lactation), measures of survival (ie, turnover and death rates <60 DIM), metabolic indicators (eg, first milk test fat-to-protein ratios), udder health indicators (eg, first milk test somatic cell count new infection rates), calf survival (ie, stillbirth rate), and records of health events with a consistent definition (eg, incidence of displaced abomasum).[2] These metrics facilitated the identification of herd design and management approaches that resulted in improved performance.

Simultaneously, over the last 15 years, there has been unprecedented interest in the impact of facility design on cow behavior and how that in turn can affect health and milk production. Although poor nutrition and feeding was often blamed for poor transition, the author's group at the University of Wisconsin-Madison, School of Veterinary Medicine began to realize the importance of facility design. Cook and Nordlund[3] reviewed the approaches to housing and management that were becoming commonplace at that time and, based on herd troubleshooting experiences, began to question them. Chief among our concerns were the amount of lying and feeding space provided and the number of group changes that cows were exposed to during transition. It was not uncommon to find cows moved between 5 different groups during the period from 21 days before to 21 days after calving, and dry cows were accommodated in pens with restricted bunk space in the belief that they would simply find a way to consume the nutrients they required because they were no longer spending time out of the pen milking. In essence, the needs of the cow as a highly complex and social animal were forgotten. This article summarizes the science accumulated over the last 15 years to support the current recommendations for housing the cow in transition.

THE WISCONSIN BLUEPRINT

Using surveys of herds with differing levels of transition performance, Nordlund and Cook developed a simple blueprint for transition barn design in 2006 based on 4 key criteria:

1. Provide sufficient bunk space 21 days before and after calving for all the cows to eat at the same time.
2. Provide a soft lying surface for nonlame and lame cows to gain adequate rest.
3. Provide sufficient stalls per cow of appropriate dimensions or a bedded pack area to allow all the cows to rest at the same time.
4. Avoid regrouping cows during the critical 2 to 7 days before calving when optimizing dry matter intake (DMI) is already challenged.

This blueprint was made available through the Web site at https://thedairylandinitiative.vetmed.wisc.edu/ and used by the dairy industry in the Upper Midwest and elsewhere to construct new facilities for transition cows. When coupled with excellent feeding management and well-trained care-givers who could identify and treat sick cows effectively, the blueprint achieved the goal of improving early lactation cow performance and cow health during the postpartum period.

In 2004, DeVries and colleagues[4] elegantly demonstrated the impact of reduced bunk space on subordinate cow feeding behavior during the period after fresh feed delivery. In what would turn out to be a series of studies on transition cows assigned to calibrated total mixed ration feeding bins in a controlled environment, Huzzey and colleagues[5] were the first to show reduced dry matter intake (DMI) in prefresh cows that subsequently developed metritis after calving in a competitive feeding situation when compared with control cows that remained healthy postpartum. This work supported the view that even dry cows needed access to the bunk alongside all of their herd mates, especially when fresh feed was delivered to maximize DMI.

At the same time, the Cook and colleagues[6] had shown the impact of a soft bedded surface on lame cow behavior and promoted the use of deep sand bedded freestalls; not only during lactation but also during transition when a comfortable bedded pack could be used for the same purpose. Deep loose bedding promotes longer lying bouts, requiring fewer bouts to be taken each day, which results in fewer times that the cow must rise and lie down.[7] Deep sand also provided traction and secure footing to facilitate rising and lying movements, mainly for lame cows with sore feet because it allowed them to maintain a normal pattern of resting behavior.[8] Subsequently, lameness has been identified as a risk factor for postpartum health problems in multiple studies.[9–11] This is likely due to extended periods of forced rest and reduced feeding time during the period immediately after the delivery of the calf.[12,13]

The need for normal patterns of rest also necessitated the requirement for 1 resting space per cow in the blueprint. Although there were, and continue to be, fewer data to support this request, studies have demonstrated the loss in lying time that occurs at elevated stocking rates.[14] Bach and colleagues[15] were able to show the impact on milk production of elevated numbers of cows per stall in 47 dairy herds fed a common ration. These studies continue to support the view that transition cows have enough challenges to deal with, without having to compete for a place to lie down.

The evidence for avoiding regrouping 2 to 7 days before calving is somewhat confusing. Schirmann and colleagues[16] were able to show that regrouping cows during the transition period resulted in a 9% reduction in DMI in the moved cows on the day of the move compared with the previous baseline, confirming for the first time that regrouping had an impact during transition. However, not all studies have been supportive of the avoidance of regrouping at this time. Coonen and colleagues[17] failed to show a significant impact of social stability during the dry period on DMI, blood nonesterified fatty acids concentrations, or early lactation milk production. Similarly, Silva and colleagues[18,19] found no significant effect on milk production, health, blood metabolites, or immune function when comparing an all-in-all-out transition grouping strategy with a movement scheme in which regrouping occurred once per week. However, a later study did show significantly reduced displacements from the bunk between cows and altered feeding time in the all-in-all-out group, notably within 1 day of regrouping.[20] At face value, these studies do not seem to support the stable group concept put forward in the blueprint. However, a closer look at these studies and subsequent work provides some insight on the lack of observed effects. In the study by Coonen and colleagues,[17] cows were managed in comfortable deep bedded loose housing with space for all of the cows to eat and rest at once, while the study by Silva and colleagues[18] used Jersey cows housed in deep bedded freestalls with a minimum of 2.2 ft (0.66 m) of bunk space per cow. So, it is possible that the facility design, in particular the comfortable lying space and feed access provided, reduced the impact of group changes in these well-controlled studies. Indeed, Talebi and colleagues[21] demonstrated that there is a significant mitigating effect of stocking density on regrouping stress, and it is likely that an experimental situation fails to incorporate all the challenges and variations faced by cows transitioning on commercial dairy farms. The avoidance of regrouping stress remains part of the author's blueprint in the belief that there remains sufficient evidence for a potential negative effect on the transition cow, particularly when other criteria of the blueprint are not met.

ADDITIONAL DESIGN ELEMENTS

Transition facilities for dairy cows must also meet the needs of the cow at the point of calving. (See Kathryn L. Proudfoot's article, "Maternal Behavior and Design of The Maternity Pen," in this issue.) The need for a quiet place to calve is easily forgotten in the design process, with maternity areas often located near the busiest areas of the farm. However, there is evidence that isolation of this area from the rest of the dairy should be attempted so that it is calm and quiet, and approaches that allow individual cows to isolate themselves from the rest of the group should be explored.[22]

Over the past decade, dairy producers have coalesced around 2 main approaches to calving management. With the first approach, termed just-in-time calving, the cow is moved to the maternity pen at the point of calving. With the second, the short-stay maternity approach, cows are limited to an approximately 2-day stay in the calving pen. A third approach is still used by some farms in the industry with longer stays in large-group maternity pens of 3 or more days. However, this approach promotes increased social turmoil, constant regrouping, and is less desirable overall.

Considerable debate also revolves around the design of the feed bunk, with the 2 options being headlocks or a simple post-and-rail design that does not delineate separate feed spaces for each cow. Huzzey and colleagues[23] were able to show reduced rates of displacement from the bunk between cows fed at a headlock-fitted feed bunk compared with a post-and-rail design. Similarly, Endres and colleagues[24] showed that a headlock barrier enabled subordinate cows to maintain feeding times alongside more dominant herd mates compared with a post-and-rail design. This observation has particular importance in a mixed parity group of prefresh cows. Anecdotally, transition performance improved with the use of headlocks during the prefresh and postfresh periods, particularly when heifers and mature cows are grouped together. The theory is that the headlock affords the subordinate cow some protection from dominant cows while feeding. At issue is the requirement for heifers to have experienced headlocks before joining the prefresh group if they are to be used in this area. Even if heifers are accustomed to using headlocks, some producers will provide a bunk with sections of both designs to ensure all cows have access to feed at this critical period (**Fig. 1**).

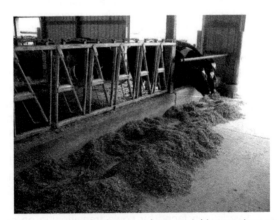

Fig. 1. Use of headlocks in the prefresh pen reduces social interactions at the bunk. Heifers that are unaccustomed to this bunk design benefit from prior training during the rearing period and having part of the prefresh area fitted with a post-and-rail design to ensure that all cows have access to feed.

Although the focus of heat abatement strategies is often on the lactating cow, the benefits of cooling have been amply demonstrated for the dry cow and for the survival and subsequent performance of the calf.[25–27] The provision of fast-moving air (>200 ft/min or 1 ms^{-1}) in the cows' resting space and sufficient air exchange to remove the heat from the barn are just as important for the dry cows as for lactating cows. (See Mario R. Mondaca's article, "Ventilation Systems for Adult Dairy Cattle," in this issue.)

The provision of controlled lighting has also received some interest during the dry period, with a positive milk response achieved through short-day photoperiods (8 hours of light and 16 hours of dark).[28,29] However, the implementation of such an approach is challenging in naturally ventilated barns and, although it has been attempted in larger mechanically designed facilities, around-the-clock calving and work patterns make the approach difficult to successfully implement.

CORRECT GROUP SIZING

It is easy to suggest to the farm that they provide sufficient space to accommodate the transition cows but actually designing a fixed-sized facility to accommodate a biological process that is far from consistent over time is a significant challenge. The main problem is that the average herd rarely achieves an average rate of calving at any particular time. **Fig. 2** shows the number of cows and heifers calving per week over 2 years for an example herd. Surges in calving occur from time to time and occur for different parity groups at different periods. In some herds, a surge may be a rebound from poor fertility during periods of heat stress, whereas in others it might relate to the synchronization of breeding in heifers. It is obvious that if the facility is designed around the average rate of calvings, the pens will be overstocked half the time and, during calving surges, the system will be put under extreme duress because both the resting space and feeding area will be significantly compromised.

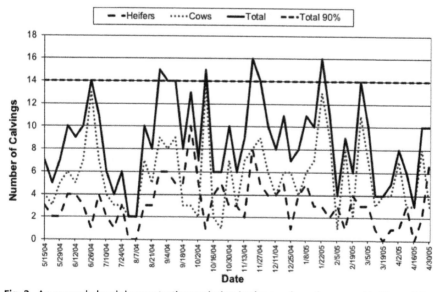

Fig. 2. An example herd demonstrating variation in the number of cows and heifers calving per week over 2 years. The horizontal dashed line represents the 90th percentile of the weekly calving rate of cows and heifers.

Correct sizing of transition cow pens requires an understanding of target duration of stay in each pen, calving rate, and cow flow between different groupings. For this discussion, it is assumed that cows transition from a far dry group, typically 60 days before calving, to a prefresh (or close-up) group, from 21 to 30 days before calving until the day of calving. Then, they deliver in a maternity pen and then move into a fresh pen for the first 21 days of lactation.

The prefresh and maternity area is the most significant bottleneck to cow flow through the transition facility. These pens are unique on the farm in that the cow ultimately decides when she leaves them rather than the herd manager. Exit depends on the timing of birth. Further complicating design is the variation in gestation period. Although Holstein cows may average 280 days pregnant, there are approximately 14 days variation in due dates between cows within a herd. With this variation, pen stays of 14 days or less cannot be recommended if cows are to adjust to a new diet or new surroundings. Therefore, the author recommends entry into the prefresh pen 21 to 30 days before the due date.

Based on estimates of calving rate variation over time, the author has recommended using 120% to 150% of the average rate of calving to overbuild these important pens. This range seems to be the best predictor of the 90th percentile of the calving rate, which is the cutpoint above which only 10% of the weeks exceed the threshold. In general, the longer the duration of stay, the lower the multiplier used because there will be some averaging of cow flow from week to week as they enter the pen. The author recommends building for 120% of the average weekly calving rate for pen stays greater than 30 days, 130% for stays of 22 to 29 days, 140% for stays of 3 to 21 days, and 150% for pen stays of 2 days or less.

For a herd with 1000 total average cows (milking and dry), a rule of thumb suggests that they will calve 10% more cows per year ($1000 \times 110/100/365$ days = 3.01 cows and heifers per day on average). For a 21-day prefresh stay the author recommends accommodation for 87 cows and heifers ($3.01 \times 1.4 \times 21 = 87$ cows and heifers).

Although this approach leads to the construction of pens that will be understocked part of the time, it has merit because it avoids the severe overstocking that may occur during calving surges. Unlike a lactating cow pen, where 1 stall and 1 feed space affects 1 cow for a lactation cycle, a transition cow pen and feed space affects multiple cows and multiple lactation cycles. This defrays the cost because it is a cost per cow in the herd rather than a cost per stall.

APPROACHES TO PREFRESH COW HOUSING

Dairy owners have implemented the blueprint for transition barn design in a variety of different ways to suit their management style and farmstead layout. Over the last decade, 3 main approaches to prefresh pen housing have emerged:

1. Traditional
2. Sequential fill
3. All-in-all-out.

Traditional

Traditional is the most common approach. A single pen is built to accommodate a 21-day to 30-day pen stay for cows and heifers, and is typically paired with just-in-time calving with an individual or group calving pen. In smaller herds, the pen may accommodate cows for the entire dry period in 1 group. The freestall pen is 2-row layout with

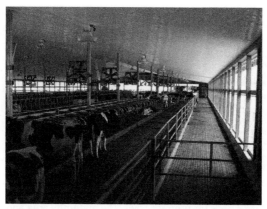

Fig. 3. A traditional prefresh pen layout with a 2-row head-to-head stall design, separate pens for prefresh heifers and prefresh mature cows, with connection to the maternity area though a drover's lane on the outside of the pen. This lane also facilitates viewing cows in the stalls for signs of labor without the need to enter the pen.

crossovers every 12 to 15 stalls to ensure sufficient bunk space. Crossovers are typically 14-ft (4.3-m) wide to allow for the waterer and plenty of room for cow flow around it. Shared crossovers may be installed with a 26-ft (7.9-m) space between the stalls and a centrally located waterer with access from both sides. These pens can be divided with gates at the waterer or opened to provide more space if needed.

Without a drover's lane on the nonfeed alley side of the pen, a head-to-tail layout is preferred so that each recumbent cow can be seen from the feed alley for signs of labor. Alternatively, with a drover's lane, a head-to-head or tail-to-tail layout may be used because the caregiver can walk around the perimeter of the pen. With this approach, cows do not need to be disturbed by a person entering the pen unless there is a cow in labor (**Fig. 3**).

Heifers and mature cows may be grouped separately from each other in dedicated prefresh pens. The advantage is that stalls can be sized more closely to the size of the animal using them, and separate rations may be fed if desired.

Sequential Fill

The sequential fill approach is becoming more common in larger herds with more than 1000 cows and is also paired with just-in-time calving, although it can be adapted for other maternity pen strategies. It has the singular advantage that it focuses the attention of workers on a smaller group of cows immediately adjacent to the maternity area.

The prefresh area is sized for a 21-day pen stay and, rather than being operated as a single pen for the entire stay, it is divided into 3 weekly fill pens. Separate lines of pens may be provided to split heifers and mature cows if the herd is large enough (**Fig. 4**).

The pen furthest from the maternity area is filled with a group of cows starting 21 days before the due date. This group displaces the group that was in this pen to the adjacent pen. They will now be 14 days before the due date and they in turn displace the resident group in the next pen immediately adjacent to the maternity area. These cows will be within 7 days of due date and will receive most of the attention from the maternity pen workers because they will be the actively calving group. The last pen will, of course, not be empty when the next group wishes to enter so it should be oversized by 10% to 15% to accommodate the cows who have not yet calved and must join the incoming group. This system creates the risk of regrouping

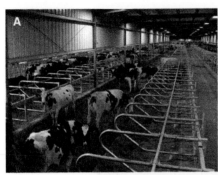
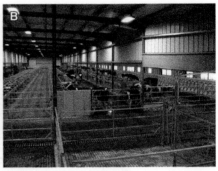

Fig. 4. (*A*) A sequential fill prefresh layout for a 2500-cow dairy herd. There are 3 pens separated by gates on 1 side of the drover's lane for prefresh heifers and on the right side of the drover's lane, there are 3 pens for prefresh cows. The maternity area and office can be seen at the end of the third pen. Cows are moved between the pens once a week toward the maternity area. (*B*) The sequential fill prefresh area viewed from the maternity end of the pens.

within 7 days of calving in a small percentage of the cows. However, the negative impacts of regrouping are less on the resident cows compared with the cows being moved into the pen and are further lessened by the provision of adequate space.[16,21]

Pen design is for the traditional prefresh pen (see previous discussion). Exits to the drover's lane between pens are important to facilitate cow flow. In this design, the last pen before calving can be a freestall or a loose bedded pack area, which can double as a calving pen. This concept has also been used for large dry lot dairy herds in which the prefresh dry lot is divided into 3 separate areas with movement between the pens toward the calving center as the due date approaches.

With multiple pens, it is important to be able to single-handedly move cows around the facility via the drover's lane. In these designs, 1 to 2 stalls are omitted to add an access point and gate to allow for easy transfer of cows to a different pen or to the maternity area (**Fig. 5**).

All-In-All-Out

The All-in-all-out system is the least common approach to transition cow management but it can be adapted to a system using only bedded packs (**Fig. 6**) or freestalls

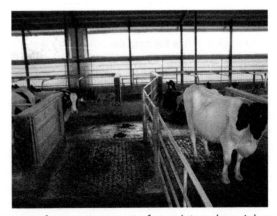

Fig. 5. A pen access gate for easy movement of cows into a drover's lane for movement to another pen or to the maternity area.

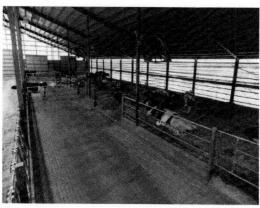

Fig. 6. An all-in-all-out prefresh area for a 700-cow dairy with 5 loose housed straw bedded pack pens for 10 prefresh cows grouped together 30 days before calving. Each group is socially stable with no new cows added to the group for the entire period. Cows calve in the pen or in an adjacent maternity area.

combined with a maternity pen (**Fig. 7**). The duration of stay can be modified to accommodate only the prefresh period or the entire dry period using pens sized to match the approximate weekly average calving rate. Each pen would be filled and the cows would remain in a socially stable group for the entire prefresh or dry period. In bedded pack systems, the cows may calve in the pen itself or in a separate maternity pen.

THE MATERNITY PEN

A maternity pen, the pen in which the cow delivers her calf, may be designed as an individual or group pen. (See Kathryn L. Proudfoot's article, "Maternal Behavior and Design of the Maternity Pen," in this issue.) High design priorities include pens with adequate space (typically 100–150 sq ft [9.3–13.9 sq m] per cow), a soft surface that preferably has straw bedding,[30] easy access for cleaning, close proximity to

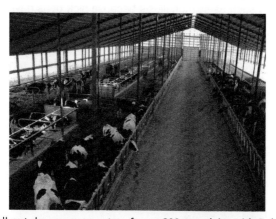

Fig. 7. An all-in-all-out dry cow pen system for an 800-cow dairy with 5 deep sand bedded freestall pens for 30 cows housed together for the 45-day dry period. Each group is socially stable, with no new cows added to the group for the entire period. The outside drover's lane is used to transfer cows to the maternity area.

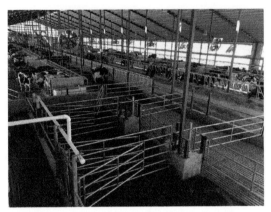

Fig. 8. Individual maternity pens located close to the prefresh area with a viewing area above the pens and gating to assist the cow if necessary.

the prefresh area, avoidance of high-traffic areas, and options for isolation of individuals from the rest of the group (**Fig. 8**).

Ideally, pens should have a means to milk the cow easily to harvest colostrum soon after birth (**Fig. 9**), and a clean and warm adjacent area for the calf to be moved to once it has been licked off, out of sight of the dam. Food and water should also be provided.

THE COLOSTRUM PEN

During the immediate postpartum period, the cow needs a comfortable low-stress area to recover from delivery. Mature cows treated with dry cow antibiotic therapy will also have a milk withhold, necessitating segregation of the milk to avoid a residue violation. In some herds, these cows join a fresh pen or other lactating cow pen and the milk is segregated at milking time. In others, these cows will join a separate colostrum pen for a few days until they clear antibiotic residue testing. In others, this pen is a hospital pen, also populated by sick cows under antibiotic treatment. Obviously, mixing sick cows with cows immediately postpartum is a potential risk factor for the spread of diseases such as salmonellosis because sick pens have been repeatedly shown to be areas with high rates of contamination[31,32]; however, many herds seem to tolerate and manage the risk without obvious issues.

The author's preference is to maintain a group bedded pack area adjacent to the maternity area solely for cows under residue withdrawal, and to manage sick and

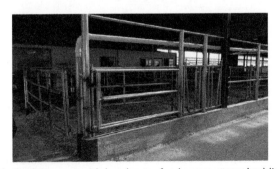

Fig. 9. An individual calving pen with head gate, feed access, straw bedding, and a vacuum line for harvesting colostrum in the pen.

lame cows in a separate hospital area that is physically separated from these high-risk cows. Priorities for sick cow housing include making sure that animals do not share a water source with fit cows and that the sick pen is located at the end of a manure scrape alley to avoid moving contaminated manure through well-cow pens.

One further nuance that may need to be addressed in the immediate postpartum period is a change to the current standard of separating the calf from the dam at or very soon after birth. This approach does not sit well with informed consumers, who may demand a change in cow and calf management for the first few days of life in the not too distant future.[33] Different approaches to maintaining cow–calf contact before weaning have been reviewed,[34] and there are some promising approaches emerging involving contact for part of the day. The addition of a restricted nursery area for calves that is connected to an intermediate area where recently calved cows can be moved from the colostrum pen to nurse their calves is a viable approach that requires more research to investigate long-term health implications. To succeed, the calf-rearing area must be hygienically managed with supplemental milk feeding with no access for the cows. A combination of rails, finger gates, and curbs may suffice to achieve this goal; however, to the author's knowledge, this approach is still not field-tested in the United States.

APPROACHES TO FRESH COW HOUSING

Fresh or postfresh pens receive cows leaving the maternity area or from a separate colostrum area where the cow's milk has been segregated for a few days after calving. The idea for a separate fresh pen is to put the cows that are at high risk of periparturient disease in a separate place on the farm so that they may be monitored closely and perhaps fed a separate ration from the lactating cows.

It is known that the median days in milk for the onset of a displaced abomasum is approximately 12 days after calving, so the author does not recommend an average fresh pen stay of less than 14 days and prefers a stay of 21 to 30 days. Fit cows that are milking well may be moved out earlier, whereas cows off to a slow start may remain in the pen longer.

Space allowance in the fresh pen is critical because regrouping will be occurring on a daily basis as cows leave the maternity pen. The fresh pen is typically sized to accommodate 1.3 to 1.4 times the weekly average rate of calving in the herd.

The fresh pen could be a bedded pack area or freestalls with a 2-row layout. Because this is a pen where cows are examined frequently by caregivers, the feed bunk should be fitted with 30-inch (76-cm) wide headlocks to facilitate access between cows. Because total lockup time should be limited to as short a time as possible, the headlocks should be grouped into small clusters (maximum 10–15 cows) that can be locked and unlocked separately so that cows that have been screened and treated can be let go as soon as possible rather than having them wait for the whole group to be processed.

Appropriately sized, deep loose bedded stall surfaces are of particular importance for the fresh cows recovering from calving, which seems particularly challenging for lame cows.[10,13] Indeed, it may be possible to create a separate high-risk group of fresh cows. This high-risk group of mature cows, as defined by Vergara and colleagues,[10] consists of individuals that are parity 3 or greater, lame, and cows that have suffered a calving problem, such as a twin birth, stillbirth, or dystocia. It may be preferable to house this subset of fresh cows on a bedded pack and adopt management strategies to facilitate recovery, such as a reduced milking frequency (maximum of 2 times per day) to maximize the time available for rest, and routine dosing of oral calcium[9,35] and glucose precursors.[36]

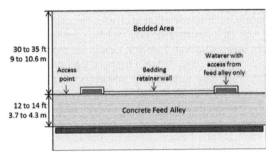

Fig. 10. Basic layout for a bedded pack area suitable for dry cows, a group maternity area, or for fresh cows.

BEDDED PACKS OR LOOSE HOUSING DESIGN

Bedded packs or loose housing are used in transition cow barns for dry cows, maternity areas, and for cows in the immediate postpartum period. They can be managed aerobically (so-called compost barns) or anaerobically. These pens have been associated with excellent cow comfort and low rates of injury.[37] Typically, aerobic beds use fine dry wood sawdust bedding and are composted over approximately 6 months by stirring twice a day to a depth of 8 to 12 inches (20–30 cm), with the aim of generating a minimum temperature of 140 °F (60 °C). By contrast, anaerobic beds typically use fresh dry straw added daily to a bed that accumulates in layers over 4 to 6 weeks before removal and replacement. The layers compact, become moist, and decompose, which removes oxygen from the bed. The basic design of each of these systems is very similar (**Fig. 10**). The area should be rectangular, with the longest side adjacent to the feed bunk, and divided lengthwise to create a 12-ft to 14-ft (3.7–4.3-m) wide concrete apron next to the bunk and a bedded area typically no more than 30 to 35 ft deep (9–10.6 m). So it does not drift onto the concrete apron, the bedding must be contained by the use of a bedding retainer, the size and shape of which depends on the type of bedded pack being constructed. For anaerobic beds, a low curb is all that is required, whereas for aerobic compost beds, the retaining wall is built higher to allow for the accumulation of bedding over an extended period. Water access should only be possible from the concrete apron, not from the bedded area.

SUMMARY

This article attempts to summarize the research supporting an approach to transition cow housing that optimizes access to feed, provides each cow a comfortable place to rest, uses a grouping and movement strategy that minimizes regrouping stress during the critical period in late gestation, and that provides a quiet place to calve. Producers have adopted a variety of strategies to achieve these goals and, as a result, early lactation health and performance has improved when combined with excellent ration design and feed delivery, and thorough screening of cows for signs of disease.

ACKNOWLEDGMENTS

The author would like to acknowledge the assistance and support of Dr Kenneth Nordlund who led the development of the Transition Cow Index and worked tirelessly to help develop the ideas represented in this article. The author would also like to acknowledge the funding support for the Dairyland Initiative at https://thedairylandinitiative. vetmed.wisc.edu/home/housing-module/supporters/.

REFERENCES

1. Schultz KK, Bennett TB, Nordlund KV, et al. Exploring relationships between Dairy Herd Improvement monitors of performance and the Transition Cow Index in Wisconsin dairy herds. J Dairy Sci 2016;99(9):7506–16.
2. Nordlund KV, Cook NB. Using herd records to monitor transition cow survival, productivity, and health. Vet Clin North Am Food Anim Pract 2004;20(3 SPEC. ISS.):627–49.
3. Cook NB, Nordlund KV. Behavioral needs of the transition cow and considerations for special needs facility design. Vet Clin North Am Food Anim Pract 2004;20(3 SPEC. ISS.):495–520.
4. DeVries TJ, von Keyserlingk MAG, Weary DM. Effect of feeding space on the inter-cow distance, aggression, and feeding behavior of free-stall housed lactating dairy cows. J Dairy Sci 2004;87(5):1432–8.
5. Huzzey JM, Veira DM, Weary DM, et al. Prepartum behavior and dry matter intake identify dairy cows at risk for metritis. J Dairy Sci 2007;90(7):3220–33.
6. Cook NB, Bennett TB, Nordlund KV. Effect of free stall surface on daily activity patterns in dairy cows with relevance to lameness prevalence. J Dairy Sci 2004;87(9):2912–22.
7. Gomez A, Cook NB. Time budgets of lactating dairy cattle in commercial freestall herds. J Dairy Sci 2010;93(12):5772–81.
8. Cook NB, Nordlund KV. The influence of the environment on dairy cow behavior, claw health and herd lameness dynamics. Vet J 2009;179(3):360–9.
9. Oetzel GR, Miller BE. Effect of oral calcium bolus supplementation on early-lactation health and milk yield in commercial dairy herds. J Dairy Sci 2012; 95(12):7051–65.
10. Vergara CF, Döpfer D, Cook NB, et al. Risk factors for postpartum problems in dairy cows: Explanatory and predictive modeling. J Dairy Sci 2014;97(7): 4127–40.
11. Neves RC, Leno BM, Stokol T, et al. Risk factors associated with postpartum subclinical hypocalcemia in dairy cows. J Dairy Sci 2017;100(5):3796–804.
12. Huzzey JM, von Keyserlingk MAG, Weary DM. Changes in feeding, drinking, and standing behavior of dairy cows during the transition period. J Dairy Sci 2005; 88(7):2454–61.
13. Calderon DF, Cook NB. The effect of lameness on the resting behavior and metabolic status of dairy cattle during the transition period in a freestall-housed dairy herd. J Dairy Sci 2011;94(6):2883–94.
14. Fregonesi JA, Tucker CB, Weary DM. Overstocking reduces lying time in dairy cows. J Dairy Sci 2007;90(7):3349–54.
15. Bach A, Valls N, Solans A, et al. Associations between nondietary factors and dairy herd performance. J Dairy Sci 2008;91(8):3259–67.
16. Schirmann K, Chapinal N, Weary DM, et al. Short-term effects of regrouping on behavior of prepartum dairy cows. J Dairy Sci 2011;94(5):2312–9.
17. Coonen JM, Maroney MJ, Crump PM, et al. Short communication: Effect of a stable pen management strategy for precalving cows on dry matter intake, plasma nonesterified fatty acid levels, and milk production. J Dairy Sci 2011;94(5): 2413–7.
18. Silva PRB, Moraes JGN, Mendonça LGD, et al. Effects of weekly regrouping of prepartum dairy cows on innate immune response and antibody concentration. J Dairy Sci 2013;96(12):7649–57.

19. Silva PRB, Dresch AR, Machado KS, et al. Prepartum stocking density: Effects on metabolic, health, reproductive, and productive responses. J Dairy Sci 2014; 97(9):5521–32.
20. Lobeck-Luchterhand KM, Silva PRB, Chebel RC, et al. Effect of prepartum grouping strategy on displacements from the feed bunk and feeding behavior of dairy cows. J Dairy Sci 2014;97(5):2800–7.
21. Talebi A, von Keyserlingk MAG, Telezhenko E, et al. Reduced stocking density mitigates the negative effects of regrouping in dairy cattle. J Dairy Sci 2014; 97(3):1358–63.
22. Proudfoot KL, Jensen MB, Weary DM, et al. Dairy cows seek isolation at calving and when ill. J Dairy Sci 2014;97(5):2731–9.
23. Huzzey JM, DeVries TJ, Valois P, et al. Stocking density and feed barrier design affect the feeding and social behavior of dairy cattle. J Dairy Sci 2006;89(1): 126–33.
24. Endres MI, DeVries TJ, von Keyserlingk MAG, et al. Short communication: effect of feed barrier design on the behavior of loose-housed lactating dairy cows. J Dairy Sci 2005;88(7):2377–80.
25. do Amaral BC, Connor EE, Tao S, et al. Heat-stress abatement during the dry period: does cooling improve transition into lactation? J Dairy Sci 2009;92(12): 5988–99.
26. Tao S, Dahl GE. Invited review: heat stress effects during late gestation on dry cows and their calves. J Dairy Sci 2013;96(7):4079–93.
27. Dahl GE, Tao S, Monteiro APA. Effects of late-gestation heat stress on immunity and performance of calves 1. J Dairy Sci 2016;99(4):3193–8.
28. Dahl GE, Buchanan BA, Tucker HA. Photoperiodic effects on dairy cattle: a review. J Dairy Sci 2000;83(4):885–93.
29. Auchtung TL, Rius AG, Kendall PE, et al. Effects of photoperiod during the dry period on prolactin, prolactin receptor, and milk production of dairy cows. J Dairy Sci 2005;88(1):121–7.
30. Campler M, Munksgaard L, Jensen MB, et al. Short communication: Flooring preferences of dairy cows at calving. J Dairy Sci 2014;97(2):892–6.
31. Peek SE, Hartmann FA, Thomas CB, et al. Isolation of Salmonella spp from the environment of dairies without any history of clinical salmonellosis. J Am Vet Med Assoc 2004;225(4):574–7.
32. Fossler CP, Wells SJ, Kaneene JB, et al. Cattle and environmental sample-level factors associated with the presence of Salmonella in a multi-state study of conventional and organic dairy farms. Prev Vet Med 2005;67(1):39–53.
33. Ventura BA, von Keyserlingk MAG, Schuppli CA, et al. Views on contentious practices in dairy farming: The case of early cow-calf separation. J Dairy Sci 2013; 96(9):6105–16.
34. Johnsen JF, Zipp KA, Kälber T, et al. Is rearing calves with the dam a feasible option for dairy farms?—Current and future research. Appl Anim Behav Sci 2016; 181:1–11.
35. McArt JAA, Oetzel GR. A stochastic estimate of the economic impact of oral calcium supplementation in postparturient dairy cows. J Dairy Sci 2015;98(10): 7408–18.
36. McArt JAA, Nydam DV, Oetzel GR. A field trial on the effect of propylene glycol on displaced abomasum, removal from herd, and reproduction in fresh cows diagnosed with subclinical ketosis. J Dairy Sci 2012;95(5):2505–12.
37. Barberg AE, Endres MI, Salfer JA, et al. Performance and welfare of dairy cows in an alternative housing system in Minnesota. J Dairy Sci 2007;90(3):1575–83.

Ventilation Systems for Adult Dairy Cattle

Mario R. Mondaca, PhD

KEYWORDS

- Ventilation • Dairy • Economic • Microclimate

KEY POINTS

- The most common types of ventilation systems are natural, tunnel, cross, and hybrid ventilation.
- Ventilation needs to provide appropriate airspeeds at the stall, adequate ventilation rate, and a methodology to operate effectively year-round.
- The cost of different types of mechanical ventilation systems is similar making the choice between systems dependent on the location of the barn, herd size, and preferences of the owner.

INTRODUCTION

Ventilation is the provision of fresh air to a space. It is a necessary part of confinement housing to avoid the buildup of temperature, humidity, and harmful gases in animal housing beyond safe levels[1] and to eliminate areas of still air.[2] Although the cost of ventilation is significant, the cost of inadequate ventilation is much higher due to poor performance, heat stress, and respiratory disease in dairy cattle.

There are theoretic and practical limits for pathogen removal[3] and cooling due to ventilation, and these concepts are addressed throughout ventilation design options used in the dairy industry. This article highlights the difference between barn-level ventilation and cow-level ventilation, and various system design parameters for typical ventilation systems are addressed. Finally, the challenges and costs of maintaining a ventilation system, as well as the estimated costs of installing and operating typical ventilation designs are described.

The most common point of confusion in the dairy industry is the difference between recirculation and ventilation. Ventilation is when fresh air enters the barn whereas recirculation is when the same air in the barn is sped up, typically through the use of a fan. Circulation fans are commonly found in dairy barns to mix air within the

Disclosure Statement: Parts of this article are based in part on work supported by the USDA National Institute of Food and Agriculture under Grant No. WIS02011.
Department of Medical Sciences, School of Veterinary Medicine, University of Wisconsin, 2015 Linden Drive, Madison, WI 53706, USA
E-mail address: mondacaduart@wisc.edu

barn and/or provide fast-moving air for summertime cooling, but they do not provide ventilation.

Another point of confusion is the difference between ventilation and cooling. Cooling is the transfer of thermal energy via sensible or latent heat transfer processes. A sensible heat transfer process is one in which heat transfer occurs due to a temperature gradient without a change in phase, like cold water running on your hand, while a latent heat transfer process occurs due to change in phase, such as sweat evaporating off skin.

Because sensible heat requires a gradient of temperature to cool or heat the animal, if the air is the same temperature as the cow, it will not be cooled or warmed. Meanwhile, latent heat needs a humidity gradient to occur because most latent heat is removed through evaporation of water (eg, animal panting, cooling wet-pads, soakers, foggers). If the air is saturated with water, meaning the relative humidity is very high, the potential temperature reduction is only 30% to 40% that of dry environments.[4]

The most a ventilation system can achieve alone is to have the temperature, humidity, and gas inside the building reach the same levels as the outside air.

OVERALL VENTILATION DESIGN

Natural ventilation depends on the natural wind speed and direction, and temperature differences in the air to create the pressure differentials that drive air in and out of the barn. Openings in a natural barn can be either inlets or outlets depending on the direction of the air and the pressure gradients generated at the openings.

Mechanical ventilation uses positive pressure, negative pressure, or a combination of both. Negative-pressure ventilation uses exhaust fans to draw air out of the barn, creating a negative pressure inside compared with the outside.

A positive-pressure system pushes air into the barn, creating a positive pressure inside when compared with the outside. Positive-pressure tube ventilation systems are an example of such a system, and some versions are beginning to combine a positive-pressure system with a matching negative-pressure system, creating a so-called "neutral-pressure" barn.

Mechanical ventilation systems are typically defined using 3 key design metrics: air changes per hour (ACH), barn cross-sectional area airspeed, and air flow per animal unit (**Fig. 1**). They each address a different aspect of the ventilation design, and all 3 should be considered when evaluating a system.

Natural ventilation systems are not easily defined, although some studies have attempted to quantify natural ventilation rates.[5–7] Instead, natural systems rely on

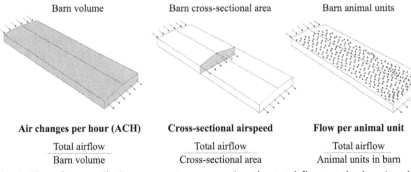

Barn volume	Barn cross-sectional area	Barn animal units
Air changes per hour (ACH)	**Cross-sectional airspeed**	**Flow per animal unit**
Total airflow / Barn volume	Total airflow / Cross-sectional area	Total airflow / Animal units in barn

Fig. 1. Three key ventilation parameters comparing the total flow to the barn's volume, cross-sectional area, and number of animals.

the barn dimensions, orientation, and spacing to capitalize on ventilation created by thermal buoyancy and natural wind patterns.

VENTILATION SYSTEMS
Natural Ventilation

Natural ventilation is the most common system on mid-size to small-size farmsteads.[8] Natural ventilation relies on 2 main factors to provide ventilation in a building. One is the thermal buoyancy created by the warm air around the animals, which rises and exits through an open ridge, which is called the "chimney" or "stack" effect. Hotter air has a lower density and tends to rise, whereas colder air drops. This creates a natural flow pattern that is mainly temperature driven. During cold temperatures, the stack effect is the main driver of ventilation.

The force of the wind into the building openings creates wind gusts and the air passing over the open ridge creates a lifting force inside the building. During warmer temperatures, large open curtain sidewalls will allow for natural wind forces to enter the barn. Although the stack effect will still occur during the summer, the large openings will be the main ventilation driver. For this reason, naturally ventilated barns need to be oriented perpendicular to prevailing summer winds. Because the air typically enters through the sidewall and exits through the ridge, it is also a benefit for airflow if the winter prevailing winds hit the eave openings.[1]

The main characteristics of naturally ventilated barns are an open ridge, open eaves, adequate interior roof slope, freedom from wind shadows, and an east to west orientation. To maximize natural ventilation, it is important to have an insulated smooth ceiling with a 3:12 or 4:12 pitch and an open ridge of 2 inches (5 cm) for every 10 ft (3 m) of barn width, with a minimum ridge opening of 6 inches (15 cm). The eave openings on each sidewall should be half of the ridge opening, ensuring the total sidewall opening is the same as the ridge during cold temperatures. Sidewalls are usually 13 to 16 ft (4–5 m) high fitted with curtains that are completely opened in the summer to capture as much of the prevailing winds as possible. The eave openings can be either built into the barn's structure or be controlled with a split curtain sidewall.

The provision of adequate ventilation and cooling in naturally ventilated buildings that house dairy cattle is challenged by the wide variety of different building structures in the farmstead. Wind shadows refer to areas of disturbed airflow downstream of an obstruction, such as an adjacent building structure. A common source of wind shadows in large naturally ventilated facilities is another barn in an H-configuration (**Fig. 2**). As seen in **Fig. 2**, the barn downstream receives a much lower airflow than the one directly facing the incoming winds. It takes approximately 5 to 10 times the height of the obstruction for the airflow to return to their original airspeeds.

Practically, most natural ventilated facilities are being constructed at 100 ft (30 m) separation distance to prevent as much wind shadow as possible. Although recommendations on separation distances are higher than that,[1] 100 ft (30 m) or shorter are commonly found because of limited space on the farmstead, and how far cows, workers, and manure have to travel between buildings.

Mechanical Ventilation

Mechanical ventilation relies on exhaust fans, intake fans, or both to provide fresh air in the facility. A significant advantage over natural systems is that the barn orientation and layout are not as limited by the surrounding structures. Mechanical systems also have a lower ceiling than natural systems and can be placed closer together to a minimum of 60 ft (18 m) for proper water drainage. A drawback to fully mechanical

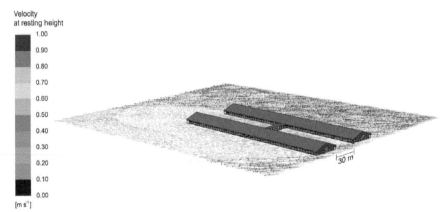

Fig. 2. Computational fluid dynamics results of natural ventilated barns separated by 30-m distance and the resulting velocity vectors at 1 m s^{-1} in a 45° direction.

systems is that there is no natural ventilation option, so a backup generator is necessary in case of emergency.

There are 2 main types of mechanical ventilation systems currently in use in the dairy industry: tunnel and cross ventilation. In general, tunnel ventilation is when the air flows parallel to the feed lane, and cross ventilation is when the air flows perpendicular to the feed lane (**Fig. 3**).

Tunnel-ventilated barns

The main changes implemented in tunnel barns compared with natural barns are a reduction in roof pitch and changes to the sidewalls. Typically the pitch will be half or one-third of that used in natural barns, often 1:12 or 2:12. Some systems are also designed with a false ceiling, giving the inside structure a flat ceiling almost flush with the sidewall height to reduce the flow area and increase airspeed. Depending on where the feed lanes are, the sidewalls may be a few ft lower than natural barns and only a small section of the barn will have curtain sidewalls, enough to provide inlet airspeeds of at least 500 ft min^{-1} (2.5 m s^{-1})[9] at the maximum ventilation rate.

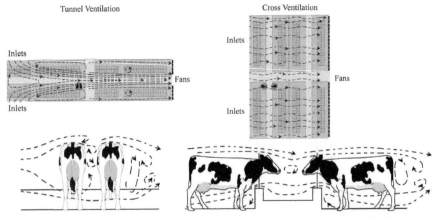

Fig. 3. Typical flow profiles for tunnel-ventilation (*left*) and cross-ventilation (*right*) systems; tunnel ventilation flows (*left*) parallel to the feed lane. Cross-ventilation (*right*) flows perpendicular to the feed lane.

In tunnel-ventilated barns, the fastest airspeeds will be at the feed lane, followed by the pen alleys, and then the stall microenvironment. Achieving appropriate air speeds in the stall microenvironment is difficult if only exhaust fans are used. This is due to a number of structural components that restrict and redirect the airflow away from the stalls; mainly walls or waterers at the cross-overs. These effects can be demonstrated using a computational fluid dynamics model (**Fig. 4**) of a tunnel barn.

The dark blue areas in the model have airspeeds below 200 ft min^{-1} (1 m s^{-1}) and are typically found at the end of the barn farther from the fans, after the inlets, and in the stalls behind the cross-over walls.

Hybrid barns

Although technically hybrid barns refer to any barn with a combination of natural and mechanical ventilation, most hybrid barns refer to tunnel-style barns with either an adjustable ridge or ridge cupola fans. The idea behind these systems is to have a mechanical system during the summer to provide a consistent supply of fresh air and heat abatement, and an ability to switch to a natural-style ventilation system during the winter months, capitalizing on the sidewalls for even distribution of fresh air. In hybrid barns, the roof may be pitched as a tunnel barn, with cupola fans used to assist air movement up toward the ridge.

Cross-ventilated barns

Cross-ventilated barns have the lowest roof pitch: typically 0.5:12. The sidewalls are often higher, especially if the feed lanes are located on the edges of the barn, to allow for overhead doors and feed trucks. When cows are feeding or resting, their orientation is such that the cows do not block the airflow from each other because of the air traveling perpendicularly to the feed lanes. One sidewall holds the fans and the opposite sidewall is an adjustable curtain or a wet-pad to serve as an inlet.

Cross-ventilated barns are commonly designed for 2 main reasons: lower cost and lower barn footprint per stall. Cross barns have the benefit of economies of scale, as most of the herd is housed under a single facility, which saves both space and building materials. Cross-ventilated barns work well with 8 to 12 rows of stalls, but air quality issues can arise as more rows of stalls are added.

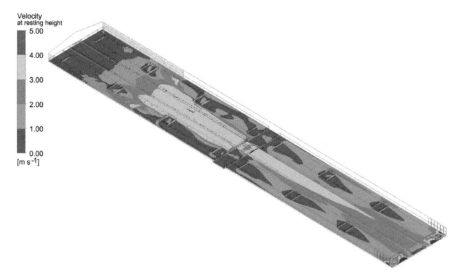

Fig. 4. Computational fluid dynamics model of a tunnel-ventilated barn at 41 ACH.

The key design features of the ventilation systems described in this article are summarized in **Fig. 5.**

Based on the wide variation in barn design and the challenges of providing fresh air at an appropriate speed for the climate, ventilation and cooling systems should be designed to also meet the following more general priorities:

1. Provide air movement at the appropriate speed in the stall microenvironment
2. Provide sufficient air exchange to remove heat, noxious gases, and moisture from the barn
3. Ensure that the system works well across all seasons

PROVIDE AIR MOVEMENT AT THE APPROPRIATE SPEED IN THE STALL MICROENVIRONMENT

The barn can be split into 3 key microenvironments that need to be ventilated: the overall barn, the pen, and the stall (**Fig. 6**).

The priority under conditions of heat stress is to provide fast-moving air within the stall microenvironment because the increased airspeed at the cow's body improves both sensible and latent heat transfer by mixing the air in the stall.[10,11] When heat stressed, adult cows lying in freestalls undergo body temperature increases of approximately 1.1°F (0.6°C)[12] per hour and soon reach body temperatures at which the cow must stand to cool, reducing resting time and putting the cow at increased risk for lameness and other health challenges.[13] Furthermore, cows prefer fast-moving air when they are hot,[14] and for cow barns we have traditionally failed to provide sufficient fast-moving air to help keep the cow cool in her resting space.[15]

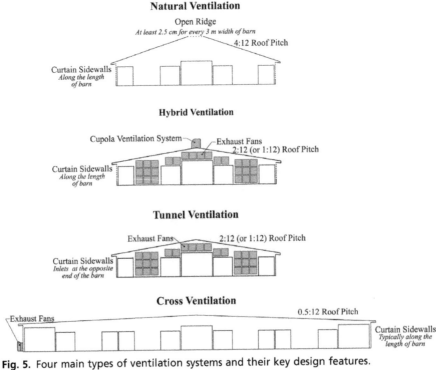

Fig. 5. Four main types of ventilation systems and their key design features.

Barn environment   Pen microenvironment

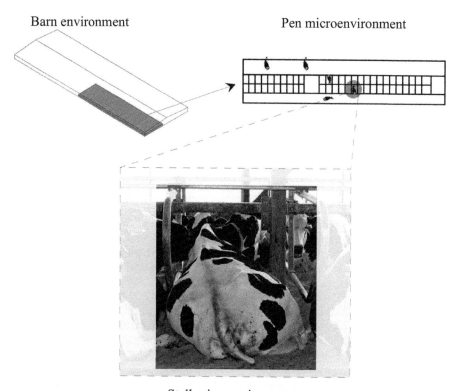

Stall microenvironment

Fig. 6. Various environments within the dairy barn: barn-level environment, pen microenvironment, and stall microenvironment.

Unfortunately, air is "lazy" in that it will follow the path of least resistance. The barn is littered with potential obstructions, such as feed curbs, stall loops, waterers, other cows, and concrete walls, which will redirect the flow away from the cow's resting space. The challenge is using barn-level design numbers (ACH, cross-sectional airspeed, and flow/animal, see **Fig. 1**) to evaluate the different pen and stall microclimates (see **Fig. 4**).

Minimum Cooling Airspeed

Although the temperature humidity index (THI) is a good measure of the heat stress a cow might experience,[7] it does not include an airspeed effect. There is surprisingly little information on what airspeed is necessary to provide adequate cooling. A series of psychroenergetic studies[16] published as bulletins at the University of Missouri evaluated the heat and mass transfer for various breeds of cattle. In bulletin 552,[17] the respiration rate of Holstein cattle was found to decrease with increasing airspeeds. At temperatures below 95°F (35°C), increasing airspeed resulted in a lower respiration rate, but the decrease in respiration rate when increasing airspeed from 40 to 433 ft min^{-1} (0.2–2.2 m s^{-1}) was much higher than the decreased respiration rate when airspeed was further increased from 433 to 787 ft min^{-1} (2.2–4.0 m s^{-1}). Findings from these series of experiments are still being used as a reference for heat generation for adult lactating cows in standards,[18] even though milk production per cow has dramatically increased since 1959. Similar diminishing returns of faster-moving air were found on cows with wetted skin under various airspeeds.[11] There was a significant difference in respiration rate and temperature between cows cooled with fans and water to the control, but no significant difference was found between the cows cooled at different airspeeds. The benefits of increasing from still air to 200 ft min^{-1} (1 m s^{-1}) appear much greater than the benefits of increasing airspeeds beyond 400 ft min^{-1} (2 m s^{-1}).

A heat stress model designed for cattle[19] was modified to consider Holstein cows. The new heat stress model[10] found that air velocities of 167 ft min^{-1} (0.85 m s^{-1}) can help cows increase their threshold temperature (temperature at which the respiration rate rose above 53% of the maximal respiratory rate). Further increasing airspeed to 295 ft min^{-1} (1.5 m s^{-1}) increased the threshold temperatures and reduced the negative effects of high humidity to practically zero. Similarly, there was a significant difference of air temperature between still air and 200 ft min^{-1} (1 m s^{-1}) but no significant difference between 200 ft min^{-1} (1 m s^{-1}) and 400 ft min^{-1} (2 m s^{-1}).[11]

Although the specifics of the heat and mass balance between the cow and its environment have changed significantly since 1959, the underlying diminishing returns between airspeed and heat stress markers (respiration rate, vaginal temperature, and skin temperature) have remained a constant finding in the limited studies performed. Therefore, we define the minimum cooling airspeed (MCAS) required for cows as 200 ft min^{-1} (1 m s^{-1}). Airspeeds should be at a minimum 200 ft min^{-1} (1 m s^{-1}) with little reported benefit of exceeding 400 ft min^{-1} (2 m s^{-1}), and be evenly distributed through the microenvironment of the stall, particularly in high humidity environments.

Achieving Minimum Cooling Airspeed

Panel fans

Panel, or recirculation fans, are great options for providing MCAS in the stall's microenvironment. These fans are typically 48 to 54 inches (1.2–1.4 m) in blade diameter and are recommended to be spaced at approximately 24-ft (7.3-m) intervals. The traditional recommendations of spacing fans 10 blade diameters apart are erroneous, as MCAS is not achieved for a sufficient proportion of the resting area.[15] The stalls immediately after a fan are commonly the areas with the lowest airspeed. It is the area farthest from the previous fan that does not receive the MCAS of the fan directly above them (**Fig. 7**).

The fan's air jet will not reach the cows immediately (see **Fig. 7**). This means that when fans are 48 ft (14.6 m) apart, the fan has to cover 68 ft (20.6 m): the distance between fans plus the first 20 ft (6 m) of the next fan. At 24 ft (7.3 m) apart (approximately 5 diameters of the fan in **Fig. 7**), the fan has to provide fast-moving air for 43 ft (13.3 m) (~50 ft [15 m] before the jet billows in **Fig. 7**).

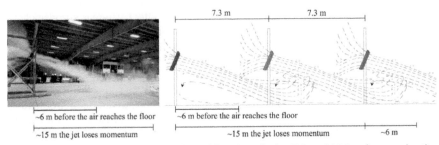

Fig. 7. A 54-inch fan smoking trial (*left*) and fans installed at 7.3 and 14.6 m from each other (*right*). If the red fan was not included, the black fan's jets would not reach the 6-m zone of still air in front of the blue fan.

This is all dependent on the fan angle and size, which should be aimed toward the resting space enough to increase the airspeed. With so many variations in barn, stall, and fan design, this angle is best determined by aiming the previous fan toward the space underneath the next fan. An anemometer could be used to measure the air-speeds at the resting height, particularly a few stalls after the fan to ensure there is over-lap between them and most cows have proper airflow while resting. Another option is large, louvered fans commonly known as "cyclone" fans. These are 72 inches (1.8 m) in diameter and usually provide good results when installed at 60-ft (18.3-m) intervals.

There is some debate as to how to position the recirculation fans. All of the options shown in **Fig. 8** provide adequate airspeeds at the resting area, but there are pros and cons. More frequent fan installation provides a more even distribution of airspeeds, but at the cost of doubling the necessary wiring for installation.

A similar trade-off exists when considering panel fans against larger cyclone fans (**Fig. 9**). One large cyclone fan covers a similar number of stalls compared with 2-panel to 3-panel fans. This reduces the wiring costs and maintenance by two-thirds, although the panel fans will likely achieve more evenly distributed resting airspeeds, and depending on fan choice, operate at similar running cost. Whatever the fan cho-sen, however, they are typically turned on at 65 to 68°F (18.3–20.0°C).

In many naturally ventilated barns, producers have installed circulation fans (typically panel fans) to consistently improve the airspeed at the resting area. Due to the signif-icant consequences of heat stress,[13,20] the number of recirculation fans used in a nat-ural ventilation system is similar to those found in mechanical ventilation systems.

For tunnel-ventilated barns, there are 3 main zones where airspeeds in the resting area tend to be low: the end-wall opposite to the exhaust fans, the area after the inlets, and the stalls after the cross-overs (see **Fig. 4**). Increasing the ventilation rate has diminishing returns for improving the airspeeds in these areas and there is a recent trend for tunnel ventilation to use fans over the stalls similar to natural ventilation sys-tems to provide fast-moving air. The concept is to have the exhaust fans provide enough ventilation to remove excess heat while the fans over the stalls provide MCAS (see **Fig. 9**).

In cross-ventilated barns, using panel fans is a relatively new idea, although some systems have begun using variable frequency drives (VFDs) combined with panel fans as a replacement for baffles to improve the airflow distribution during the winter and provide cooling in the summer.

High-volume low-speed fans

There is little information about the use of high-volume low-speed (HVLS) fans in dairy barns to provide fast-moving air. As their name implies, these systems move large vol-umes of air at low speeds. The lack of information on their performance in dairy barns makes it difficult to recommend specific design choices. However, through clinical

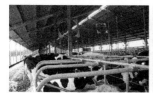
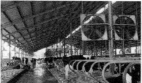
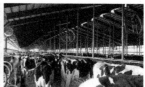

Fig. 8. Natural ventilation barns equipped with a panel fan every support post (*left*), 2 panel fans side by side over head-to-head stalls and a panel fan over single-row stalls every other support post (*middle*), and alternating fans every other support post over head-to-head stalls (*right*).

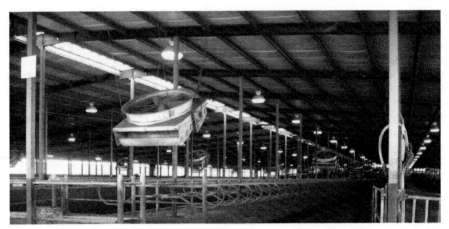

Fig. 9. Hybrid-ventilated barn with cyclone fans over the stalls to provide fast-moving air in the stall microenvironment and a closed ridge with a cupola system.

experience, we have found that 20-ft (6-m) HVLS fans should be installed at a 40-ft (12.2-m) spacing interval. Installations at 60 ft (18.3 m) do not provide MCAS throughout the resting area. These fans, however, are a good choice to de-stratify the environment within the barn (useful during cold winters).

Positive-pressure tube ventilation systems

More commonly considered a winter ventilation system for calf barns, some producers have used the idea of installing positive-pressure tube ventilation systems (PPTV) above the stalls to direct fresh air and MCAS over the cows (**Fig. 10**). Similar to the HVLS fans, they provide a good distribution and help de-stratify the air, but unlike the HVLS fans, this system also ventilates. Unfortunately, the air jets from these systems are extremely susceptible to any wind pressure and there is very little research on their potential use for heat abatement.

PPTV systems are not recommended for typical freestall facilities, but are a good choice for retrofitted stanchion, tie stall, or other systems in which ventilation is severely limited.

Baffles

Baffles are devices used to redirect the flow of air from the headspace above the cows toward the microenvironment of the stall (**Fig. 11**) and are generally considered a staple in cross-ventilated barns. Although variation exists, baffles are typically located along the building support posts, which are usually along the middle of head-to-head stalls. Baffles work well to provide MCAS at the stall level, but have issues during the winter months, as warmer air tends to get trapped in-between the baffles, accumulating humidity and heat. To prevent trapping of air, retractable baffles that can be adjusted in the winter are a potential solution, or circulation fans can be used to help mix the air. Baffles are designed at a minimum height of 7 ft (2.1 m) from the stall surface to avoid animals and machinery from reaching and damaging them.

The airspeed increase due to baffles tends to be short-lived and is generally easily disrupted by other restrictions to the airflow created by cows, concrete curbs, and so forth. This means tunnel-ventilated barns require a much higher number of baffles to provide MCAS in the cow resting area. Each time the flow is redirected, it is also

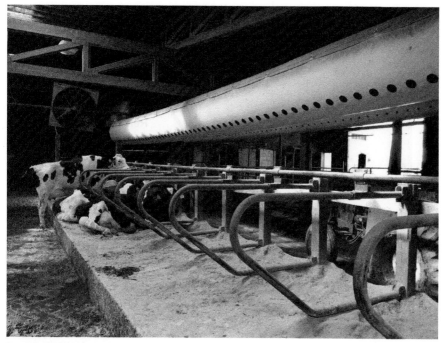

Fig. 10. PPTV system for adult cows.

restricted, and pressure is added to the system,[21] lowering exhaust efficiency. For this reason, baffles are typically not recommended for tunnel-ventilation systems. In cross systems, the ideal baffle placement is over the inlet side of the head-to-head stall platform, or the middle of the platform.

Although designs vary from barn to barn, baffle opening height is typically designed to generate 510 ft min^{-1} (2.6 m s^{-1}) in the area underneath the baffle.[22]

PROVIDE SUFFICIENT AIR EXCHANGE TO REMOVE HEAT, NOXIOUS GASES, AND MOISTURE FROM THE BARN

The main purpose of a ventilation system is to maintain harmful gases, moisture, and temperature at safe levels throughout the year (**Fig. 12**). The minimum ventilation

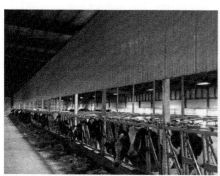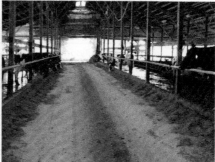

Fig. 11. Baffles installed in a cross-ventilated (*left*) and a tunnel-ventilated (*right*) retrofit barn.

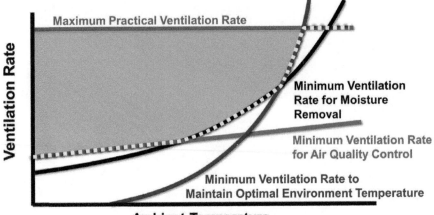

Fig. 12. The ideal ventilation design curve. (*Adapted from* Christianson LL. Ventilation - energy and economics - Figure 14.2. In: Hellickson MA and Walker JN, editors. Ventilation of agricultural structures. St. Joseph (MI): American Society of Agricultural Engineers; 1983. p. 336; with permission.)

required to maintain each of these factors changes with the seasons. Typical design values for mechanical ventilation are 4 ACH during the winter and 40 to 60 ACH, 500 ft min^{-1} (2.54 m s^{-1}) cross-sectional area airspeeds, and 1500 ft^{3} min^{-1} (2550 m^{3} h^{-1}) per cow during the summer. However, some producers are designing systems up to 100 ACH[18] for summertime cooling.

Similar to the MCAS, the required ventilation rate for adult cows is not well defined. A wide range of recommendations and standards exists (**Table 1**). The standards[18]

Table 1
Mechanical ventilation summer recommendations

m^{3} h^{-1} per Animal Unit	ft^{3} m^{-1} per Animal Unit	Source	Animal Unit	Specified For	ACH
113	66	Shen et al,[32] 2013	600 kg cow	Humidity balance	2
463	272	Shen et al,[32] 2013	625 kg cow	dT <3°C in 27°C outside conditions	8
535	315	MWPS-1,[33] 1983	453 kg cow	Hot weather rate	9
798	470	Holmes et al,[34] 2013	635 kg cow	Hot weather rate	13
1700	1000	Tyson et al,[35] 2014; Gooch & Stowell,[36] 2003	—	Summer rate	29
2549	1500	Tyson et al,[35] 2014	—	Summer rate	43
1787	1052	MWPS-1,[33] 1983	453 kg cow	Alternative hot weather rate	30
2383	1403	Nordlund[37]	—	Minimum hot weather rate	40
3574	2104	Holmes et al,[34] 2013	635 kg cow	Alternative hot weather rate	60
5957	3506	Stowell et al,[38] 2003	—	Hot weather rate	100

Abbreviation: ACH, air changes per hour.

use a heat and mass balance methodology to avoid a 1.8 to 3.6°F (1–2°C) increase in temperature between the inlet and outlet of the barn. The relative humidity should be below 80% and the inside surfaces should have enough insulation to avoid reaching dew-point temperatures at 80% relative humidity to avoid condensation.

Each ventilation system should be individually evaluated, as average recommendations make assumptions of production, weight, location, and flow distribution that will not accurately represent every microclimate.[23] Unfortunately, these recommendations and standards are all at a barn-level resolution, which has not been properly related to the microenvironment of the pen or the microenvironment of the stalls.

One of the main reasons for these discrepancies is that freestall barns tend to have a tall ceiling and ridge. It is not uncommon for ceilings to go as high as 26 ft (8 m) or higher, meaning the stall microclimate is limited to approximately 20% of the total flow area, depending on the pen location. Because most heat and mass transfer processes (eg, cow panting, sweating, ammonia from manure) occur within the microenvironment of the pen, it is important that the ventilation system is able to reach these areas.

A recent trend for tunnel-ventilation systems is to use a ventilation rate of 40 ACH, as it is usually enough to meet the temperature difference standards in mild climates. Regardless of the ventilation rate, it is recommended that local sources of airspeed, like fans over the stalls, are used in tunnel ventilation because the ventilation rate has diminishing returns on minimizing low airspeed areas after 40 ACH.

Unlike mechanical ventilation, it is difficult to estimate and control specific ventilation rates for natural barns. Instead, if the building is located, oriented, and designed with the overall recommendations, the system should perform well, although inconsistencies are common due to natural wind patterns.

ENSURE THAT THE SYSTEM WORKS ACROSS ALL SEASONS

A ventilation system needs to be designed so that it performs well across all seasons. This will vary significantly between climatic regions because the ventilation system needs to serve the workers, the facility, and the cows equally. Improper management of the system through the various climatic changes is the most common issue with ventilation systems in the dairy industry. It is very common to find excellent winter systems that perform poorly during the heat of the summer, particularly in natural systems without fans over the stalls. Meanwhile, large mechanically ventilated facilities face the opposite problem where summer ventilation is optimal, but there are significant distribution and condensation issues during the winter.

Because dairy cattle are cold tolerant, the goal in the winter is to maintain adequate moisture and gas concentration levels in the air to avoid respiratory disease rather than keeping the animals warm. The ventilation rate must be high enough to ensure adequate air quality but low enough to prevent as much freezing and condensation within the barn as possible. Typically, producers use 4 ACH as the minimum winter ventilation rate and 40°F (4.4°C) as the winter temperature set-point for minimum ventilation, but some producers use 8 ACH at 40°F (4.4°C) and 4 ACH farther down at 20°F (−6.6°C). As ambient temperature increases, the minimum ventilation rate required to maintain adequate environmental temperature and moisture levels increases and eventually, the maximum practical ventilation rate is achieved, typically at 40 to 60 ACH (see **Fig. 12**).

In the summer, the main goal of ventilation is to ensure that natural and manmade cooling processes are occurring as efficiently as possible by exhausting excess heat and preventing thermal buildup in the facility. In general, cows are considered to be in a comfortable environment in temperatures between 40 and 68°F (4.4 and

20°C), and the most common set-point for the ventilation system to operate at the maximum summer rate is 68°F (20°C); however, some producers are beginning to shift the set-point to 65 °F (18.3 °C) because of the high costs associated with heat stress.[24] The THI, which is a number that combines temperature and humidity impact on the cow, is the most commonly used measure of heat stress for dairy cows. A THI of 68 is where cows typically begin to show signs of heat stress.[25]

One of the most important factors for adequate natural ventilation a producer can control is having a well-insulated barn. During cold temperatures, a well-insulated barn will conserve heat and maintain warmer surface temperatures on the inside, improving the stack effect and preventing condensation. During hot temperatures, a well-insulated barn will reduce heat gain from solar radiation and convection effects, reducing the ventilation needed to maintain a comfortable environment.

Almost every newly installed mechanical ventilation system now includes a transition methodology between the summer and winter conditions. A mechanical ventilation system uses a combination of temperature, and more recently humidity, sensors, and a controller that operates fans and adjusts the sidewall curtain openings to ensure adequate inlet openings during the various ventilation stages.

Fans should be operated from a control system that monitors temperature within the barn (pen), and inlets and fans should be evenly distributed to equalize airflow patterns between regions of the barn as much as possible. This should be planned with a detailed wiring and control map of which fans are used and that are switched off at various intervals across the seasons. The advent of VFDs has allowed even natural ventilation systems to include a transition methodology in which the circulation fans will operate at minimum speeds to mix the air in the winter and speed up as temperature increases to provide cooling.

There is little information on what the ventilation rate should be during mild weather. It is recommended to stage the ventilation system every 3.6°F (2°C),[7] but the ramping functions are more usually dependent on the number of fans and how the fans were wired during installation. The most commonly found methodology to stage the ventilation system from winter to summer is to use a linear ramping function. Once a minimum and maximum ventilation rate is designed, a straight line is drawn between them to determine the different stages. The specifics of how many stages and whether VFDs are used depend on the fan manufacturer, builder, and producer.

Each ventilation system has different challenges as the seasons change. One issue with tunnel barns is the temperature and humidity difference between the inlet and the outlet of the barn, which is influenced by barn length. Barns should be no longer than 600 ft (183 m) long because a significant drop in air quality can be observed after 600 ft (183 m), particularly in the winter. A similar problem is found in cross-ventilated barns that are too wide.

Hybrid systems provide the most flexibility across seasons, but tend to have the highest installation cost due to combining 2 or more ventilation systems, as well requiring curtain sidewalls along the length of the barn. Because the whole sidewall can be opened in these systems, they can ventilate in emergency situations (**Fig. 13**).

During the summer, the hybrid system will have mechanical ventilation combined with circulation fans to provide sufficient fresh air and MCAS. As the temperature drops, the mechanical system will decrease the ventilation rate until a determined set-point at which the system will transition to a natural or assisted natural ventilation system. In the assisted natural system, the exhaust system shuts off, but a series of cupola fans will turn on. Depending on the design, the cupola system will cover more than the minimum winter ventilation rate, with 1 or 2 more ventilation stages. These systems can excel in climates where temperatures fluctuate significantly

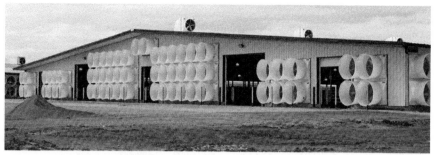

Fig. 13. A hybrid ventilation system with fans at the end-wall for summer ventilation and cupola fans for winter ventilation.

throughout the year, but are not necessary in locations with more consistent temperatures; like arid climates or year-round temperate regions.

VENTILATION SYSTEM MAINTENANCE

Proper system maintenance is just as important as proper design. Fans with poor maintenance can lose 30% to 50% of their efficiency.[26] Reactive maintenance can be costly and dangerous, as it can quickly degrade ventilation performance, degrading the cow's microenvironment along with it. Evaporative cooling systems using wet-pads require significant maintenance, as they can clog up quickly with water residue. For fans, belts should be inspected for tightness, and blades and louvers should be inspected for buildup and dust. Ideally, the farm will maintain fans that operate year-round at least twice a year and summer fans at least once a year, but these schedules should be considered the bare minimum.

ECONOMICS OF VENTILATION SYSTEMS

There is little information on the costs of ventilation systems in the dairy industry. In a survey of energy use in dairy farms,[27] ventilation was shown to account for 20% of the total energy use on farm.

A facility designed for 1008 cows housed in 4 pens was quoted by a building company and 7 ventilation designs were evaluated for operating costs. The 7 systems consisted of 2 natural barns with fans every 48 ft (14.6 m) (NAT1), every 24 ft (7.3 m) (NAT2); 2 tunnel-ventilated barns designed at 60 ACH (TUN60) and 40 ACH (TUN60) with panel fans every 24 ft (7.3 m); a hybrid system designed at 40 ACH with cyclone fans every 60 ft (18.3 m) (HYB40) and a cupola system; and 2 cross-ventilated barns, an 8-row (8CRO) and a 16-row (16CRO) barn. Previous economic models and surveys[28–30] have quoted the cost of building a new facility at $2500 per stall without including electrical costs. The total costs before including the cost of financing showed a similar range of $2300 to $2700 per stall depending on the ventilation system and layout (**Table 2**).

Overall, construction costs are similar across the range of different designs. Therefore, other factors, such as herd size, location, barn orientation, footprint per stall, cow flow, lighting, manure handling, and owner preference should be considered over the capital costs of building and installing a specific type of barn ventilation system. In general, it costs approximately twice as much to operate a mechanical system per year than a natural system, and approximately double to operate it in a hot climate as opposed to a temperate climate. However, as variable speed fans become more

Table 2
Capital costs of 7 ventilation systems amortized over 10 years, cost in USD

Ventilation System	Building Cost	Ventilation Installation Cost	Total Costs (+5% Fee)	Total Financed Cost (4.25% APR)	Total Capital Cost Per Stall Per Year
NAT1	2,156,432	62,860	2,330,257	2,902,862	289
NAT2	2,156,432	125,720	2,396,260	2,991,254	287
TUN60	2,145,902	182,095	2,444,397	3,051,344	303
TUN40	2,145,902	247,682	2,513,263	3,137,310	311
HYB40	2,309,893	273,732	2,712,806	3,386,399	336
8CRO	2,099,789	171,110	2,384,444	2,976,504	295
16CRO	3,611,588	171,110	3,971,833	4,958,044	246

common, the operating costs can be reduced by optimizing the operating schedules of the variable speed fans.[31] Fan selection has the largest effect on the cost of operating ventilation systems. Therefore, fans with a higher ventilation efficiency rating should be selected whatever the system used.

SUMMARY

A wide variety of ventilation systems can provide an excellent environment for the cow within a barn, provided they meet 3 critical design criteria; the provision of appropriate air speeds in the stall microenvironment defined as a minimum air speed of at least 200 ft min^{-1} (1 m s^{-1}); the provision of sufficient air exchange to effectively remove heat, noxious gases, and moisture from the barn, typically at least 4 ACH in the winter and 40 to 60 ACH; and the system must be designed to function well across all seasons with an effective transition methodology. Once these criteria are met, it is further essential to perform at least bi-annual fan maintenance for year-round systems.

ACKNOWLEDGMENTS

The author acknowledges Courtney Halbach for her extensive revision of this article.

REFERENCES

1. Midwest Plan Service. MWPS-33. Natural ventilating systems for livestock housing. 1st edition. Ames (IA): Midwest Plan Service; 1989. Available at: https://www-mwps.sws.iastate.edu/catalog/ventilation-livestock-housing/natural-ventilating-systems-livestock-housing. Accessed August 30, 2018.
2. Callan RJ, Garry FB. Biosecurity and bovine respiratory disease. Vet Clin North Am Food Anim Pract 2002;18(1):57–77.
3. Nardell EA, Keegan J, Cheney SA, et al. Airborne infection: theoretical limits of protection achievable by building ventilation. Am Rev Respir Dis 1991;144:302–6.
4. Berman A. Extending the potential of evaporative cooling for heat-stress relief. J Dairy Sci 2006;89(10):3817–25.
5. Bruce JM. Natural convection through openings and its application to cattle building ventilation. J Agric Eng Res 1978;23(2):151–67.
6. Wu W, Zhai J, Zhang G, et al. Evaluation of methods for determining air exchange rate in a naturally ventilated dairy cattle building with large openings using computational fluid dynamics (CFD). Atmos Environ 2012;63:179–88.

7. Bjerg B, Cascone G, Lee IB, et al. Modelling of ammonia emissions from naturally ventilated livestock buildings. Part 3: CFD modelling. Biosyst Eng 2013. https://doi.org/10.1016/j.biosystemseng.2013.06.012.

8. Brotzman R, Cook N, Nordlund K, et al. Cluster analysis of Dairy Herd Improvement data to discover trends in performance characteristics in large Upper Midwest dairy herds. J Dairy Sci 2015;98(5):3059–70.

9. Hellickson MA, Walker JN. Ventilation of agricultural structures. Monograph no. 6. St. Joseph (MI): American Society of Agricultural Engineers; 1983. Available at: https://books.google.com/books/about/Ventilation_of_Agricultural_Structures.html?id=ML9NP-RaRX4C. Accessed August 24, 2018.

10. Berman A. Estimates of heat stress relief needs for Holstein dairy cows. J Anim Sci 2005;83:1377–84. Available at: https://academic.oup.com/jas/article-abstract/83/6/1377/4803167. Accessed August 24, 2018.

11. Berman A. Increasing heat stress relief produced by coupled coat wetting and forced ventilation. J Dairy Sci 2008;91(12):4571–8.

12. Hillman PE, Lee CN, Willard ST. Thermoregulatory responses associated with lying and standing in heat-stressed dairy cows. Trans ASAE 2005;48(2):795–801.

13. Cook NB, Mentink RL, Bennett TB, et al. The effect of heat stress and lameness on time budgets of lactating dairy cows. J Dairy Sci 2007;90(4):1674–82.

14. Calegari F, Calamari L, Frazzi E. Fan cooling of the resting area in a free stalls dairy barn. Int J Biometeorol 2014;58(6):1225–36.

15. The Dairyland Initiative. Ventilation and Heat Abatement – The Dairyland Initiative. 2018. Available at: https://thedairylandinitiative.vetmed.wisc.edu/home/housing-module/adult-cow-housing/ventilation-and-heat-abatement/. Accessed August 24, 2018.

16. Yeck RG, Stewart RE. A ten-year summary of psychroenergetic laboratory dairy cattle research at the University of Missouri. Trans ASAE 1959;2(1):71–7.

17. Kibler H, Brody S. Environmental Physiology With Special Reference to Domestic Animals. 1951. Available at: http://www.asrc.agri.missouri.edu/research/bec/MO Ag Exp Bulletins/Bulletin 552 - Influence of wind on heat exchange and body temperature regulation in jersey holstein brown swiss and brahman cattle.pdf. Accessed August 24, 2018.

18. American Society of Agricultural Engineers. ASAE EP270.5 DEC1986 (R2017) Design of Ventilation Systems for Poultry and Livestock Shelters. 2017. Available at: https://elibrary.asabe.org/azdez.asp?JID=2&AID=24432&CID=s2000&T=2. Accessed August 24, 2018.

19. McGovern RE, Bruce JM. A model of the thermal balance for cattle in hot conditions. J Agric Eng Res 2000;77(1):81–92.

20. West JW. Effects of heat-stress on production in dairy cattle. J Dairy Sci 2003; 86(6):2131–44.

21. Harner JP, Smith JF. "Let it flow, let it flow" moving air into the freestall space. In: Housing of the future. Sioux Falls (SD). 2008. Available at: https://www.asi.k-state.edu/doc/dairy/moving-air-into-the-freestall-space.pdf. Accessed August 30, 2018.

22. Smith JF, Bradford BJ, Harner JP, et al. Short communication: effect of cross ventilation with or without evaporative pads on core body temperature and resting time of lactating cows. J Dairy Sci 2016;99(2):1495–500.

23. Seedorf J, Hartung J, Schröder M, et al. A survey of ventilation rates in livestock buildings in Northern Europe. J Agric Eng Res 1998;70(1):39–47.

24. St-Pierre NR, Cobanov B, Schnitkey G. Economic losses from heat stress by US livestock industries. J Dairy Sci 2003;86:E52–77.

25. Collier RJ, Zimbelman RB, Rhoads RP, et al. A re-evaluation of the impact of temperature humidity index (THI) and black globe humidity index (BGHI) on milk production in high producing dairy cows. In: Western Dairy Management Conference . Reno, Nevada. 2011. p. 113–25. Available at: http://wdmc.org/2011/A Re-Evaluation of the Impact of Temperature Humidity Index %28THI%29 and Black Globe Humidity Index %28BGHI%29 on Milk Production in High Producing Dairy Cows pg 113-126.pdf. Accessed August 30, 2018.

26. Bodman GR, Shelton DP. G95-1242 Ventilation Fans: Performance. 1995. Available at: http://digitalcommons.unl.edu/extensionhisthttp://digitalcommons.unl.edu/extensionhist/600. Accessed August 30, 2018.

27. Ludington D, Johnson E. Dairy farm energy audit summary. New York: New York State Energy Res Dev Authority; 2003. Available at: https://www.nyserda.ny.gov/-/media/Files/Publications/Research/Energy-Audit-Reports/dairy-farm-energy.pdf.

28. Ferreira FC, Gennari RS, Dahl GE, et al. Economic feasibility of cooling dry cows across the United States. J Dairy Sci 2016. https://doi.org/10.3168/jds.2016-11566.

29. Kammel DW. Building cost estimates-dairy modernization. Madison. 2015. Available at: https://fyi.uwex.edu/dairy/files/2015/11/Building-Cost-Estimates-Dairy-Modernization.pdf. Accessed August 30, 2018.

30. Tyson JT. Heat abatement techniques in dairy housing in the northeast. 2008. Available at: https://etda.libraries.psu.edu/files/final_submissions/3034. Accessed August 30, 2018.

31. Atkins I, Mondaca M, Choi C. Energy efficiency and air distribution of VFD-driven mechanical ventilation systems. In: 2016 American Society of Agricultural and Biological Engineers Annual International Meeting, ASABE, Orlando, Floria, July 17–20, 2016. https://doi.org/10.13031/aim.20162461516.

32. Shen X, Zhang G, Wu W, et al. Model-based control of natural ventilation in dairy buildings. Comput Electron Agric 2013;94:47–57.

33. Midwest Plan Service, Structures and Environment Subcommittee. MWPS-1. Structures and environment handbook. Ames (IA): Midwest Plan Service; 1983. Available at: https://www-mwps.sws.iastate.edu/catalog/construction-farm/structures-and-environment-handbook. Accessed August 30, 2018.

34. Holmes BJ, Cook NB, Funk T, et al. Dairy freestall housing and equipment. Midwest Plan Service; 2013. Available at: https://www-mwps.sws.iastate.edu/catalog/livestock/dairy/dairy-freestall-housing-and-equipment. Accessed August 24, 2018.

35. Tyson JT, McFarland DF, Graves RE. Tunnel ventilation for tie stall dairy barns. PennState Extension 2016. Available at: https://extension.psu.edu/tunnel-ventilation-for-tie-stall-dairy-barns.

36. Gooch CA, Stowell RR. Tunnel ventilation for freestall facilities – design, environmental conditions, cow behavior, and economics. In: Janni K, editor. Fifth international dairy housing. Fort Worth (TX). 2003. p. 227–34. Available at: https://elibrary.asabe.org/azdez.asp?JID=1&AID=11626&CID=dhc2003&T=2. Accessed August 30, 2018.

37. Nordlund K. Ventilating existing buildings. In Preconvention Seminar 7: Dairy Herd Problem Investigation Strategies American Association of Bovine Practitioners 36th Annual Conference, Columbus, OH, September 15–17, 2003. Available at: https://www.vetmed.wisc.edu/dms/fapm/fapmtools/9ventilation/VetsVent.pdf.

38. Stowell RR, Gooch CA, Bickert WG. Design parameters for hot-weather ventilation of dairy housing: a critical review. In: Janni K, editor. Fifth international dairy housing. Fort Worth (TX). 2003. p. 218–26. Available at: https://elibrary.asabe.org/azdez.asp?AID=11625&t=2. Accessed August 30, 2018.

Considerations for Cooling Dairy Cows with Water

Jennifer M.C. Van Os, PhD

KEYWORDS

- Heat stress • Heat abatement • Sprinklers • Soakers • Spray • Misters • Foggers
- Conductive beds

KEY POINTS

- Heat abatement should ideally be provided to all life stages of dairy cattle.
- Shade should be provided in conjunction with all cooling systems to limit additional heat gain from solar radiation.
- Soaking cools cattle when water evaporates from the skin and the surroundings (air, the ground); fluid convection from water dripping off the animal also has a role in quickly removing heat.
- To evaluate whether cooling is effective and to make adjustments, animal-based indicators (respiration rate, panting) should be collected in addition to environmental measures (air temperature, temperature humidity index).
- Cows willingly use and prefer soakers compared with shade alone for cooling and insect deterrence, although they avoid exposing their heads to spray.

INTRODUCTION

Heat stress creates costly problems for the US dairy industry on the order of $850 million to $1.5 billion annually[1] owing to reduced dry matter intake (DMI), milk production,[2] fertility,[3] and increased cull and death rates.[4–6] High-producing cows are most vulnerable to heat stress and because per-cow production levels are increasing over time, the current economic losses associated with heat stress may be even greater. Additionally, heat stress negatively affects cattle health and welfare,[7] which are topics of increasing societal concern. Furthermore, climate change models predict increasing average temperatures and more frequent heat waves in the coming decades.[8] Therefore, managing heat stress is a critical issue affecting the long-term sustainability of US dairy production.

The author has nothing to disclose.
Department of Dairy Science, College of Agricultural and Life Sciences, University of Wisconsin-Madison, 1675 Observatory Drive, Madison, WI 53706-1205, USA
E-mail address: jvanos@wisc.edu

HOW COOLING WORKS: OVERVIEW OF HEAT EXCHANGE

Cattle gain heat in environmental conditions of high air temperature and humidity and from exposure to solar radiation. They dissipate heat both within their bodies (by conduction from the core to the surface through the tissues, and by convection through blood movement and vasodilation) and to their surroundings (heat is removed from the body through air movement or when in contact with a cooler surface). Because these nonevaporative (sensible) mechanisms of heat exchange occur in proportion to the temperature gradient between the animal and its surroundings, the rate of heat loss decreases at higher ambient temperatures. In contrast, evaporative (latent) heat loss does not depend on a temperature gradient; water is converted from liquid to vapor using energy from the animal and/or its surroundings. High skin temperature stimulates peripheral thermal receptors and triggers the natural evaporative cooling responses of elevated respiratory rates, panting, and sweating.[9]

In addition, cattle show several behavioral adaptations that reduce metabolic heat production (**Box 1**). Physical and muscular activity produce heat and increase body temperature,[10] and cattle show decreased activity in summer, including estrous behavior.[11–13] Feeding and digestion, particularly ruminal fermentation, also generate considerable body heat. According to 50-year-old estimates, heat production doubles when cattle lactate.[9] Given the subsequent increases in individual milk yield, this difference may be even higher today. Therefore, decreases in DMI and milk yield (often with a 1–2 day lag following hot weather events)[14,15] and reduced reproductive performance, which occur when cattle are heat stressed, can be understood as adaptive responses to restore thermal balance.

Cows also show behaviors to reduce heat gain by seeking shade[16,17] and to dissipate heat by spending more time near water sources,[18–20] which may be due to a cooler microclimate[19,21] or to splash themselves with water.[22] Time spent drinking[23] and water intake[24] also increase in warmer weather, which helps replenish respiratory and cutaneous water losses from panting and sweating.[25] In warmer conditions, cows also spend less time lying down.[17,20,26] Normally, dairy cattle are highly motivated to spend half of their day lying down[27] and lying time is commonly used as an indicator of cow comfort. In warm weather, respiration rate and body temperature increase during lying events and decrease when cattle stand up,[28,29] likely because standing exposes more surface area for convective heat loss[22,26,28,30] or increases the efficiency of respiration.[21]

For high-producing dairy cows, however, these intrinsic mechanisms for dissipating heat are sometimes insufficient and body temperature can increase above the normal

---

Box 1
Physiologic and behavioral responses of cattle to heat stress

- Vasodilation
- Elevated respiratory rate and panting
- Sweating
- Reduced activity
- Reduced feeding behavior and DMI
- Reduced milk yield and reproductive performance
- Shade and water seeking, increased water intake
- Reduced lying time and increased standing

range (hyperthermia). To help cattle cope with heat stress, dairy producers can provide resources to dissipate body heat (eg, fans or water spray) and to limit heat gain (ie, shade). Indeed, 94% of US dairies provide at least 1 of these heat abatement resources.[31] The importance of shade provision cannot be overstated. During the day, if shade is lacking, the effectiveness of heat dissipation can be counteracted by heat gain. Furthermore, threats to animal welfare encompass not only impaired biological functioning but also include concerns about the animals' emotional experiences and potential distress, as well as opportunities to express important behaviors.[32] Shade-seeking is part of the natural behavioral repertoire of cattle and they highly value this resource.[33] Shade should be provided in conjunction with other cooling methods.

UNDERSTANDING HEAT STRESS: WHEN TO INTERVENE?

Although all heat abatement methods require an initial capital investment, fans and water spray also involve ongoing expenses for energy and water, and producers must decide when to activate these devices. The economic benefits of providing heat abatement to reduce losses to production, reproduction, and survival are easily recognized.[1] To optimize animal welfare, however, earlier intervention may be required to help cattle cope before obvious problems occur; understanding this rationale requires a more detailed exploration of the definition of heat stress.

Heat stress and thermal comfort in homeothermic animals are often conceptualized in relation to ambient conditions, metabolic heat production, and outcomes such as milk yield. Homeothermy refers to core body temperature remaining within the normal range, and hypothermy and hyperthermy are deviations below and above this range, respectively. Thermoneutrality refers to a narrower range of conditions (bounded by lower and upper critical ambient temperatures) in which metabolic heat production remains stable (**Fig. 1**). Definitions of heat stress and thermal comfort, however, vary in the literature. This author favors the 50-year-old interpretation by Bianca,[9] who described thermal comfort within an even narrower range in which the physiologic and behavioral defense mechanisms associated with heat exchange (see previous discussion) are not yet activated (see **Fig. 1**). Based on this concept, cattle can be identified as beginning to experience heat stress based on vasodilation occurring; followed by sweating, increasing respiratory rate, and panting; behavioral changes to reduce heat gain and increase heat dissipation; and, finally, by behavioral strategies such as reduced feed intake to lower heat production.[9]

In the subsequent decades, however, many investigators have equated thermal comfort with thermoneutrality and have defined heat stress as occurring above the upper critical temperature[34] or when production losses begin to appear.[35] Many thermal indexes have been developed from models describing the relationships between environmental conditions and cattle responses, primarily in terms of production losses. The most common is the temperature humidity index (THI), which combines air temperature and relative humidity.[36] Many studies have aimed to identify break points or thresholds at which increases in THI result in marked changes in body temperature,[37] milk yield,[38] milk quality (ie, somatic cell score),[39] or mortality.[5] Based on such studies, THI values of 72 or, more recently, 68 are frequently used as thresholds for heat stress.

Defining heat stress with THI thresholds has several limitations. First, environmental variables besides temperature and humidity also contribute to heat exchange, and indexes have been developed evaluating a more comprehensive suite of environmental variables (eg, heat load index, which adds air speed and black globe temperature to incorporate the effects of radiation) for their effects on body temperature.[40] Second, when ambient heat increases, there is a lag before body temperature increases and

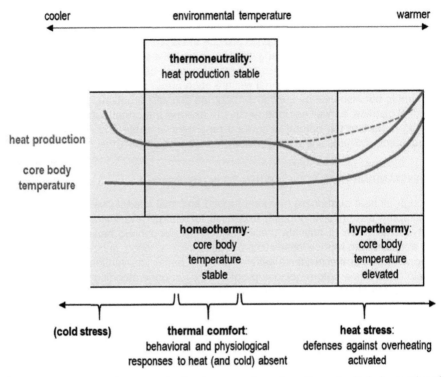

Fig. 1. Heat stress can be conceptualized as occurring when the animal's behavioral and physiologic defense mechanisms against overheating are activated. These responses begin before the animal's core body temperature has begun to increase and before changes in metabolic heat production occur (while both homeothermy and thermoneutrality, respectively, are maintained). The blue and orange lines represent core body temperature and metabolic heat production, respectively. As heat stress begins, metabolic heat production may initially decrease as a result of adaptive behavioral responses (eg, reduced feed intake) and will eventually increase, along with core body temperature, when the defense mechanisms become insufficient. Responses to cold environmental conditions are not depicted. (*Data from* Bianca W. Thermoregulation. In: Hafez ESE, editor. Adaptation of domestic animals. Philadelphia: Lea & Febiger; 1968. p. 97–118.)

production declines.[14] More recent models incorporate increased respiration rate and skin temperature (eg, equivalent temperature index of cattle),[41] which precede elevated body temperature and are more sensitive indicators of the need for heat abatement. Third, cattle may begin to feel discomfort and experience negative effects in conditions cooler than predicted by THI thresholds for production losses. Consistent with Bianca's[9] earlier interpretation of heat stress, cows seek cooling under thermoneutral conditions: they make some voluntary use of spray overnight[21,42] and show clear preferences for water spray starting in the morning, several hours before the daily peak in ambient temperature,[42] as well as on days with mild conditions.[43]

On commercial dairy operations, water-based cooling systems are commonly activated either manually or based on a single air temperature sensor, usually at or around 21° to 24°C (70°–75°F), which may not capture the variety of microclimates that cows experience. Ideally, the criteria for activating heat abatement should be adjusted by observing the animals on a given farm. Measuring animal responses is important, not only because farms vary in their facilities and management but also because individual cattle respond differently within the same environment depending on breed, milk production, pregnancy or health status, plane of nutrition,[9] and coat characteristics, along with factors such as social status, which could affect access to drinking water, cooler microclimates, and heat abatement. Nonetheless, it can be challenging for producers to identify cows experiencing heat stress and in need of additional intervention, and for animal welfare assessment programs to establish criteria for verifying the effectiveness of a farm's heat abatement strategies. For example, the Welfare Quality program in Europe designates thermal comfort as a requirement for good cattle housing; however, no measure has been established to assess this principle.[44]

Conspicuous, noninvasive indicators (**Box 2**) to identify heat stress include signs of panting, such as drool, an extended tongue, or an open mouth.[45,46] However, panting is associated with markedly elevated respiration rates (100 breaths per minute on average),[45,46] and identifying an increase in respiration rate earlier would be a more sensitive indicator. Recording respiration rate can be labor-intensive, however, because this measure needs to be observed at least every 90 minutes to accurately determine changes over time.[46] In addition, for a continuous variable, establishing precise cutoffs for intervention is challenging. In summer, cows with 24-hour access to cooling had average respiration rates of 50 breaths per minute,[21,42] whereas cows given a choice after being deprived of cooling began to show preferences for high-output sprinklers when their respiration rates reached approximately 60 breaths per minute.[43] In an experiment testing respiration rate monitors in a tunnel-ventilated barn with evaporative cooling pads, a THI of 68 corresponded to approximately 60 breaths per minute.[29] Based on these patterns, along with suggestions in the older literature,[47] a threshold of 60 breaths per minute could be used as the minimum respiration rate for cooling intervention. In the near future, technological advancements may allow for more automated detection of heat stress using physiologic and behavioral indicators, and for automatic activation and adjustment of heat abatement resources.

BENEFITS OF DIRECT LOW-PRESSURE SOAKING

Cooling spray is delivered in the form of either high-pressure foggers or misters with fine droplets or low-pressure soakers or sprinklers with coarse droplets, and at least

---

Box 2
Early indicators of the need for heat abatement

- The zone of thermal comfort is narrower than the thermoneutral zone.

- Heat stress begins before metabolic rate and body temperature increase and before production problems appear.

- THI thresholds are commonly used; however, cooling should ideally be adjusted based on animal indicators.

- Rising respiration rate is an early, noninvasive indicator of heat stress and should be measured every 90 minutes to track changes.

- Cows begin to prefer high-output soakers when their respiration rates reach 60 breaths per minute.

- Panting (drool, open mouth, and/or extended tongue) is a sign cattle are clearly heat stressed and is associated with respiration rates of 100 breaths per minute.

one of these methods is used in 62% of US milking herds of 500 head or more.[31] Fogging or misting results in indirect cooling of cattle by injecting the air with very fine water droplets, which evaporate and lower the temperature of the surrounding microclimate. This method is more commonly used successfully in lower-humidity climates such as the southwest United States,[48] whereas in higher-humidity climates, the air has less capacity for water to evaporate (ie, a reduced water vapor gradient) for latent heat loss.

Low-pressure soakers also cool the air[42,43,49,50] because all nozzles output a range of droplet sizes, including smaller droplets that evaporate before landing on cows. The main cooling mechanism of soakers, however, occurs by wetting cows directly and using energy from their body heat to evaporate the water. To allow time for water to evaporate from the cows between spray applications, low-pressure soaking systems are typically run on preset on-off cycles. Sprinkler nozzles are commonly mounted either above the feed bunk and angled to spray cows' backs intermittently while they eat, overhead in the holding area while they wait to be milked, or over the parlor exit lane (eg, Edstrom Cool Sense; Avidity Science, Waterford, WI, USA) to automatically activate spray as cows walk underneath. The author has also observed some dairies showering cows in the parlor itself during milking (**Fig. 2**).

Direct soaking has been well-documented to effectively reduce core body temperature in heat stressed cows (**Box 3**). Core body temperature typically shows a diurnal pattern with a nadir early in the morning and a peak in the late afternoon or evening.[9] In warm weather, the evening peak in vaginal temperature can be more than 1°C higher than the early morning measurements[20,42,49,51,52]; however, when cattle have access to intermittent feed bunk soakers, the daily peak is suppressed.[20,42] Across days, body temperature can increase by 1.6°C for each 10°C increase in air temperature; however, the magnitude of this relationship was halved when cows had access to feed bunk soakers.[20,42] In studies with a discrete spraying session (similar to holding pen soaking), body temperature reached a nadir between 30 and 60 minutes after spraying stopped[49,51,53] and remained lower than unsprayed controls for 1.5 to 4 hours afterward.[49,51,54] High airspeeds (either from wind or forced air from fans) enhance the effectiveness of spray for keeping body temperature suppressed[20,55] and for reducing respiration rate[56] by aiding in evaporation and moving heat away from the cow's body and immediate surroundings.

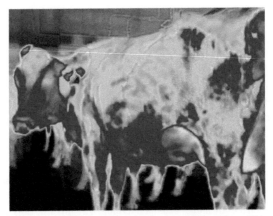

Fig. 2. Infrared photograph of a lactating Holstein cow exiting the milking parlor following low-pressure soaking by an overhead shower.

Box 3
Benefits of direct soaking of cows using low-pressure, high-flow sprinklers

- Reduced body temperature, respiration rate, and skin temperature
- Increased feeding time and DMI
- Increased milk yield
- Reduced insect-avoidance behaviors

The annual economic losses to the US dairy industry were estimated at $1.5 billion if cows were housed with only shade; however, this figure was reduced by 43% when the models included water spray and fans.[1] Indeed, when cows have access to soakers, both feeding time[42] and DMI increase in many studies,[52,57,58] and daily milk yields have been reported to be 1.5 to 3.7 kg higher.[20,59,60] Although the bulk of the research on cooling has focused on lactating cows, there is also a large body of evidence that heat stress in dry cows negatively affects their future productivity, fertility, and immune function,[61] as well as the performance, health, and survival of their offspring.[2,62] Because soakers and fans can mitigate these effects, recent models have indicated that providing heat abatement to dry cows is profitable.[61] However, there has been little attention to date on the potential benefits of spraying young calves and heifers. Beef steers (10 months old) with no previous cooling experience preferred feed bunks with sprinklers compared with those without, especially in warmer weather.[63] Based on this finding, a logical prediction is that younger dairy cattle would also seek out cooling. On commercial dairy operations, although economic constraints are important considerations, ideally, all life stages of cattle should be provided with heat abatement.

CONSIDERATIONS FOR SPRAY APPLICATION

Most dairies soak cows with potable water, and the amount used varies widely among farms (eg, 4.5–25.7 L/h per cow).[64] In the coming decades, water is predicted to become increasingly limited.[8] Therefore, in addition to mitigating heat stress, reducing water footprint is a major sustainability concern for the US dairy industry.[65] Many recommendations can be found for how much water to apply for cooling[66–69] but, until recently, evidence was lacking from peer-reviewed studies on live cattle. Earlier research used simulations,[70–72] and the single study comparing different sprinkler flow rates soaked cows in the bedded area, which does not reflect common industry practice.[73] Recent studies in a low-humidity climate varied the total amount of water applied by manipulating either the sprinkler flow rate or application duration. These studies demonstrated that soakers remove heat through additional mechanisms besides evaporation from the skin and coat and provided the first empirical evidence for the amount of water needed to cool cows effectively.

Because latent heat loss does not rely on a temperature gradient between the animal and its environment, discussions about soaking typically focus on the cooling that occurs through evaporation from the animal after the water is turned off. Industry publications recommend that cows should be "soaked to the hide along the topline while not getting wet to the point of having water running off the sides"[74] and that "sprinklers should wet the back and then stop the cycle to allow the water to evaporate prior to another cycle beginning."[69] Additionally, dripping water has been associated with speculative concerns about mastitis,[53] although no studies have shown a direct link. However, when water (which is typically cooler than the skin) drips from the body, this removes heat. Along with the cooler microclimate that results when droplets evaporate from the ground and in the air, dripping water generates rapid reductions in skin temperature and respiration rate, which were reduced relative to unsprayed controls after a single spray application of 3 minutes (using ≥ 1.3 L/min)[55] or 90 seconds (using 4.9 L/min).[56] Longer spray applications (up to 13 minutes) resulted in greater reductions in these measures,[56] and body temperature was reduced at the end of single, continuous spray applications of 10 or 12 minutes,[16,43] before the coat had time to begin drying. These results demonstrate that the cooling contributions of fluid convection and a cooler microclimate (indirect evaporation) should not be discounted.

Although minimizing water use is an important concern, enough water should be applied to generate effective cooling. A single 12-minute spray application of 4.8 L[43] or 4 repeated spray applications of 1.2 L[55] were insufficient to reduce body temperature. Furthermore, relative to those lower-flow nozzles, higher-output sprinklers better cooled the microclimate[43] and reduced respiration rate.[43,55] Nonetheless, applying more water results in a pattern of diminishing returns for cooling. In a lower-humidity climate, the optimal quantity seems to be approximately 4 L per spray application (which can cool 2–3 adjacent cows at the feed bunk) when water was applied 4 or 5 times per hour.[20,55] Regardless of whether cows are soaked only enough to wet the back or if water drips from their sides, the coat takes 14 to 16 minutes to dry, on average.[56] Drying time is reduced in warmer or windier conditions,[56] supporting the common practice of spraying more frequently when air temperatures increase. These findings also suggest that although a single spraying session has the potential to suppress body temperature for a while afterward,[43,49,51] spray applications should be less than 15 minutes apart to generate consistent cooling throughout the day (**Box 4**).

In terms of nozzle selection, some investigators have expressed concerns about smaller water droplets landing on the hair coat instead of soaking through to the skin. Some have speculated that smaller droplets may form an insulating barrier of water on the surface of the hair coat, trapping heat and exacerbating heat stress.[48,75] This idea, however, may be a misinterpretation of earlier statements that when droplets rest on the coat instead of reaching the skin, evaporation will transfer heat away from the coat rather than from the body surface, resulting in less efficient cooling.[2,53] A recent study evaluated the cooling effects of droplet size within a given flow rate, with the prediction that larger droplets would cool more effectively because they are less likely to evaporate before landing (although this could cool the microclimate, similar to misting) and might better penetrate the hair coat. Despite 1.2-fold to 1.5-fold

---

Box 4
Guidelines for low-pressure soaking at the feed bunk

- Contrary to popular belief, empirical evidence shows cooling benefits when water drips from the coat.

- Sufficient water should be used to generate effective cooling; however, adding more reaches a point of diminishing returns.

- Using 4 L of water in each spray application (to soak 2–3 adjacent cows) at a frequency of 4 to 5 times per hour works well in lower humidity climates.

- The coat dries in 15 minutes or less in lower humidity climates, and spray should be applied at least this frequently, especially in warmer weather.

- At a given sprinkler flow rate, droplet size does not affect cooling. However, lower-flow nozzles may increase spray drifting into the feed.

differences in the average droplet diameter, no effects of droplet size were detected.[55] Nonetheless, smaller droplets have the potential downside of drifting into the feed instead of landing on the cows. Because lower-flow nozzles output smaller droplets on average,[76] this could be a reason to choose higher-flow nozzles. To further reduce the risk of spray drift, producers should mount nozzles as low as possible while still remaining out of reach of the cows (**Fig. 3**A) to prevent damage (**Fig. 3**B) and maintain proper function (**Fig. 3**C).

BEHAVIORAL RESPONSES TO WATER SPRAY

Three-quarters of US dairy cows are kept in freestalls or drylots.[31] In these loose housing systems, cows can choose when to stand under soakers at the feed bunk. Variability in cattle behavior can moderate both cooling effectiveness and the water wasted by sprinklers. Earlier research on spraying cows with water focused primarily on physiologic and production outcomes. Several studies in the past decade have improved the understanding of how cattle respond behaviorally to spray. In addition to cooling, sprinklers also seem to provide benefits for cows in terms of insect deterrence. Overall, cattle use and prefer sprinklers; however, this depends on ambient conditions and shade provision, and they avoid exposing their heads to spray.

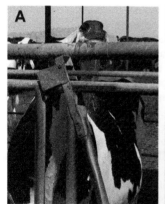
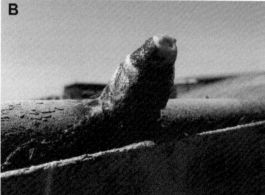
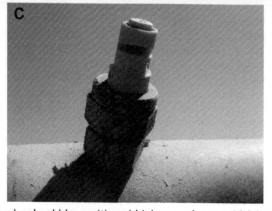

Fig. 3. Soaker nozzles should be positioned high enough to avoid (*A*) cattle interference and prevent (*B*) damage. They should be examined and maintained regularly to ensure they are (*C*) intact, clean, and properly functioning.

Besides cooling cows, sprinklers reduce fly avoidance behaviors, presumably because they deter insects. Cattle typically show a suite of avoidance behaviors in response to flies,[77] and when cows stand under spray they show fewer tail flicks,[16,43,49] hoof stamps,[16,49] and skin twitches.[43] Although research is needed to quantify insect load and confirm whether spray repels flies, this potential benefit, rather than cooling, could be the primary explanation for why 41% of cows' visits to a pressure-activated shower were less than 1 minute long.[21]

Although cows obtain both cooling and insect deterrence benefits from sprinklers, they avoid exposing their heads to the spray. When cows stand in the rain or under sprinklers, they protect their heads by either lowering[16,49,78] or keeping them out of the spray radius.[16,42] In addition, when high-output nozzles (which generate greater spray impact than lower-flow nozzles)[79] are mounted at the feed bunk, cows change their visit patterns and the timing of when they approach and leave the area to avoid walking through the spray.[20] When cows do walk through the spray, they lower their heads,[20,79] especially with high-output nozzles.[79] Cows' head-specific avoidance of spray may be explained by the greater sensitivity of the ears in response to nonnociceptive stimuli relative to the trunk.[79] In these studies when cows walked through spray only briefly they did not show overall avoidance of spray.[20,79] However, when cows do not have the option to remove their heads from the spray radius, such as in the premilking holding area, this could create a short-term conflict for animal welfare in which cows obtain cooling benefits but may simultaneously experience discomfort.

Despite protecting their heads from spray, cows willingly use[20,21,42] and prefer[42,43,63] sprinklers in most studies. To date, a single experiment found that pastured dairy cows did not prefer sprinklers, in part because air temperature was at least 5C lower than in other studies (24-hour average 18C).[16] In these conditions, the sprinklers may have generated more cooling than the cows needed. Indeed, when cows are sprayed in the morning[51] or on cooler days,[49] body temperature temporarily increases afterward, suggesting compensation to conserve heat. Comparing across days within studies, cows spent more time using a pressure-activated shower or soakers at the feed bunk,[20,21,42] and their preference for soakers compared with shade alone was more marked on warmer days or when their respiration rate or body temperature was higher.[42,43,63]

Cattle use of sprinklers also depends on the availability of shade, an important resource to them.[33] Even in mild temperatures (24-hour average 18C), cows preferred shade compared with none.[16] Furthermore, compared with unshaded sprinklers, cows preferred shade alone,[16] and they showed wide individual variation in use of an unshaded shower.[21] When cows did not face this tradeoff and were given choices that were both shaded, they clearly preferred feed bunks with soakers to those without.[42] Shading the feed bunk enhances cooling by reducing the heat that both the cows and the water pipes gain from solar radiation; the latter effect could help maintain a larger temperature gradient between the water and the skin. On many drylot operations, shade is provided in the corral but not over the feed bunk,[64] and it is important to combine soakers with shade.

CURRENT CHALLENGES AND FUTURE DIRECTIONS

A pitfall of soakers is their use of potable water, an increasingly limited resource. Current sprinkler systems are typically activated in timed cycles and inevitably waste water at times. In both the premilking holding area and at the feed bunk, cow density varies throughout the day, and sprinklers activate intermittently regardless of cattle presence. A potential technological solution to save water would be to engineer a

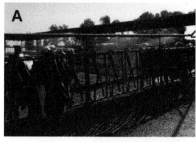
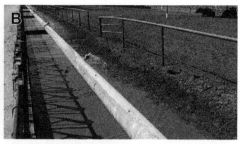

Fig. 4. Current systems for soaking cows activate spray along the entire feed bunk automatically using timers, resulting in wasted water when there are (*A*) few or (*B*) no cows at the feed bunk.

sensor system that activates spray nozzles when cows are detected, thus avoiding spraying the ground in empty areas of the holding pen, when few cows are present at the feed bunk (**Fig. 4**A), or when they are away for milking or elsewhere in the home pen (**Fig. 4**B).

The proof of concept has already been demonstrated with automated parlor exit-lane showers (eg, Edstrom Cool Sense), which activate spray as individual cows walk underneath. This method of delivery potentially reduces water waste by only spraying when cows are detected. Ideally, however, the spray should activate with a slight delay to avoid spraying the head, contrary to older recommendations to "begin water application as the head passes through."[80] In the decade since that suggestion was published, a growing body of evidence from behavioral studies (see previous discussion) has supported producers' anecdotes of cows avoiding spray on their heads and balking when approaching spray. More research is needed to evaluate how soaking cows when they have little control over the body parts that are sprayed, such as in the premilking holding pen (**Fig. 5**), affects animal welfare and behavior.

In the holding area, an alternative to overhead soaking is to wet cows from underneath. Some dairies use floor-mounted udder washing sprinklers in the holding pen

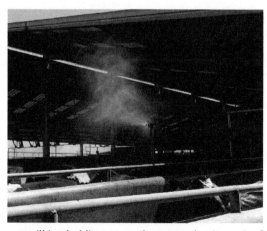

Fig. 5. Soaking the premilking holding area, where cow density varies from tightly packed to empty, presents challenges for creating consistent cooling and can result in wasted water and spraying the cows' heads, which the animals often try to avoid exposing to spray.

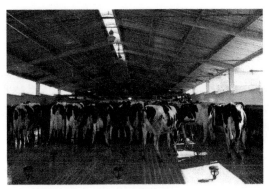

Fig. 6. Some dairies in low-humidity climates use floor-mounted udder-wash systems in the premilking holding area, which may also provide a source of cooling.

(**Fig. 6**), and older studies suggest that soaking the udder may reduce body temperature[51,81] to a degree similar to when spraying the back[82]; however, the duration of this cooling effect is unknown. Udder washing sprinklers are uncommon in regions with higher relative humidity because insufficient drying before milking can lead to bacterial contamination of the teat ends.[83] With overhead sprinklers, some researchers have likewise expressed speculative concerns about excess water running onto the teats,[53] although no studies to date have found an increase in mastitis associated with sprinkler provision.[84] Rather, milk somatic cell score[39] and mastitis incidence[85] are higher overall in summer, and these measures should be included in future studies comparing the costs and benefits of spraying the udder and the back.

Another cooling solution that would both save water and avoid spraying cows' heads is to install pipes under the lying area to recirculate chilled water and transfer heat away from cows when they lie down on the cooled surface.[86] Conductive cooling beds have shown some promise for reducing heat stress[87,88]; however, the technology is currently experimental and the real-world costs and benefits are untested. In addition, the reduction in lying time cows show in warmer weather[19,26,89] is not mitigated by the provision of either cooled beds[88] or sprinklers.[20,21,42,90] Rather than improving lying time, providing feed bunk soakers results in a shift in the location where cows stand: they spend less time standing in the bedded area and more time standing (without eating) at the feed bunk.[42] In some loose housing systems, the feed apron is concrete, whereas the bedded area has softer footing (eg, drylots or freestalls where cows can stand fully in the stalls). Both standing on concrete[91–93] and wet flooring[94,95] have been established as risk factors for lameness. Therefore, research is needed to understand the relationships between heat stress, soaker use, and hoof health.

SUMMARY

Heat stress begins before production problems appear, and the best defense is direct soaking of cattle using low-pressure, high-output nozzles in combination with shade and fans. Soakers can reduce body temperature, respiration rate, and skin temperature, increase feeding time, DMI, and milk yield, and sprinklers also reduce insect-avoidance behaviors. In warm weather, cattle willingly use and prefer sprinklers compared with shade alone; however, they avoid exposing their heads to spray. Although potable water use is a relevant sustainability concern, sufficient water should be used to generate effective cooling. In addition to evaporation, soaking cools cows when water drips from the coat. Decisions about when to activate soakers and how much water to use are best made by collecting animal indicators (eg, respiration rate, panting) along with environmental measures (air temperature, relative humidity). Ideally, all life stages of dairy cattle should have access to heat abatement.

REFERENCES

1. St-Pierre NR, Cobanov B, Schnitkey G. Economic losses from heat stress by us livestock industries. J Dairy Sci 2003;86:E52–77.
2. Hahn GL. Management and housing of farm animals in hot environments. In: Yousef MK, editor. Stress physiology of livestock. Boca Raton (FL): CRC Press, Inc; 1985. p. 151–74.
3. De Rensis F, Scaramuzzi RJ. Heat stress and seasonal effects on reproduction in the dairy cow: a review. Theriogenology 2003;60:1139–51.
4. Stull CL, McV Messam LL, Collar CA, et al. Precipitation and temperature effects on mortality and lactation parameters of dairy cattle in California. J Dairy Sci 2008;91:4579–91.
5. Vitali A, Segnalini M, Bertocchi L, et al. Seasonal pattern of mortality and relationships between mortality and temperature-humidity index in dairy cows. J Dairy Sci 2009;92:3781–90.
6. Morignat E, Perrin J-B, Gay E, et al. Assessment of the impact of the 2003 and 2006 heat waves on cattle mortality in France. PLoS One 2014;9:e93176.
7. Polsky L, von Keyserlingk MAG. Invited review: effects of heat stress on dairy cattle welfare. J Dairy Sci 2017;100:8645–57.
8. Rosenstock T, Smukler S, Cavagnaro T. California agricultural landscapes and climate change. In: Cavagnaro T, Jackson L, Scow K, editors. Climate change: challenges and solutions for California agricultural landscapes. Sacramento (CA): California Climate Change Center; 2006. p. 3–12.
9. Bianca W. Thermoregulation. In: Hafez ESE, editor. Adaptation of domestic animals. Philadelphia: Lea & Febiger; 1968. p. 97–118.
10. Mader TL, Davis MS, Kreikemeier WM. Case study: tympanic temperature and behavior associated with moving feedlot cattle. PAS 2005;21:339–44.
11. Pennington JA, Albright JL, Diekman MA, et al. Sexual activity of Holstein cows: seasonal effects. J Dairy Sci 1985;68:3023–30.
12. De Silva AWMV, Anderson GW, Gwazdauskas FC, et al. Interrelationships with estrous behavior and conception in dairy cattle. J Dairy Sci 1981;64:2409–18.
13. Gwazdauskas FC, Lineweaver JA, McGilliard ML. Environmental and management factors affecting estrous activity in dairy cattle. J Dairy Sci 1983;66:1510–4.
14. Spiers DE, Spain JN, Sampson JD, et al. Use of physiological parameters to predict milk yield and feed intake in heat-stressed dairy cows. J Therm Biol 2004;29: 759–64.
15. West JW, Mullinix BG, Bernard JK. Effects of hot, humid weather on milk temperature, dry matter intake, and milk yield of lactating dairy cows. J Dairy Sci 2003; 86:232–42.
16. Schütz KE, Rogers AR, Cox NR, et al. Dairy cattle prefer shade over sprinklers: effects on behavior and physiology. J Dairy Sci 2011;94:273–83.
17. Tucker CB, Rogers AR, Schütz KE. Effect of solar radiation on dairy cattle behaviour, use of shade and body temperature in a pasture-based system. Appl Anim Behav Sci 2008;109:141–54.

18. Widowski T. Shade-seeking behavior of rotationally-grazed cows and calves in a moderate climate. In: Proc Int Livest Env Symp, May 21–23, 2001. Louisville, KY: American Society of Agricultural Engineers.

19. Schütz KE, Rogers AR, Poulouin YA, et al. The amount of shade influences the behavior and physiology of dairy cattle. J Dairy Sci 2010;93:125–33.

20. Chen JM, Schütz KE, Tucker CB. Cooling cows efficiently with water spray: behavioral, physiological, and production responses to sprinklers at the feed bunk. J Dairy Sci 2016;99(6):4607–18.

21. Legrand A, Schütz KE, Tucker CB. Using water to cool cattle: behavioral and physiological changes associated with voluntary use of cow showers. J Dairy Sci 2011;94:3376–86.

22. Ansell RH. Extreme heat stress in dairy cattle and its alleviation: a case report. In: Clark JA, editor. Environmental aspects of housing for animal protection. London: Butterworths; 1981. p. 285–306.

23. Shultz TA. Weather and shade effects on cow corral activities. J Dairy Sci 1984; 67:868–73.

24. Mader TL, Fell LR, McPhee MJ. Behavior response of non-Brahman cattle to shade in commercial feedlots. Livest Env Iron 1997;5:795–802.

25. Silanikove N. Effects of heat stress on the welfare of extensively managed domestic ruminants. Livest Prod Sci 2000;67:1–18.

26. Cook NB, Mentink RL, Bennett TB, et al. The effect of heat stress and lameness on time budgets of lactating dairy cows. J Dairy Sci 2007;90:1674–82.

27. Jensen MB, Pedersen LJ, Munksgaard L. The effect of reward duration on demand functions for rest in dairy heifers and lying requirements as measured by demand functions. Appl Anim Behav Sci 2005;90:207–17.

28. Hillman PE, Lee CN, Willard ST. Thermoregulatory responses associated with lying and standing in heat-stressed dairy cows. Trans ASAE 2005;48:795–801.

29. Atkins IK, Cook NB, Mondaca MR, et al. Continuous respiration rate measurement of heat-stressed dairy cows and relation to environment, body temperature, and lying time. Trans ASABE 2018;61:1475–85.

30. Igono MO, Johnson HD, Steevens BJ, et al. Physiological, productive, and economic benefits of shade, spray, and fan system versus shade for Holstein cows during summer heat. J Dairy Sci 1987;70:1069–79.

31. United States Department of Agriculture. Facility characteristics and cow comfort on U.S. dairy operations, 2007. Fort Collins (CO): UDSA-Animal and Plant Health Inspection Service-Veterinary Services, Centers for Epidemiology and Animal Health; 2010.

32. Fraser D, Weary DM, Pajor EA, et al. A scientific conception of animal welfare that reflects ethical concerns. Anim Welf 1997;6:187–205.

33. Schütz KE, Cox NR, Matthews LR. How important is shade to dairy cattle? Choice between shade or lying following different levels of lying deprivation. Appl Anim Behav Sci 2008;114:307–18.

34. Yousef MK. Principles of bioclimatology and adaptation. In: Johnson HD, editor. Bioclimatology and the adaptation of livestock. New York: Elsevier; 1987. p. 17–31.

35. Berman A, Meltzer A. Critical temperatures in lactating dairy cattle: a new approach to an old problem. Int J Biometeorol 1973;17:167–76.

36. Kelly CF, Bond TE. Bioclimatic factors and their measurement. In: National Research Council, editor. A guide to environmental research on animals. Washington, DC: National Academies Press; 1971. p. 7–92.

37. Dikmen S, Hansen PJ. Is the temperature-humidity index the best indicator of heat stress in lactating dairy cows in a subtropical environment? J Dairy Sci 2009;92:109–16.
38. Bohmanova J, Misztal I, Cole JB. Temperature-humidity indices as indicators of milk production losses due to heat stress. J Dairy Sci 2007;90:1947–56.
39. Lambertz C, Sanker C, Gauly M. Climatic effects on milk production traits and somatic cell score in lactating Holstein-Friesian cows in different housing systems. J Dairy Sci 2014;97:319–29.
40. Gaughan JB, Mader TL, Holt SM, et al. A new heat load index for feedlot cattle. J Anim Sci 2008;86:226–34.
41. Wang X, Gao H, Gebremedhin KG, et al. A predictive model of equivalent temperature index for dairy cattle (ETIC). J Therm Biol 2018;76:165–70.
42. Chen JM, Schütz KE, Tucker CB. Dairy cows use and prefer feed bunks fitted with sprinklers. J Dairy Sci 2013;96:5035–45.
43. Chen JM, Schütz KE, Tucker CB. Sprinkler flow rate affects dairy cattle preferences, heat load, and insect deterrence behavior. Appl Anim Behav Sci 2016; 182:1–8.
44. Welfare Quality. Welfare quality assessment protocol for cattle. Lelystad (Netherlands): Welfare Quality Consortium; 2009.
45. Gaughan JB, Mader TL. Body temperature and respiratory dynamics in unshaded beef cattle. Int J Biometeorol 2014;58:1443–50.
46. Tresoldi G, Schütz KE, Tucker CB. Assessing heat load in drylot dairy cattle: refining on-farm sampling methodology. J Dairy Sci 2016;99:8970–80.
47. Webster J. Environmental physiology and behaviour. In: Webster J, editor. Understanding the dairy cow. Boston: Blackwell Scientific Publications; 1993. p. 91.
48. Mitlöhner FM, Morrow JL, Dailey JW, et al. Shade and water misting effects on behavior, physiology, performance, and carcass traits of heat-stressed feedlot cattle. J Anim Sci 2001;79:2327–35.
49. Kendall PE, Verkerk GA, Webster JR, et al. Sprinklers and shade cool cows and reduce insect-avoidance behavior in pasture-based dairy systems. J Dairy Sci 2007;90:3671–80.
50. Frazzi E, Calamari L, Calegari F. Productive response of dairy cows to different barn cooling systems. Trans ASAE 2002;45:395–405.
51. Araki CT, Nakamura RM, Kam LWG, et al. Diurnal temperature patterns of early lactating cows with milking parlor cooling. J Dairy Sci 1985;68:1496–501.
52. Gaughan JB, Davis MS, Mader TL. Wetting and the physiological responses of grain-fed cattle in a heated environment. Aust J Agric Res 2004;55:253–60.
53. Flamenbaum I, Wolfenson D, Mamen M, et al. Cooling dairy cattle by a combination of sprinkling and forced ventilation and its implementation in the shelter system. J Dairy Sci 1986;69:3140–7.
54. Brown-Brandl TM, Eigenberg RA, Nienaber JA. Water spray cooling during handling of feedlot cattle. Int J Biometeorol 2010;54:609–16.
55. Chen JM, Schütz KE, Tucker CB. Cooling cows efficiently with sprinklers: physiological responses to water spray. J Dairy Sci 2015;98:6925–38.
56. Tresoldi G, Schütz KE, Tucker CB. Cooling cows with sprinklers: spray duration affects physiological responses to heat load. J Dairy Sci 2018;101:4412–23.
57. Strickland JT, Bucklin RA, Nordstedt RA, et al. Sprinkler and fan cooling system for dairy cows in hot, humid climates. Appl Eng Agric 1989;5:231–6.
58. Morrison SR, Prokop M, Lofgreen GP. Sprinkling cattle for heat stress relief: activation temperature, duration of sprinkling and pen area sprinkled. Trans ASAE 1981;24:1299–300.

59. Flamenbaum I, Wolfenson D, Kunz PL, et al. Interactions between body condition at calving and cooling of dairy cows during lactation in summer. J Dairy Sci 1995; 78:2221–9.

60. Her E, Wolfenson D, Flamenbaum I, et al. Thermal, productive, and reproductive responses of high yielding cows exposed to short-term cooling in summer. J Dairy Sci 1988;71:1085–92.

61. Ferreira FC, Gennari RS, Dahl GE, et al. Economic feasibility of cooling dry cows across the united states. J Dairy Sci 2016;99:9931–41.

62. Dahl GE, Tao S, Monteiro APA. Effects of late-gestation heat stress on immunity and performance of calves. J Dairy Sci 2016;99:3193–8.

63. Parola F, Hillmann E, Schütz KE, et al. Preferences for overhead sprinklers by naïve beef steers: test of two nozzle types. Appl Anim Behav Sci 2012;137:13–22.

64. Tresoldi G, Schütz KE, Tucker C. Cow cooling on commercial drylot dairies: a description of 10 farms in California. Calif Agric 2017;71:249–55.

65. von Keyserlingk MAG, Martin NP, Kebreab E, et al. Invited review: sustainability of the us dairy industry. J Dairy Sci 2013;96:5405–25.

66. Brouk MJ, Smith JF, Harner JP. Effectiveness of cow cooling strategies under different environmental conditions. In: West Dairy Man Conf, March 12–14, 2003. Reno, NV: Western Dairy Management Conference.

67. Brouk MJ, Armstrong D, Smith J, et al. Evaluating and selecting cooling systems for different climates. In: West Dairy Man Conf, March 9–11, 2005. Reno, NV: Western Dairy Management Conference.

68. Washington State University Veterinary Medicine Extension. Ag animal health spotlight: heat stress. Pullman (WA): Washington State University; 2008.

69. Bailey T, Sheets J, Bryan M. Mechanics of heat abatement. Greenfield (IN): Elanco Animal Health; 2012.

70. Kimmel E, Arkin H, Broday D, et al. A model of evaporative cooling in a wetted hide. J Agr Eng Res 1991;49:227–41.

71. Gebremedhin KG, Wu BX. Simulation of sensible and latent heat losses from wet-skin surface and fur layer. J Therm Biol 2002;27:291–7.

72. Arkin H, Kimmel E, Berman A, et al. Heat transfer properties of dry and wet furs of dairy cows. Trans ASAE 1991;34:2550–8.

73. Means SL, Bucklin RA, Nordstedt RA, et al. Water application rates for a sprinkler and fan cooling system in hot, humid climates. Trans ASAE 1992;8:375–9.

74. Edstrom. Edstrom: cooling systems for dairy cattle. Waterford (WI): Edstrom Industries; 2011.

75. Armstrong DV. Heat stress interaction with shade and cooling. J Dairy Sci 1994; 77:2044–50.

76. Doble SJ, Matthews GA, Rutherford I, et al. A system for classifying hydraulic and other atomisers into categories of spray quality. In: Proc Brit Crop Protection Conf Weeds, November 18–21, 1985. Brighton, UK: British Crop Protection Council.

77. Dougherty CT, Knapp FW, Burrus PB, et al. Stable flies (*Stomoxys calcitrans* l.) and the behavior of grazing beef cattle. Appl Anim Behav Sci 1993;35:215–33.

78. Tucker CB, Rogers AR, Verkerk GA, et al. Effects of shelter and body condition on the behaviour and physiology of dairy cattle in winter. Appl Anim Behav Sci 2007; 105:1–13.

79. Chen JM, Schütz KE, Tucker CB. Sprinkler flow rate affects dairy cattle avoidance of spray to the head, but not overall, in an aversion race. Appl Anim Behav Sci 2016;179:23–31.

80. Collier RJ, Dahl GE, VanBaale MJ. Major advances associated with environmental effects on dairy cattle. J Dairy Sci 2006;89:1244–53.

81. Araki CT, Nakamura RM, Kam LWG, et al. Effect of lactation on diurnal temperature patterns of dairy cattle in hot environments. J Dairy Sci 1984;67:1752–60.
82. Gebremedhin KG, Lee CN, Larson JE, et al. Cooling cows: the udder way. In: 9th Int Livest Env Symp, July 8–12, 2012. Valencia, Spain: European Society of Agricultural Engineers.
83. Galton D, Petersson L, Merrill W, et al. Effects of premilking udder preparation on bacterial population, sediment, and iodine residue in milk. J Dairy Sci 1984;67:2580–9.
84. Aggarwal A, Upadhyay R. Heat stress and animal productivity. New Delhi (India): Springer India; 2013.
85. Bernabucci U, Lacetera N, Baumgard LH, et al. Metabolic and hormonal acclimation to heat stress in domesticated ruminants. Animal 2010;4:1167–83.
86. Mondaca M, Rojano F, Choi CY, et al. A conjugate heat and mass transfer model to evaluate the efficiency of conductive cooling for dairy cattle. Trans ASABE 2013;56:1471–82.
87. Perano KM, Usack JG, Angenent LT, et al. Production and physiological responses of heat-stressed lactating dairy cattle to conductive cooling. J Dairy Sci 2015;98:5252–61.
88. Ortiz XA, Smith JF, Rojano F, et al. Evaluation of conductive cooling of lactating dairy cows under controlled environmental conditions. J Dairy Sci 2015;98:1759–71.
89. Zähner M, Schrader L, Hauser R, et al. The influence of climatic conditions on physiological and behavioural parameters in dairy cows kept in open stables. Anim Sci 2004;78:139–47.
90. Overton MW, Sischo WM, Temple GD, et al. Using time-lapse video photography to assess dairy cattle lying behavior in a free-stall barn. J Dairy Sci 2002;85:2407–13.
91. Vokey FJ, Guard CL, Erb HN, et al. Effects of alley and stall surfaces on indices of claw and leg health in dairy cattle housed in a free-stall barn. J Dairy Sci 2001;84:2686–99.
92. Cook NB. Prevalence of lameness among dairy cattle in Wisconsin as a function of housing type and stall surface. J Am Vet Med Assoc 2003;223:1324–8.
93. Somers JGCJ, Frankena K, Noordhuizen-Stassen EN, et al. Prevalence of claw disorders in Dutch dairy cows exposed to several floor systems. J Dairy Sci 2003;86:2082–93.
94. Borderas TF, Pawluczuk B, de Passillé AM, et al. Claw hardness of dairy cows: relationship to water content and claw lesions. J Dairy Sci 2004;87:2085–93.
95. van Amstel SR, Shearer JK, Palin FL. Moisture content, thickness, and lesions of sole horn associated with thin soles in dairy cattle. J Dairy Sci 2004;87:757–63.

Designing Automated Milking Dairy Facilities to Maximize Labor Efficiency

Jouni Pitkäranta, MSc[a], Virpi Kurkela, DVM[b], Virpi Huotari, MSc[b],
Marjo Posio, MSc[b], Courtney E. Halbach, MBA[c],*

KEYWORDS

- Automatic milking systems • Labor efficiency • Barn layout • Robot layout
- Grouping

KEY POINTS

- Barn design affects labor efficiency, and the barn should be designed around the unique management style of the farmer.
- Layout of the robot, the number of robots per pen, dedicated handling areas, and how cows are grouped influence cow flow and barn efficiency.
- Deep, loose-bedded stalls; a minimum of 24 in (61 cm) feed bunk space per cow; solid concrete floors with automatic manure scrapers; a well-designed footbath; a dedicated fresh pen with voluntary access to the robot; excellent gating for easy sorting of cows; and a stocking rate of 55 cows per robot are preferred.

INTRODUCTION

Automatic milking systems (AMS) have become commonplace in Europe since the installation of the first units in the early 1990s in the Netherlands. In these units, groups of 50 cows to 70 cows are milked by a robotic arm installed in a milking box located in the cow pen, which records teat placement of each cow, attaches the milking unit, and harvests the milk without the need for human intervention. More recently, they are becoming popular in the United States and Canada due to difficulties associated with sourcing high-quality labor on farms to milk cows in conventional parlors.

Disclosure Statement: 4dBarn Oy provides facility design consultation services to dairy farmers and is not affiliated with any manufacturer of automatic milking systems. Their recommendations are independent of robot manufacturers and are based solely on company experience.
[a] 4dBarn Oy, Ketojenkatu 8, Seinäjoki 90100, Finland; [b] 4dBarn Oy, Kauppurienkatu 23, Oulu 90100, Finland; [c] The Dairyland Initiative, University of Wisconsin–Madison, School of Veterinary Medicine, 2015 Linden Drive, Madison, WI 53726, USA
* Corresponding author.
E-mail address: Courtney.halbach@wisc.edu

The potential benefits of AMS units include a reduction in labor to run the dairy and an increase in milk production from a higher milking frequency.[1] Salfer and colleagues[2] noted that milk production per cow and labor savings were the main management factors determining whether AMS units were more profitable to operate than conventional herds. These benefits are often realized in smaller herds of 60 milking cows to 120 milking cows that typically milked 2 times a day in a tiestall facility or a small parlor.[3] Salfer and colleagues[4] observed that 57% of AMS installations in the Upper Midwest transitioned from aged tiestall facilities. Some dairy herds in the United States, however, are building on a larger scale, sometimes with 20 or more box robots per farm to accommodate 1000 or more milking cows. These herds are asked to replace conventional parlor milking management achieving high milk production with 3-times-a-day milking with robotics, where increased milk production may not be realized. Additionally, the presumed benefits of labor reduction may be lessened because workers must visit multiple pens of cows to complete chores and fetch cows that have failed to milk at the robot within a predetermined period of time.[3] Rather, there is a shift in labor away from the daily stresses of milking toward farm management and data analysis in herds with AMS units. Good farm managers and those with realistic expectations of the AMS system may see some relief in labor through flexible working hours, but someone must still be on-call at all times due to continuous milking around the clock.

Barn design and layout intuitively have an impact on labor efficiency and cow well-being. In conventional milking herds, barn design is vitally important to the overall performance of the herd.[5,6] Recent evaluation of records from more than 600 North American AMS units suggests that overall performance is disappointing. Herds averaged only 70 lb (32 kg) of milk per cow per day, with 2.9 milkings per day,[7] which compares unfavorably with the high performing conventionally milked herds evaluated by Cook and colleagues[8] in the Upper Midwest, with milk yields in excess of 90 lb (41 kg) milk per cow per day. In the cluster analysis by Tremblay and colleagues,[9] a Midwest group of Holstein breed herds with AMS units faired not much better, averaging 78 lb (35 kg), whereas a similar group of herds surveyed by Salfer and colleagues[4] averaged 73 lb (33 kg). One reason for this performance gap may be lameness control. Although the high-performing conventional herds surveyed by Cook and colleagues[8] averaged only 13% lameness prevalence, studies from AMS units in North America suggest that lameness is affecting approximately 15% to 31% of cows in these herds.[4,10,11] Other research[12–14] has shown that lameness has a significant impact on the frequency of visits to the AMS unit[12–14] for milking, thereby undermining the overall performance of the herd and making lameness prevention a high priority for AMS design and management.

Aspects of AMS facility design that may be detrimental to lameness control and high milk production include too many cows per robot, mattress-bedded stalls, slatted floors, lack of sufficient bunk space and a separate fresh pen for heifers and cows, poor ventilation and cooling, and limited footbath use. Design elements that are known to be vitally important to the success of conventional milking herds are even more important for AMS herds. Salfer and colleagues[4] showed that lameness in Upper Midwestern AMS herds is less in herds using sand bedding compared with those with mats and mattresses, mirroring Cook and colleagues'[8,15] findings in conventional milking herds. In addition, Deming and colleagues[16] stressed the importance of providing sufficient bunk space to cows in AMS units. More specific to AMS design and milk production, Tremblay and colleagues[7] showed that milk production per robot was higher in free-flow systems compared with guided-flow systems—where cows must enter the robot to be milked before accessing the feed bunk.

These findings suggest that elements of barn design in AMS units can drive the overall health and production of the herd, and this is the focus of the remainder of this article.

KEYS TO SUCCESS

The barn can be considered a tool for improving labor efficiency, cow production, and cow welfare. There are several design elements that need to be met to achieve these goals. These include:

- A comfortable, deep, loose-bedded freestall designed for the size of the cows using them
- Access to food and water—a minimum of 24 in (61 cm) of bunk space per cow with headlocks for animal handling and 3.5 in (9 cm) of accessible water trough perimeter per cow
- Ten-ft to 12-ft (3.1–3.7 m)–wide stall alleys, 14-ft (4.3 m)–wide feed alleys, and 14-ft–wide crossovers between the feed and stall alleys with appropriately grooved concrete to allow for safe, clear access to the robots
- Sufficient open area in front of the robot(s), with minimal congestion for cows entering and leaving the robot area
- A traffic system for ease of sorting cows and convenient gating for a single person to move cows
- An adequately sized fetch pen that is easily accessible
- A functional footbath location to minimize the impact on robot visits but operate independent of the caregiver
- A designated fresh pen for heifers and mature cows, with 24-hour access to the robot and 30 in (76 cm) bunk space per cow
- Separation pens for treatment cows and lame cows and for cows in heat, with facilities for handling, examination, and treatment
- Easy access to the robot from the maternity area
- Excellent ventilation and cooling

The authors favor 55 cows per robot, housed in pens with deep, loose-bedded freestalls and solid, grooved concrete floors with automatic scrapers and well-designed footbaths in the robot exit lane. Whether a free-flow or guided-flow approach is used, the design of the access area is critical to avoid bullying and limited access to the milking machine.

LABOR EFFICIENCY

4dBarn Oy, an independent consulting service headquartered in Finland, specializes in designing AMS facilities to maximize labor efficiency. Since their inception, they have conducted a survey looking at labor efficiency on 53 AMS farms located in Finland, Sweden, Denmark, the Netherlands, Great Britain, and the United States, with 5 robot manufacturers represented in the survey. A portion of the survey looked at time spent completing various tasks during a farmer's morning work routine, and the data collected were used to determine labor minutes per cow and milk produced per labor hour.

Findings from 4dBarn's unpublished (Pitkäranta and colleagues, 2018) survey showed a wide variation in labor minutes per cow across all 53 farms (**Fig. 1**). The average time spent per cow was 5.1 minutes, with the most efficient farm clocking in at 1.5 minutes per cow and the least efficient farm maxing out at 13.8 minutes per cow. The most time-consuming tasks included fetching, cleaning stalls, and taking care of calves on milk.

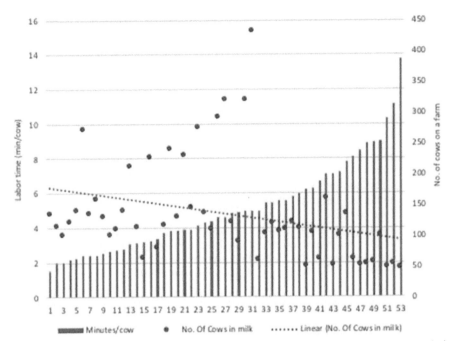

Fig. 1. Labor time observed on 53 farms ranging in herd size. Labor minutes per cow varied among herds of similar size.

Labor efficiency was calculated based on the amount of milk produced per labor hour by dividing the total milk in the bulk tank by the total daily labor hours, which included working with calves, heifers, and cows as well as feeding. Farms with only 1 AMS unit ranged between 37 gallons and 124 gallons (140–470 L) of milk whereas farms with 2 AMS units varied from 53 gallons to 248 gallons (201–939 L), and farms with more than 3 AMS units ranged from 91 gallons to 235 gallons (345–890 L of milk) (**Fig. 2**). These numbers show that high labor efficiency can be achieved on farms with as few as 2 AMS units.

The findings from the labor survey have led to the following observations and recommendations for AMS facility design.

Fetch Cows

As discussed previously, fetching cows is time consuming. On average, 8% of the cows in the pen need to be fetched on a daily basis,[10] but the fetch rate can be as high as 42%.[17]

Fetch cows often include early and late lactation cows, lame cows, and sick cows. Motivations for not wanting to visit the robot may be contributed to poor facility design, the number of cows per robot, pellet allowances in the robot, balance of the partial mixed ration at the feed bunk, and cows that have been trained to visit the robot only with human interaction. The fetching process can be improved with proper gate placement and properly designed fetch pens that have a split entry so that the farmer does not have to wait for the fetched cow to enter the robot while cows from the main milking group continue to have access to the robots. Higher production per minute the cow spends in the robot and higher production per robot have been associated with barns that have a split-entry fetch pen.[18] The fetch pen should provide 20 sq ft to 30 sq ft (1.9–2.8 m²) per cow and be sized to accommodate 4 cows to 6 cows per robot.

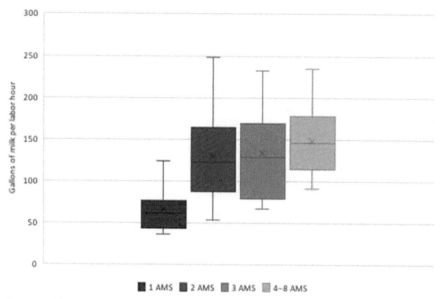

Fig. 2. High labor efficiency found in herds with more than 2 AMS units can also be achieved on farms with 2 AMS units.

However, with excellent facility design and management, the number of fetch cows per robot can be reduced to 1 cow to 3 cows per robot.

ANIMAL TRAFFIC SYSTEMS

There are 3 types of AMS cow traffic systems currently used in the United States — free-flow, guided-flow, and semi guided-flow. In a free-flow system, cows have the ability to freely visit the robot, feed bunk, and resting space at any time. Voluntary robot attendance is driven by the availability of a specialized, high-quality feed pellet in combination with a mixed ration at the feed bunk. Plenty of space in front of the robot, wide alleys, stalls designed for the cow's body weight, and excellent gating are key facility components in making a free-flow system work well.

Strong preferences toward a specific traffic system are held among robot manufacturers and farmers. Proponents of free-flow systems claim better cow welfare due to the cow's ability to freely move about the pen whereas proponents of guided-flow systems profess greater labor efficiency due to less time fetching cows[19-21] and greater robot capacity due to preselection of cows. Social dominance at the robot takes precedence in guided-flow systems. There is a greater likelihood of timid cows being trapped in the commitment pen for longer periods of time[22] without access to feed, water, and a lying space due to dominant cows pushing them away from the robot entry or exit sort gate. Ways to accommodate timid cows and increase cow flow around the robot are to add a lane the length of a cow at the robot entrance so that a dominant cow cannot push a cow away from the side, and to have 2 sort gates attached to the commitment pen rather than 1 to relieve congestion at the gate. One sort gate would be dedicated to sorting cows from the resting area to the commitment pen for feed or milk access, whereas the other sort gate would sort cows from the commitment pen to the feeding area. Guided-flow systems, however, become more challenging to manage with larger pen sizes. When there is more than 1 robot per pen, cows exit from the robot back into the commitment pen where they then have to find the sort gate to let themselves out.

This creates a crowded commitment pen and a roadblock to animal traffic through the sort gates. One way to reduce overcrowding in the commitment pen is to install the robots in a tollbooth layout where cows exit away from the robot entrance.

ROBOT POSITIONING

Robot orientation and space around the robot can help drive visits to the AMS units. Footbath location, cow traffic and behavior, sorting options, and plans for expansion should be discussed when determining the position of the robot(s). Six common robot positions have emerged, each with their advantages and disadvantages, but the key to making any of the positions work well is to provide plenty of space around the robots, especially when cow traffic increases with the number of robots in the pen. Also, laying out the robots so that there is a protected entry area in front of the robot with a dedicated exit to the main group allows for better cow flow and creates a positive robot visit experience for the cow.

Side Installation

Installing robots on the side of the barn, parallel to the pen, is commonly seen in North America (**Fig. 3**). Side installations offer many advantages such as easy access to the robot room with the option of putting multiple robots next to each other, are cheaper to build, cater well to retrofit setups, work in both free- and guided-flow traffic systems, and the robots are out of the way of manure alleys. When there are multiple robots in a

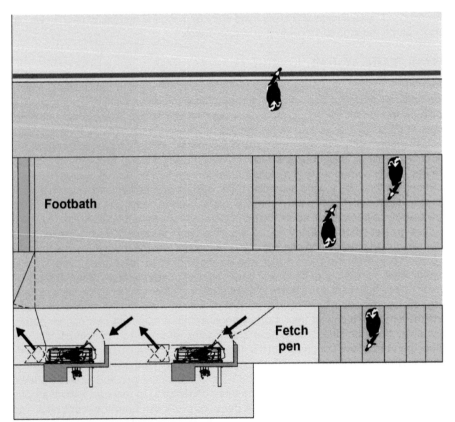

Fig. 3. Example of a side installation where 2 robots are installed on the side of the barn.

pen that face the same direction, cows can be sorted from the first robot into a holding area where they pass through the second robot into a designated handling area. This is less than ideal, however, because unproductive time in the second robot adds up with cows waiting to be sorted.

In regard to ventilation, robots installed on the side of the barn complement tunnel-ventilated facilities because the robot rooms do not obstruct air flow in the pen, but robots placed on the side in naturally ventilated facilities decrease the sidewall opening, thus creating a dead spot in front of the robot.

Disadvantages to side installations include limited sorting capabilities, increased cow traffic in front of the robots due to cows entering and exiting in the same area, and no 24-hour access for a second group placed behind the robots. Additionally, determining where to locate the footbath is challenging. Typically, the footbath is placed in the holding area, the area directly in front of the robots, next to a row of stalls or in a robot exit lane.

Crossway Installation

Robots placed crossway or perpendicular to the pen are often designed for efficient work routines and robot access (**Fig. 4**). Despite the advantages of having robots in 1 room and the ability to have cows exit in the same direction toward the feed alley, crossway installations block air flow in tunnel-ventilated facilities, give few options for cow separation, and make the design of manure scrapers difficult, creating large areas that require manual scraping. New installations are orienting the robots to face each other to allow cows to be sorted into a separation pen. This layout has cows exiting into the middle of the holding area, increasing cow traffic around the

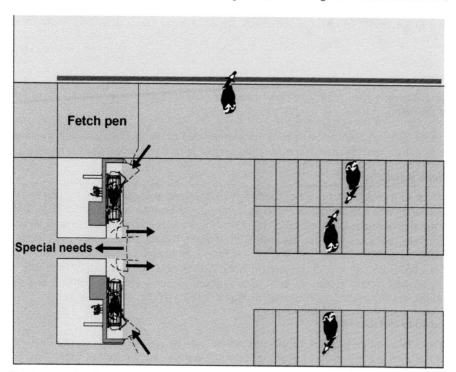

Fig. 4. Example of a crossway installation where 2 robots are installed perpendicular to the stalls in the pen.

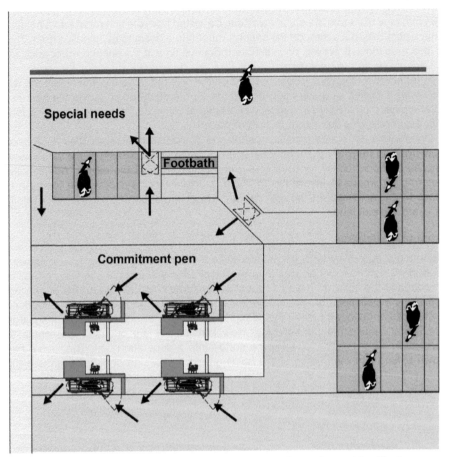

Fig. 5. Example of an island installation where 2 robots are located as an island in the center of the barn.

robots. This robot location does provide increased bunk space per cow if the feed bunk is extended through the robot area, but locating the footbath is challenging.

Island Installation

Similar to a crossway, the robot room can be designed with the robots parallel to the feed lanes with a large room located as an island in the center of the barn (**Fig. 5**). This orientation reduces the obstruction to air flow in a tunnel ventilation system and allows automatic scrapers to clean the area in front of the robots. As with sideway installations, the ability to sort directly from the robots is limited, and the area in front of the robots can become congested. Hence, this arrangement is typically built with a guided-flow gating system in front of the robots allowing separation into a special needs pen, exit through a footbath, or return to the main lactating cow group.

L-shaped Installation

In an L-shaped installation, robots are placed parallel and perpendicular to the pen, typically on a head-to-head stall platform to keep the manure alleys open (**Fig. 6**). This setup allows for cows to be separated from both robots, and a second group of cows may have 24-hour access to the robots. For this design to work, there needs

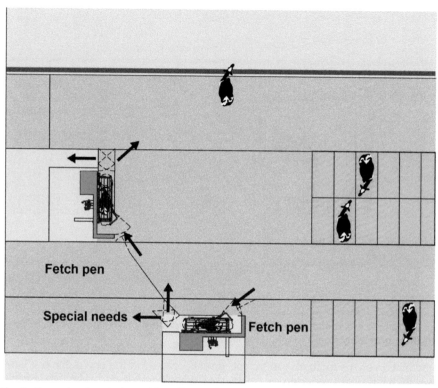

Fig. 6. Example of an L-shaped installation showing 1 robot installed on the side and the other perpendicular to the stalls.

to be a large open area in front of the robots to reduce overcrowding in the holding area. This can be achieved by making the distance to the nearest stall 26 ft to 33 ft (8–10 m). Unfortunately, the downside to this open area is that it frequently needs manual scraping. Robots can be placed facing each other, away from each other, or in the same direction. If robots are placed facing in the same direction, there needs to be a significant distance between the robot rooms because cow traffic increases with cows entering and exiting the robot in the same area. This layout requires multiple robot rooms, but does provide extended bunk space into the robot area. It is one of the most challenging layouts for footbath location, with too many facilities relying on footbaths in the furthest crossover from the robot area and routing of cows through the bath at bedding time. In some instances, the footbath is located in the exit lane of the robot nearest to the feed bunk, but for this setup to work, cows need to be directed from the other robot(s) into the fetch pen to the robot nearest the feed bunk. Similar to a crossway, the perpendicular robot room blocks air flow in a tunnel ventilation system, and the side installation limits the side wall inlet for natural ventilation, necessitating the need for appropriately located recirculation fans to facilitate air flow.

Tollbooth Installation

Cows enter the robot aligned in parallel with the freestall alleys and exit into a lane at the rear of the robot(s) running perpendicular to the freestall alleys in a tollbooth layout (**Fig. 7**). As the cows exit, they can be directed into a breeding pen, into a sick pen, through a footbath, or to a trim area, or permitted to return to the freestall area. Cows return to the pen away from the robot entry point, relieving congestion in this

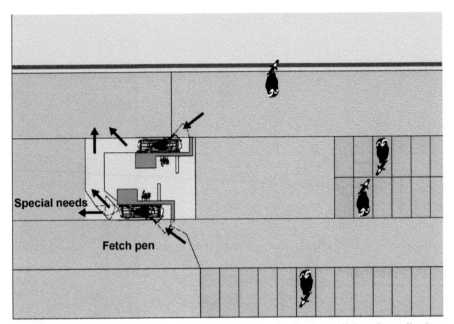

Fig. 7. Example of a tollbooth installation where the robots are parallel to the stalls. Cows exit the robots away from the robot entrance.

important area. The footbath can be conveniently located at the end of the exit lane, away from the robots, reducing the risk that the footbath may impact robot attendance. A separate group of cows can have access to the robot at the opposite end of the exit lane. Bunk space is extended around the robot area with this layout, but similar to the crossway installation, the robot rooms block air flow in a tunnel ventilation system. There are concerns regarding congestion in the lane exiting the robot with this layout, but these are reduced by ensuring that the lane is no more than 44 in (112 cm) wide.

Herringbone Installation

A relatively new concept in robot positioning is the herringbone layout where the robots are placed parallel to the stalls and slightly angled (**Fig. 8**). Cows enter the robot(s) in the holding area located on the freestall side of the robots and exit into a protected feed alley allowing for natural cow flow out of the robot toward the feed bunk and separation from cows waiting to be milked. Herringbone layouts lend themselves well to 3-row pens because feed bunk space extends in front of the robot, providing additional feeding space per cow. Cows are typically more motivated to attend the robot when the feed bunk is visible from the robot. Additional advantages to this layout include the ability to sort cows into a separation pen with 24-hour access to the robot, automatic manure removal in the holding area, and the ability to direct cows through a footbath when cows return to the pen from the protected feed area. Disadvantages to this layout include the blocking of air flow in a tunnel ventilation system and obtaining clean and safe access to the robot rooms.

FOOTBATH LOCATION

Lameness is a significant problem in AMS herds with lameness prevalence ranging between 15% and 31%.[4,10,11] Cows that are more lame have fewer visits to the robot,[12-14] which results in greater rates of fetching.[12] In 41 facilities in Canada,

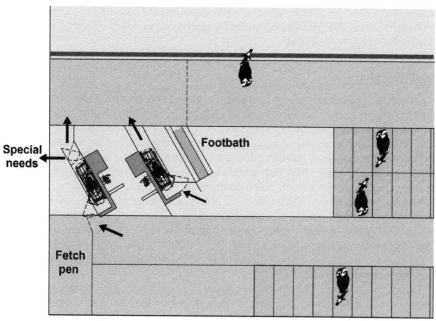

Fig. 8. Example of a herringbone layout where the robots are parallel with the stalls and slightly angled to facilitate cow flow through the robots.

lame cows were compared with non-lame cows and were found to produce 3.5 lb (1.6 kg) less milk per day, had 0.3 fewer milkings per day, and were 2.2 times more likely to be fetched.[10]

Footbath regimes are an integral component of infectious hoof disease control in freestall dairy systems,[23] but are often forgotten in AMS facility design. Topical application of antibacterials such as copper sulfate, formalin, zinc compounds, and other disinfectants have been shown to aid in the control of digital dermatitis (heel warts) by preventing the reversion of chronic lesions back into active painful stages of the disease.[23] Thus, the footbath is an essential herd management tool for making the AMS unit successful, but 30% of herds in the Upper Midwest do not even operate a footbath and of those herds that do, only 27% of them bath at a frequency more than three times per week[4]; 71% of footbaths were located at the robot exit area,[4] yet many producers claim that this positioning has a negative impact on robot attendance with little scientific evidence to support this claim. In some units, the footbaths are located in a crossover alley at the opposite end of the pen where caregivers have to route cows manually through the bath when bedding. This approach is disruptive and time consuming, is not done frequently enough (3 or more times per week is suggested), and is not recommended.

Wherever the footbath is located, it is imperative that it operates independent of the caregiver and ideally is set up to automatically select cows for bathing to avoid cows being bathed repeatedly after each robot visit. One way is to create an alternative exit from the robots that is only used on footbathing days with the bath sufficiently distant from the immediate robot area so as not to have a negative impact on attendance. For this design, the tollbooth and herringbone layouts carry an advantage over other designs. An option for guided-flow systems is to locate the footbath in the exit lane out of the robot area; alternatively, it may be located as cows exit the feeding alley when they return to the resting area.

HANDLING COWS

A dedicated handling area where cows can be sorted from the robot allows for efficient treating, breeding, and trimming of cows. Typically, these handling areas are located at the end or side of the barn out of the way of robot traffic for easy access by the hoof trimmer and have a chute adjacent to the pen. Headlocks are an essential facility component for easy cow handling and are preferred over post-and-rail for the main milking group and fresh cows. **Fig. 9** shows an example of a handling chute designed for easy animal access with an office on the side.

Pushing first-lactation heifers through the robots post-calving is often a time-consuming task that could be lessened with the use of a heifer training gate in the heifer pen. The gating system, which mirrors that of the robot, is placed in a crossover (**Fig. 10**). Heifers are manually walked through the training gate and exit in the direction of the feed bunk. The best time to push heifers through the training gate is after fresh feed has been delivered.

Gating is the essence of barn functionality and one of the main determinants of labor efficiency. The idea behind gate design is that no matter the herd size, 1 person is able to complete all daily tasks independently such as fetching, treating, and moving cows between groups. In free-flow traffic systems, having the ability to close off crossovers with gates makes fetching cows easier. One-way gates are important for moving cows to the fetch pen or treatment area and prevent fetched cows from escaping, and can help direct reluctant cows into the robot. If there are concerns that gates will be in the way most of the time, but are needed for certain tasks, gates that lift up and down are a good option. **Fig. 11** shows an example of a lifting gate that is used to make fetching cows easier.

Robot companies offer 2-way and 3-way sort gates for cows exiting the robot. These gates allow managers to automatically program if a cow is sent back to the milking group or placed in a separation pen. One of the main benefits of automatic sort gates is that they can allow fresh cows, located in a separate pen, 24-hour access to the robots in the main milking pen via a split entrance. Manual separation gates

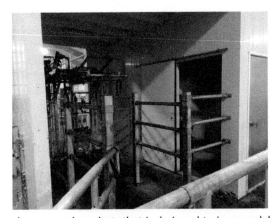

Fig. 9. A handling chute near the robots that is designed to improve labor efficiency.

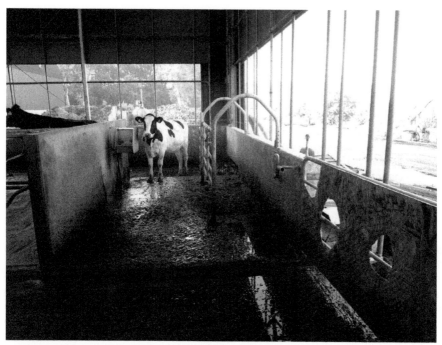

Fig. 10. Gating systems that mirror those around the robot can be placed in heifer pens to train them to visit the robot prior to calving.

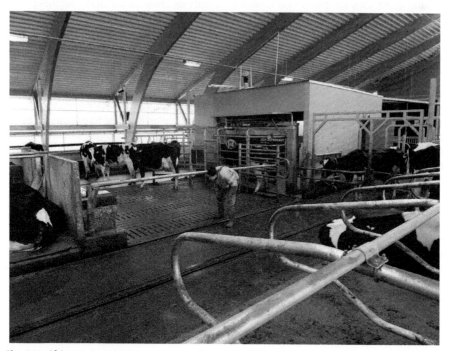

Fig. 11. Lifting gates are a good option for areas where a gate is not always needed, but is useful to have when fetching cows.

work well for moving separated cows into the fetch pen. Once milked, these cows exit through a sort gate and are directed back to the separation pen.

PEN ELEMENTS
Grouping

Milk production per robot is influenced by milk production per cow, making the number of cows supported by each robot an important decision in AMS facility design. Unfortunately, no threshold for cows per robot has yet been determined. Theoretically, with robot units operating for 20 hours per day to 22 hours per day and serving approximately 8 cows per hour, each unit could support 50 cows to 70 cows depending on the milking interval. In North American surveys, herds typically average 49 cows per robot to 56 cows per robot,[7,10,11,24] lower than the 60 cows per robot to 70 cows per robot often recommended by manufacturers. As the number of cows per robot increases above 60, visits to the robot decrease and the number of fetch cows increases because of longer milking intervals.[20] Clinical experience on farms shows that decreasing the number of cows per robot decreases the fetch rate, supporting a design average of approximately 55 cows per robot.

Once the number of AMS units has been decided, the next decision is how many robots per pen. Studies have reported greater production per robot in 2-robot to 3-robot pens compared with single-robot pens,[7,18] and increases in labor efficiency have been observed with these layouts. Having 2 or more robots per pen also ensures that cows can continue milking if 1 of the robots requires maintenance and provides timid cows another option for accessing a robot. At some point, as more robots are added, the size of the pen may become limiting due to increased walking distances for cows and challenges with locating cows when fetching.

Labor time increases for each milking group that is added to a facility as observed in 4dBarn's unpublished (Pitkäranta and colleagues, 2018) survey looking at labor efficiency. If each milking pen is viewed as a working unit, it makes sense that managing 110 cows split between 2 pens with each pen having its own robot is more time consuming than managing 1 pen of 110 cows with 2 robots.

Several factors go into deciding how cows are grouped. Mainly, cows are grouped by size or lactation. Doing so limits the potential for bullying behavior from the older, larger cows toward the younger, smaller cows, and makes it easier to design the free-stall to accommodate the cows using them. In parlor herds, grouping animals by stage of lactation has proved economically advantageous.[25] When the stalls are appropriately sized, labor, such as cleaning the stalls, can be reduced, and cow lying times can be maximized.

It is generally accepted that fresh cows up to approximately 21 days postpartum benefit from having their own pen and that being milked 3 times per day leads to greater milk production than 2 times a day milking.[26,27] Fresh cows with only manual access to the robots are more likely to be milked twice per day depending on labor availability. Therefore, AMS herds should prioritize 24-hour access to the robot for a separate group of fresh cows and heifers to optimize early lactation performance. On larger dairies, there is an opportunity to house fresh heifers and mature cows separately.

Additional groups that should have convenient access to the robot, whether automatically or manually, are the special needs cows and maternity cows. The first milking after calving can be done in the AMS unit or in the maternity pen with a bucket. Once milked, the route to the AMS unit or fresh cow pen must be short and straight to allow 1 person to guide the cow without causing undue stress.

Feed Bunk Location

The provision of adequate feed space is widely believed to be an essential component to high milk production in conventional herds, and the topic is reviewed in Trevor J. DeVries's article, "Feeding Behavior, Feed Space, and Bunk Design and Management for Adult Dairy Cattle," in this issue. Some AMS unit designers claim that because robot-milked cows can set individual schedules, there is less need for bunk space to accommodate the entire group. This belief is especially true in guided-flow systems because access to the feed bunk is controlled by smart gates. Because robot attendance is spread throughout the day for each individual cow, an argument can be made that there is less pressure on bunk attendance after rigid milking times and hence less of a need to provide sufficient bunk space for all of the cows to eat at the same time. This belief drives the use of 3 or more rows of stalls per pen, thereby off-setting the higher costs of an AMS facility.

It is known, however, that fresh feed delivery drives bunk attendance and intake in conventional herds.[28] If cows do not get to eat when all the other cows are eating, they do not return to the bunk and eat more later on. Forage and feed intake in guided-flow systems is less than that observed in semi guided-flow and free-flow traffic systems,[19,29] and Deming and colleagues[16] identified the importance of providing sufficient bunk space to optimize milk per cow. In free-flow systems, limited bunk access when fresh feed is delivered may have an impact on performance whereas in guided-flow systems, sorting of the ration by cows feeding early on after feed delivery limits the performance of cows accessing the bunk later in the delivery cycle.

With AMS units, most fresh cows enter the main cow group often immediately after milk residues have cleared, and transitions may be particularly challenging for fresh heifers as they adapt to milking through a robot. In several AMS herd troubleshooting experiences, disappointing early lactation performance in primiparous cows has been seen as a significant component of poor herd milk production performance. A minimum bunk space per cow of 24 in (61 cm) for the main lactating cow groups, and a separate fresh cow group with additional feed space (30 in [76 cm] per cow) for periparturient cows and heifers to transition is recommended. Pens with 2 rows and even 3 rows of stalls per pen may accomplish this goal when crossovers and space in front of the robot are accounted for in the feed bunk dimensions.

As the number of rows in the pen increases, the question of where to locate the feed bunk arises. In typical parlor herds, the feed bunk is located in the center of the barn with pens on either side. With robotic herds, it is important to consider animal handling and robot location within the pen in relation to the feed bunk. Pens that are parallel to each other with perimeter feeding lend themselves well for herd expansion and increased labor efficiency due to less distance between pens. Additional advantages of perimeter feeding include cow stalls located away from sidewalls, out of the sunlight, and increased bunk space per cow. Rather than having feed alleys along the perimeter of the pen, the feed bunk can be placed on the sidewall with a section of the wall that opens for the mixer to deliver feed (**Fig. 12**).

Manure Removal

An effective manure handling system is a vital component to maintaining high standards of udder and hoof cleanliness and hoof health. Common manure removal methods in AMS herds include automatic V-shaped scrapers, manual scrape options, slatted floors with robot manure scrapers, and more recently, vacuum systems. Although slatted floors are common in AMS units in Europe, they increase the risk of white line disease[30] and pose ventilation challenges in a diverse climate with hot

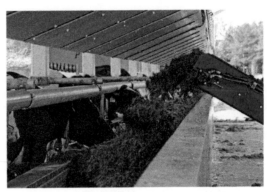

Fig. 12. A feed bunk can be installed along the sidewall with a section that opens when fresh feed is delivered in barns where the feed bunk is located on the perimeter of the pen.

summers and cold winters. Slatted floors and manure pits below the barn are also incompatible with deep-bedded sand freestalls, the use of which are consistently associated with the lowest prevalence of lameness in conventional[8] and AMS herds alike.[4]

Somewhat as expected, manual manure removal, practiced by 22% of AMS herds in the Upper Midwest, was associated with the lowest prevalence of severely dirty cows in the survey by Salfer and colleagues,[4] likely because the cows are out of the way of the manure as it is pushed out of the barn. That said, given the need to be labor efficient, V-shaped scrapers that run frequently seem the best option for robot facilities because there is little pen disturbance, and frequent manure removal lessens the buildup of manure in front of the scraper for cows to step through. V-shaped scrapers that fold-in parallel to the pen when moving backward are ideal in that they allow machinery to easily move up and down the alleys for the delivery of bedding (**Fig. 13**).

If automatic scrapers are used, there should be a manure drop every 250 ft (76 m) to reduce the depth of the manure wave that the cows must walk through as the scraper travels through the pen.

The choice of scraping or slatted floors may have an impact on the location of the AMS unit relative to the pen. AMS units at the end of a pen are usually in the way of the scraper, which leads to a large accumulation of manure around the milking area. This

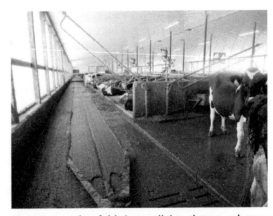

Fig. 13. An automatic V-scraper that folds-in parallel to the pen when moving backward allows for machinery to move through the pen.

has to be removed by hand or there needs to be a slatted area of flooring used to mitigate the buildup of manure.

Bedding Stalls

Sand-bedded stalls are the preferred stall surface in robot barns because they promote longer lying times[31–33] and reduce the rate of lameness,[11,15,34] thus increasing milk production per cow compared to other stall bed surfaces.[35] Although sand is known as the gold standard, many robot herds install mattresses due to the wear and tear of sand on the robot equipment and not wanting to disturb the cows to bed the stalls. As robot equipment progresses, the effects of sand on the robots is becoming less of a concern, and the benefits of sand far outweigh the small disturbance caused by bedding. If stalls are designed for the cows and properly maintained, cows quickly return to them after bedding. The best time to bed stalls is after fresh feed is delivered. In pens with 3 or more rows of stalls, cows can be gated off from the feed alley so that stalls with access to the feed bunk are bedded before the cows are released and fresh feed is delivered, opening up access to the stalls in the middle of the pen for bedding.

CONSIDERATIONS FOR RETROFITS AND LARGE HERDS

AMS units are often installed in an existing facility without thought to the change in labor and cow handling around the robot. The focus is on getting the AMS unit to milk the main milking group and not the fresh and special needs cows. The best way to add a robot to an existing dairy is to expand on the end of the barn. The expansion would house the robot(s) and have a handling area and/or sort group. This creates little disturbance and ensures adequate space around the robot. Robots can be installed in an existing pen on a platform; however, platforms are often too narrow and space is limited around the robot.

Robotic milking started as a way to solve some of the labor challenges on small herds, but it has become more difficult to find skilled and reliable labor, so large dairy farms have started to consider AMS units as an alternative means of milking. Large dairy herds are not looking to add robots to improve their lifestyle, but rather as a way to decrease labor costs. Research has yet to show, however, if there is an actual decrease in labor with this type of AMS unit and, if there is, if the decrease in labor justifies the high investment costs associated with AMS units. In the recent economic analysis by Salfer and colleagues,[2] although models for 120-cow and 240-cow units were profitable compared with conventional parlor milked herds, the breakeven labor wage for profitability for a 1500-cow AMS unit was $27 per hour compared with a similar parlor herd, suggesting that the adoption of single-box robots in larger dairy herds should proceed with caution.

SUMMARY

The goal of designing a barn with an AMS unit is to create a functional unit where work is done efficiently, and excellent cow welfare and comfort guarantee good health and productivity. To achieve this goal, time must be invested during the design process to build the barn to fit the work routines of the farmer, their management targets, and ambitions for productivity. Plenty of space around the robot; easy cow flow between the resting, feeding, and robot areas; a comfortable place to lie down; sufficient bunk space to maximize intakes; a smooth transition; easy sorting; and effective footbathing are key aspects of the barn that have to work together to succeed with an AMS.

REFERENCES

1. De Koning K, Rodenburg J. Automatic milking: state of the art in europe and north America. 2004. Available at: https://www.researchgate.net/publication/40125090. Accessed August 16, 2018.
2. Salfer JA, Minegishi K, Lazarus W, et al. Finances and returns for robotic dairies. J Dairy Sci 2017;100(9):7739–49.
3. Rotz CA, Coiner CU, Soder KJ. Automatic milking systems, farm size, and milk production. J Dairy Sci 2003;86(12):4167–77.
4. Salfer JA, Siewert JM, Endres MI. Housing, management characteristics, and factors associated with lameness, hock lesion, and hygiene of lactating dairy cattle on Upper Midwest United States dairy farms using automatic milking systems. J Dairy Sci 2018;101(9):8586–94.
5. Brotzman RL, Cook NB, Nordlund K, et al. Cluster analysis of Dairy Herd Improvement data to discover trends in performance characteristics in large Upper Midwest dairy herds. J Dairy Sci 2015;98(5):3059–70.
6. Brotzman RL, Döpfer D, Foy MR, et al. Survey of facility and management characteristics of large, Upper Midwest dairy herds clustered by Dairy Herd Improvement records. J Dairy Sci 2015;98(11):8245–61.
7. Tremblay M, Hess JP, Christenson BM, et al. Factors associated with increased milk production for automatic milking systems. J Dairy Sci 2016;99(5):3824–37.
8. Cook NB, Hess JP, Foy MR, et al. Management characteristics, lameness, and body injuries of dairy cattle housed in high-performance dairy herds in Wisconsin. J Dairy Sci 2016;99(7):5879–91.
9. Tremblay M, Hess JP, Christenson BM, et al. Customized recommendations for production management clusters of North American automatic milking systems. J Dairy Sci 2016;99(7):5671–80.
10. King MTM, Pajor EA, LeBlanc SJ, et al. Associations of herd-level housing, management, and lameness prevalence with productivity and cow behavior in herds with automated milking systems. J Dairy Sci 2016;99(11):9069–79.
11. Westin R, Vaughan A, de Passillé AM, et al. Cow- and farm-level risk factors for lameness on dairy farms with automated milking systems. J Dairy Sci 2016; 99(5). https://doi.org/10.3168/jds.2015-10414.
12. Bach A, Dinarés M, Devant M, et al. Associations between lameness and production, feeding and milking attendance of Holstein cows milked with an automatic milking system. J Dairy Res 2007;74(01):40.
13. Borderas TF, Fournier A, Rushen J, et al. Effect of lameness on dairy cows' visits to automatic milking systems. Can J Anim Sci 2008;88(1):1–8.
14. Garcia E, Klaas I, Amigo JM, et al. Lameness detection challenges in automated milking systems addressed with partial least squares discriminant analysis. J Dairy Sci 2014;97(12):7476–86.
15. Cook NB, Bennett TB, Nordlund KV. Effect of free stall surface on daily activity patterns in dairy cows with relevance to lameness prevalence. J Dairy Sci 2004;87(9):2912–22.
16. Deming JA, Bergeron R, Leslie KE, et al. Associations of housing, management, milking activity, and standing and lying behavior of dairy cows milked in automatic systems. J Dairy Sci 2013;96(1):344–51.
17. Rodenburg J, House HK. Field observations on barn layout and design for robotic milking. ASABE Publication Number. St. Joseph (MI): The American Society of Agricultural and Biological Engineers; 2007.

18. Heurkens D, Kamphuis C, Van Der Kamp A. Effects of free-stall barn layout on efficiency of Dutch dairy farms with an automatic milking system. In: Proc. Precision Dairy Farming 2016. Leeuwarden, Netherlands, June 21–23, 2016. p. 157–62.

19. Harms J, Wendl G. Automatic milking, a better understanding. In: Meijering A, Hogeveen H, de Koning CJAM, editors. The Netherlands: Wageningen Academic Publishers; 2004. p. 27–37. https://doi.org/10.3920/978-90-8686-525-3.

20. Rodenburg J, Wheeler B. Strategies for incorporating robotic milking into North American Herd Management. In: Proc. 1st North American Conf. on Robotic Milking, Toronto, Canada. Wageningen, Fort Wayne, IN, April 19–20, 2011. p. 18–32.

21. Bach A, Devant M, Igleasias C, et al. Forced traffic in automatic milking systems effectively reduces the need to get cows, but alters eating behavior and does not improve milk yield of dairy cattle. J Dairy Sci 2009;92(3):1272–80.

22. Melin M, Hermans GGN, Pettersson G, et al. Cow traffic in relation to social rank and motivation of cows in an automatic milking system with control gates and an open waiting area. Appl Anim Behav Sci 2006;96(3):201–14.

23. Cook NB. A review of the design and management of footbaths for dairy cattle. Vet Clin North Am Food Anim Pract 2017;33(2):195–225.

24. Siewert JM, Salfer JA, Endres MI. Factors associated with productivity on automatic milking system dairy farms in the Upper Midwest United States. J Dairy Sci 2018;101(9):8327–34.

25. Cabrera VE, Kalantari AS. Economics of production efficiency: nutritional grouping of the lactating cow. J Dairy Sci 2016;99(1):825–41.

26. Bach A, Busto I. Effects on milk yield of milking interval regularity and teat cup attachment failures with robotic milking systems. J Dairy Res 2005;72(1):101–6.

27. Melin M, Svennersten-Sjaunja K, Wiktorsson H. Feeding patterns and performance of cows in controlled cow traffic in automatic milking systems. J Dairy Sci 2005;88(11):3913–22.

28. Huzzey JM, DeVries TJ, Valois P, et al. Stocking density and feed barrier design affect the feeding and social behavior of dairy cattle. J Dairy Sci 2006;89(1): 126–33.

29. Melin M, Pettersson G, Svennersten-Sjaunja K, et al. The effects of restricted feed access and social rank on feeding behavior, ruminating and intake for cows managed in automated milking systems. Appl Anim Behav Sci 2007;107(1): 13–21.

30. Sogstad Å, Fjeldaas T, Østerås O. Lameness and claw lesions of the Norwegian red dairy cattle housed in free stalls in relation to environment, parity and stage of lactation. Acta Vet Scand 2005;46(4):203.

31. Tucker CB, Weary DM, Fraser D. Effects of three types of free-stall surfaces on preferences and stall usage by dairy cows. J Dairy Sci 2003;86(2):521–9.

32. Wagner-Storch AM, Palmer RW, Kammel DW. Factors affecting stall use for different freestall bases. J Dairy Sci 2003;86(6):2253–66.

33. Tucker CB, Weary DM. Bedding on Geotextile mattresses: how much is needed to improve cow comfort? J Dairy Sci 2004;87(9):2889–95.

34. Solano L, Barkema HW, Pajor EA, et al. Prevalence of lameness and associated risk factors in Canadian Holstein-Friesian cows housed in freestall barns. J Dairy Sci 2015;98(10):6978–91.

35. Rowbotham RF, Ruegg PL. Association of bedding types with management practices and indicators of milk quality on larger Wisconsin dairy farms. J Dairy Sci 2015;98(11):7865–85.

Design and Management of Proper Handling Systems for Dairy Cows

David W. Kammel, PhD[a],*, Karl Burgi[b], Jim Lewis[c]

KEYWORDS

- Dairy • Cow • Handling • System • Stress • Stockmanship • Stock person
- Stockman

KEY POINTS

- The 3 key components of a handling system are the skills of the stock person, the cow handling management plan, and the design of the handling facility.
- The dairy cow is the first consideration in the cow handling management plan and design decisions, which directly address animal welfare.
- The handling system is designed for safety of cows and stock persons.
- Minimizing stress for cows and stock persons lowers the risk of injury to both.

 Video content accompanies this article at http://www.vetfood.theclinics.com.

INTRODUCTION

A whole systems design approach to the cow handling system optimizes cow welfare and production.[1] Proper handling system design and management are inclusive of the concepts of being safe, efficient, and effective, and the result is a successful system that benefits the cows, stock persons, and the dairy business.

The design of the cow handling system and its components is based on a cow handling management plan developed by the dairy design team with the combined knowledge from a group of people that has different perspectives. The cow handling system is a tool to allow the implementation of a management plan.[2]

Disclosure Statement: D.W. Kammel has nothing to disclose. K. Burgi is owner of Sure Step Consulting International LLC. J. Lewis is owner of Stepright Stockmanship Solutions LLC.
[a] Biological Systems Engineering, University of Wisconsin, 460 Henry Mall, Madison, WI 53706, USA; [b] Sure Step Consulting International LLC, 420 Commerce Avenue, Baraboo, WI 53913, USA; [c] Stepright Stockmanship Solutions LLC, E6284 821st Avenue, Colfax, WI 54730, USA
* Corresponding author.
E-mail address: dwkammel@wisc.edu

Vet Clin Food Anim 35 (2019) 195–227
https://doi.org/10.1016/j.cvfa.2018.11.003
0749-0720/19/© 2018 Elsevier Inc. All rights reserved.

Design and management are both essential for a successful cow handling system design. The 3 key components are as follows:

1. The skills of the stock person (stockmanship)
2. The cow handling management plan
3. The design of the facility

Excellent stockmanship skills can compensate for a poor cow handling facility design, but a properly designed cow handling system design enhances the opportunity to leverage excellent stockmanship skills and a cow handling management plan.

HUMAN AND COW INTERACTION

More than a century ago, W.D. Hoard wrote: "The rule to be observed in this stable at all times, toward the cattle… is that of patience and kindness. A man's usefulness in a herd ceases at once when he loses his temper and bestows rough usage. Men must be patient. Cattle are not reasoning beings…rough treatment lessens the flow (of milk). That injures me as well as the cow. Always keep these ideas in mind in dealing with my cattle." This historical concept has evolved since that time and is now represented in animal behavior research, human-animal interaction, cow handling system designs, and stockmanship training.

Human and cow interaction is a topic that is presented in several articles and book chapters.[3–8] The behavior of both cows and stock persons needs to be considered in the interaction between the 2.

LOW STRESS

The popular term "low-stress" cattle handling has been addressed by several investigators and stockmen.[9–14] Low-stress cattle handling and its benefits directly address animal welfare concerns of the consumers and the producers.

The stress on a cow or the stock person in a particular handling situation may be due to many factors, including the following[10,15]:

- Animal breed
- Temperament
- Previous handling experience
- Age
- Fitness
- Quality of the handling facility
- Situation
- Incorrect (poor) handling techniques
- Environment
  - Physical
  - Thermal
- Diet
- Health status

STOCKMANSHIP

There are several definitions of stockmanship in published works.[4,5,14,16] The term will likely continue to evolve in the future. In this discussion, the term stockmanship is considered gender neutral. A stock person might be called a caretaker or a cow person.[8] Stockmanship may be referred to as animal husbandry, or stewardship, referring to the use of good animal care practices. Stockmanship is defined here as the knowledgeable and skillful handling of livestock in a safe, efficient, effective, and proper manner.[17] Stockmanship is enhanced with proper handling facility design to minimize stress and discomfort. Stockmanship requires an understanding of the natural behavior of the dairy cow and a skill set to leverage that natural behavior in handling the cow. The practice of stockmanship encompasses a low-stress, integrated, comprehensive, and holistic approach to livestock handling.[18,19]

STOCKMANSHIP TRAINING

Stockmanship training improves cow welfare and productivity.[20–22] Proper training of stock persons is required to use the handling system to make it a safe and efficient experience. The factors that affect the level of stress of both cows and stock persons need to be taken into consideration when training and improving handling skills.[9]

Cows should be handled by a stock person with positive and calm movement. In order for the handling system to be effective, all stock persons need to be trained to handle calves, heifers, and cows in a proper manner throughout the life of the animal. Every interaction and experience between stock persons and the animal will have an influence on the animal's reaction to future situations. This interaction includes anyone whose work may require even incidental contact with the animals. The stock person should understand that every interaction with the cow contributes to its learned behavior and can be a positive or negative experience.

Stock persons need to be trained to observe, interpret, and leverage the response of an individual cow or group of cows to the stimuli that are occurring to create the desired action. It is most desirable to produce a consistent response in the same interaction and situation for the cow in every instance. Consistent practices and interactions teach the cow what is expected when they react in the desired and proper way. The reward to the cow comes in the release or reduction of the pressure placed on them. The release of pressure will likely result in obtaining a consistent and reproducible response by the cow to the specific situation and conditions. When stock persons interact with the cow in an inconsistent manner in the same situation, the cow will likely react in an inconsistent and undesirable or improper way.

Stock persons need to understand the cow's reactions to their interaction and apply certain techniques and rules to create movement. **Box 1** is a summary describing the stock person rules that are used to properly handle cows.

COW SENSES

A cow's 5 senses include sight, hearing, smell, taste, and touch.[8,10,14,23] A stock person interacts with cows primarily through the senses of sight and hearing. The other senses may also influence the reaction of a cow to a particular interaction. They may balk at an odd smell, a shadow, a difference in temperature, or a change in floor surface they are walking on. In order for a cow to respond to a situation or interaction with the stock person, one or more of its 5 senses must be stimulated.

Cows have panoramic vision of 330°. Cows need to be able to see the stock person at all times. If not, they will stop and look around to determine where the person is. The best position to allow the cow to see the stock person is at her side. A cow has a 30° blind spot, radiating 15° on either side of the tail head.[8,24] Cows are sensitive to contrasts in light and have poor depth perception, which can cause cows to balk or slow down when moving to cross a shadow or a change in surface elevation, such as a curb, trailer, or crossover. When under stress, they tend to herd and seek low-light conditions. Cows have a broader hearing spectrum than people. They can respond

---

Box 1
Stock person rules for proper cow handling management

1. The cow is always right
2. Every interaction between the stock person and cows is important
3. Do not predetermine your actions
4. Be consistent
5. Be patient
6. Work in the pressure area
   a. Work where the cow can see you
7. Apply pressure properly
   a. Place hands in pockets
   b. Apply pressure from the side
   c. Adjust position, timing, angle of approach, speed of approach according to the situation
8. Teach cows in the order
   a. Slow the cow down
   b. Stop the cow
   c. Start the cow
   d. Turn the cow
   e. Teach the animal to take pressure
9. Starting the cow movement properly is very important
10. Greater pressure is required to start movement as compared with maintaining movement
11. Less pressure is required to move and guide the cow
12. Avoid constantly stopping motion (movement)
13. Use a rocking motion to elicit a response to stop or create movement
14. Walk straight
15. Walk with cows to slow them down
16. Walk against cows to speed up
17. Walk in a forward angle to create movement

Data from Refs. [8,18,30,32]

---

to higher and lower frequencies that humans cannot perceive. Research has shown that cows have a similar, negative response to shouting as they do to hitting.

COW BEHAVIOR

Cow behavior is described by several investigators as how the cow responds or reacts to the stimuli it receives from its senses.[24–28] Stock persons cannot understand how cows think or feel; they can only observe the reaction of the cow to the situation and learn how to use that response to achieve the desired movement.[29]

Fig. 1 shows what is defined as the flight zone and pressure zone of an individual cow.[10,14,28,30] The pressure zone is the area that surrounds the flight zone. The outer edge of the pressure zone is considered a place where the cow will not move away from the stock person. A stock person within the outside edge of the pressure zone will be noticed by the cow. The cow's reaction may be indicated by a raised head or ear movement or looking in the direction of the person. The inside edge of the pressure zone is also the outside edge of the flight zone.

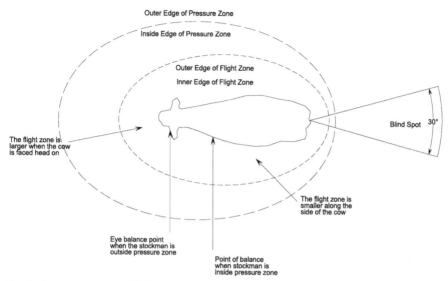

Fig. 1. Cow pressure and flight zone.

The distance from the cow to the outer edge of the flight zone is different for each individual. In general, it is a smaller zone for a dairy cow than it is for a beef cow. The distance is usually shorter on the sides of the cow as compared with the front of the animal and is shortest directly behind the cow in its blind spot. When the stock person enters the outside edge of the flight zone, the cow will move away.

Another common reference to describe how stock persons interact with a cow to achieve movement is the points of balance. The eye balance point is used when the stock person is a distance away past the outer edge of the pressure zone. The cow will notice the stock person, but it may not cause movement of the cow. The second point of balance is approximately at the shoulder of the cow and is used when the stock person is near the cow in a pen or chute.

There are leaders and followers in a group. Identifying which cows are the leaders and which are not will help when moving a group of cows. Releasing pressure on a specific cow and allowing a different cow that chooses to move forward will bring the rest of the group along. When trying to isolate an individual cow, consider moving a few cows including the individual cow away from the main group and then separate the individual cow from the group. There is a social order within the dairy herd and within each pen or group. The dominant and submissive behaviors can be observed and documented in multiple areas on the dairy, including the resting space, feed bunk area, water location, parlor entrance order, and while moving a group. Cows moving to the parlor are usually in a different rank order than when they choose to enter the parlor. Adequate time and extra space are needed at the parlor entry to allow cows to rearrange themselves according to their preference to enter the parlor.

Cows can turn equally as easily 90° to the right or left. When approaching a cow from the front, there may be a slight preference for cows to turn to the right, but cows can be trained to turn in any direction. When turning 180°, there may be a slight advantage for cows to turn to the right versus the left. When turning 180° to the right, they collapse the right side of their abdomen and turn. When turning to the left, they have to bend into their rumen, displacing the rumen, and the turn is awkward. Data on lesions from trimming records by one of the authors (K.B.) show a high incidence of lesions occur on the rear hooves. There is often a slightly higher incidence of lesions on the right rear hoof indicating that cows perhaps pivot more on the right rear hoof than the left rear hoof. There are also slight tendencies for cows to choose the left or right sides of parlors and entry into AMSs when given a choice.

TRAINING THE COW

With consistent and correct application of stockmanship practices, animals can be trained and learn to trust stock persons as leaders. This evolving concept of deliberately training cattle is not yet widely accepted or practiced.[31,32] Cows are conditioned every time they are handled. A specific cow's reaction will depend on the situation, the stock person, and any past experience. Cows can learn and remember experiences with stock persons from previous interactions. Cows can be trained to respond in a certain way when stimulated by the stock person in a specific manner. This learned behavior develops at a young age and may be recalled at specific situations later in

---

Box 2
Cow rules for proper cow handling management

1. Cows sense pressure
   i. Cows look at what is pressuring them
   ii. Cows tend to go around the pressure
   iii. Cows stop moving when the pressure is released

2. Single sources of pressure are most effective
   i. Pressure from 2 different sources produces incompatible behavior

3. Cows are herd animals

4. When a cow is isolated from a group, it becomes anxious and will tend to want to return to the group

5. Cattle are gregarious and follow each other

6. Cows prefer to walk single file

7. When blocked, cows tend to return to where they have come from

8. Cows walk in an arc around the obstruction/stock person

9. Cows move in the direction they are facing

10. Multiple experiences determine current behavioral responses

11. A cow can walk at a speed range of 1.5 to 3.1 mph (0.65–1.4 m/s)

12. A group of cows can walk at an average speed of 1.7 mph (0.75 m/s)

13. People can walk approximately 3.1-4.0 mph (1.4 -1.8 m/s)

14. Cows walk with their head down, looking where they will place their feet

15. When cows are forced into a space that is too small, they are forced to raise their heads over the tops of other cows

16. When cows cannot see where to place their feet, they slow down and take shorter strides

17. When dominant cows in a group slow down or stop, the rest of the group will slow or stop

18. Subordinate cows will not walk past dominant cows

19. Cows prefer to stand on soft surfaces as compared with concrete

20. Cows will walk slower and are more likely to slip when the concrete is covered with manure

21. Cows will stand more during heat stress

Data from Refs. [8,18,30,32]

its life. The reactions they learn will be influenced by the attitude and training of the stock person. Developing good habits and attitudes among the stock persons when handling the cow from a young calf throughout the cow's life ensures that the cow's experience is consistently positive throughout its life. **Box 2** shows the cow rules that are used to properly handle cows.

SAFETY FOR COWS AND STOCK PERSONS

Safety for both cows and stock persons is a primary goal in the design and management of the cow handling system.[33,34] There is always a risk of injury to people or animals whenever the 2 interact. That risk can be minimized with proper design and proper handling methods that address the safety of both. Whenever possible, the facility design should allow the separation of the stock person from the cow when handling the cow. Fences should allow either climbing up out of the way or rolling under the fence when necessary. Personnel passes can be incorporated into the pen fence (**Fig. 2**) or in the swing gate (**Fig. 3**) to allow easy access to the pen without opening the gate.

PROPER COW HANDLING SKILLS

A key design principle in creating an efficient handling system is the ability to create a result that is consistent and repeatable. The proximity, direction of movement, and the orientation of the stock person to the cow are variables that can result in efficient movement. The goal when handling cows is to stimulate the cow with minimal effort to illicit a specific response desired by the stock person. The combination of facility design features and the ability to stimulate and interact with the cow in a certain way will achieve the outcome desired by the stock person with minimal effort.

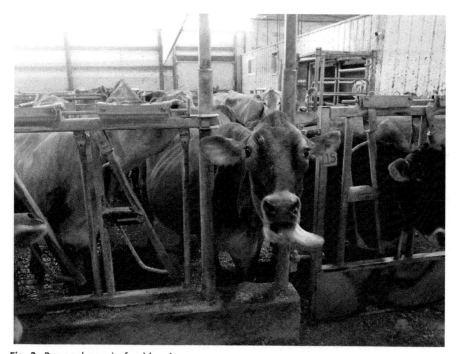

Fig. 2. Personal pass in feed barrier.

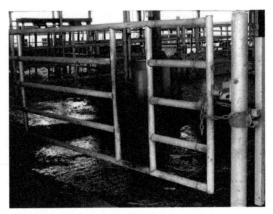

Fig. 3. Personal pass in gate.

Minimizing stress for both the cow and the stock person when interacting and handling the cows is the goal and is more efficient.

Instinctively, humans act as predators[7,28] and tend to use less effective techniques (whistling, shouting, hitting, prodding) to move livestock rather than taking advantage of the natural movement instincts of the animal.[9] In many cases, current cattle handling designs are based on the fact that the main interaction between stock persons and the cattle is fear and forcing the cow through a handling system. Grandin[10] demonstrated to the cattle industry that forcing cattle through a system caused poor flow, frustration of stock persons, and cattle injuries that cost money. She showed that working with the natural behaviors of cattle in the facility design could enhance the experience of the cattle and achieve the result desired without excessive effort and with lower stress on the cattle and people.[13]

Proper livestock handling focuses on 2 actions of "pressure" and "release."[11] Pressure is created by stimulating one or more of the 5 senses to elicit a desired response. Pressure should always be applied from where the cow can see the stock person. The alternating use of pressure and release creates controlled and desired movement of the cow. Continuous pressure may elicit a fear response in the cow, and the cow will not respond in a controlled or desired manner. It is not acceptable to use any aggressive form of handling, such as an electric prod, hitting, dragging, or yelling.

Box 3
Videos on proper handling techniques

Video 1. Moving a single cow with pressure and release.

Video 2. Sorting a single cow from a pen with pressure and release.

Video 3. Moving a group of cows with rocking motion.

Video 4. Pen settling a group of calves.

Video 5. Loading a race from a redirection pen (Bud box).

Video 6. Loading a redirection pen (Bud box).

Video 7. Loading a hoof trimming chute from a race.

The amount of pressure and the angle at which it is applied are critical in controlling what the response from the cow will be. The stock person must assess the situation, including the limitations, and react accordingly. Examples of handling techniques and the response of animals to the interactions with the stock person are shown in the videos listed in **Box 3**.

COW TIME BUDGET

Excellent cow comfort focuses on the cow's time budget and minimizing stress to provide the cow with a consistent environment throughout the day and annual life cycle.[2,35] Cows should not be forced away from the pen from rest, feed, and water for more than 3 hours total in the 24-hour day. Most of the time the cow is forced out of the pen is during the milking process. Poor design and management decisions can push the actual milking time to 4 to 5 hours per day or more, which causes additional stress on the cow by limiting her time budget for resting.

The scheduling of other procedures such as herd health check, pregnancy check, and hoof trimming, necessary in the dairy production system, should be limited to no more than one additional hour forced away from the pen on any 1 day beyond the recommended 3 hours per day.

Social disorder can occur with regrouping and can affect dry matter intake and thus production. Minimizing social stress starts with evaluating the management' plan's need to move cows. This social stress can also be minimized with proper livestock handling techniques.

COW HANDLING MANAGEMENT PLAN

The cow is the "first and foremost" consideration in the cow handling management plan and design of the cow handling system. On a dairy farm, physical interaction between cows and the stock person is required on a daily basis.

The cow handling management plan identifies and describes the necessary treatments and protocols implemented by the trained stock person. The following is a list of typical situations and reasons for restraint during required treatments:

- Artificial insemination
- Herd health checks
- Palpating/ultrasound
- Embryo transfer and flushing
- Ear tagging
- Hoof trimming or lameness treatments
- Drenching
- Injections
- Bolus
- Surgery/displaced abomasum
- Calving assistance

The cow handling management plan should document in writing the standard operating procedures (SOP) for all the cow handling situations. Typical cow handling situations for which there should be a written SOP used by trained stock persons include

- Moving an individual cow out of a group of cows
- Moving a small group of cows from the larger group

    i. To regroup
    ii. To dry off cows
    iii. To move to a transition cow pen
    iv. To move to hoof-trimming area for scheduled hoof trimming
    v. To move to hoof trimming for as-needed hoof trimming
    vi. To fetch pen for automatic milking system (AMS) units
- Moving a group of cows out of a pen
    i. To the milking facility (parlor)
    ii. To a new pen
    iii. To a new barn
- Sorting a cow from a return lane
    i. Manually
    ii. Automatically through a sort gate
- Moving cows through a race
- Moving or sorting cows through a footbath
- Pen settling
- Loading or unloading a cow or group of cows

Scheduling Cow Handling Procedures

Routine cow handling procedures should be scheduled to minimize disruption in the cow's daily time budget. Periodic cow handling procedures, such as herd health checks and hoof trimming, should be scheduled so that only one major cow handling procedure disrupts the cow's time budget on a particular day. A typical daily schedule spreads out the other cow handling tasks over a week to minimize time cows are forced away from rest, feed, and water:

Day 1: Cow dry off and close-up cow moving day
Day 2: Bedding day
Day 3: Herd health check day
Day 4: Bedding day
Day 5: Scheduled hoof trimming (varies)
Day 6: Bedding day
Day 7: Off

COW HANDLING SYSTEM DESIGN PRINCIPLES

The cow handling system design and management have 2 main principles that should be a priority when developing the handling system features.[35–40] One stock person should be able to move a group of cows or a single cow, and they should be able to isolate and restrain a cow safely and efficiently.

COW HANDLING SYSTEM DESIGN FEATURES

Most of the design information for cattle handling systems has been developed for the beef cattle industry. These practical design features and details can be adapted to the needs of the dairy cow and should be incorporated into the dairy cow handling system design to create a system that is safe for cows and people. **Box 4** shows a list of design criteria that should be considered when designing cow handling areas.

Alley Flooring

Alley floors should allow cows good traction without slipping. Concrete is the most common material used in alleys. Grooves placed in the concrete surface provide

---

Box 4
Design considerations for cow handling system

1. Consider cow behavior in the handling system design.
2. Consider safety for the stock person and cow in the handling system design.
3. Fencing should be open so that cows can see the stock person.
4. Plan every area so one stock person can perform the handling procedure.
5. Gates design, hinge point, and direction of swing should be designed to allow the cow an unrestricted access to move in the direction desired.
6. Gates should block the opening completely with no opening that suggests an exit for the cow.
7. Check cow pathway for obstructions, polished surfaces, pinch points, and sharp edges to prevent injury to cows and stock person.
8. Develop one-way traffic patterns.
9. Provide nonslip floors with grooves for traction to prevent slipping.
10. Provide soft rubber floors with grooves for traction in holding pens.
11. Use a drover alley for moving cows.
12. Consider group size when designing traffic alley widths.
13. Handling system areas should have a diffuse and uniform lighting that minimizes large contrasts between light and dark.
14. Control and maintain a suitable environment to minimize temperature extremes and good air quality.

---

grip.[35] There should be a flat surface between grooves to allow even contact between the hoof and the floor. The groove edges should be smooth and at a right angle between the groove and floor surface, and grooves are recommended to be 0.75 inch wide, 0.50 inch deep, spaced 3.25 inches on center. The groove pattern is typically placed parallel to the length of the alley and main cow traffic direction. At locations where cows are turning or changing direction, such as through cross alleys, a diamond groove pattern can be used. Grooves are usually floated into fresh concrete, but may also be cut into new or old concrete.

Rubber flooring can also be used in situations to reduce hoof wear. Cows have a preference to walk on soft rubber over concrete if given a choice. If floors are secure to walk on, healthy cows show little preference for rubber over concrete; however, a lame cow will always choose rubber over concrete because the softer surface reduces the pain of walking. Conveyor belt rubber is much harder and can become very slippery compared with more compressible natural rubber products. Rubber flooring may also be an alternative to resurfacing old smooth or slippery concrete to provide a better traction surface for the cow.

Cow Traffic Alleys

There are several types of alleys used in the dairy farmstead design. Pen alleys are used by the cows to move from resting to the feed bunk or water locations. Cows interact with other cows in the alleys while standing or moving around.

Cow traffic alleys are used to move a group of cows from the pens to the milking parlor and return to the pen. The width of the alley should be designed to allow the group to move through the alley at a speed comfortable for the group of cows in the allotted time desired by the handler, without forcing the cows to walk too fast or run.

Table 1
Cow traffic alley dimensions

Pen Size	Cow Traffic Alley Width
<150 cows	14 feet (4.3 m)
150–250 cows	16 feet (4.9 m)
250–400 cows	20 feet (6.0 m)
>400 cows	24 feet (7.3 m)

Experience gained from moving cows through lanes from pasture to the parlor in an efficient manner has been adapted to confinement traffic alley design. **Table 1** shows the dimensions for cow traffic lanes for different group pen sizes to provide adequate space for moving the cow group. Wider traffic alleys allow the cow group to move efficiently to the parlor by walking slowly so as not to contaminate the udder with splashing manure (**Fig. 4**).

Cow return alleys allow cows to exit the parlor in smaller groups or individually after being milked. The return alleys lead cows back to the cow traffic alleys, which allow cows to move back to the pen on their own initiative. There may be a single return alley with a crossover or dual return alleys depending on the parlor design. In rotary parlors, there is a single wide return alley.

Cows can be sorted automatically (**Fig. 5**) or manually on the path through the return or traffic alley. The cows may be sorted to an adjacent holding pen or an adjacent sort lane where they should only wait for a short time to be handled. Cows can be restrained with a head gate at the end of the race for subsequent treatment (**Fig. 6**). A palpation gate can be used to gain access to the rear of the cow for necessary procedures (**Fig. 7**).

Drover alleys are incorporated into the free-stall barn to allow cows to be moved from one pen to another pen without having to disrupt an adjacent pen (**Fig. 8**). The drover alley is also used to move cows to trimming areas or loading areas.

Holding Area for Milking Parlor

The holding area for a milking parlor is used to hold a pen of cows waiting to be milked. The sizing of the holding pen is dependent on the number of cows to be held for less

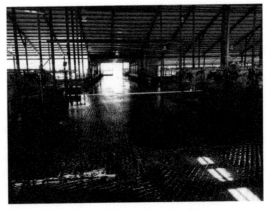

Fig. 4. Traffic alley.

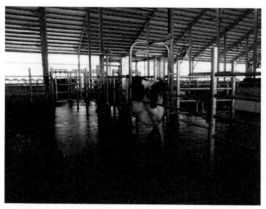

Fig. 5. Automatic sort gate.

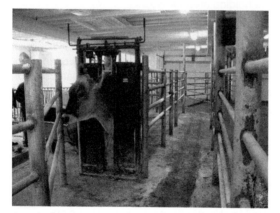

Fig. 6. Head gate at end of race.

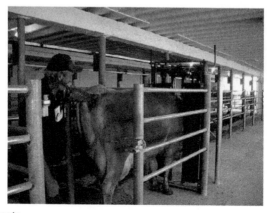

Fig. 7. Palpation gate.

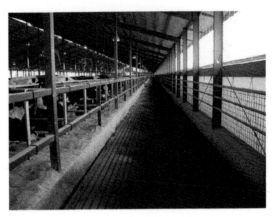

Fig. 8. Drover alley.

than an hour waiting to be milked. A minimum of 20 square feet of space per cow is recommended in the holding area for Holstein cows, to allow space available for the cows to adjust their order of entry into the parlor.

The crowd gate is managed to reduce the space available for the cows waiting in the holding area and to encourage them to move forward. A bell or buzzer can be used to train all the cows to move forward at the sound. The crowd gate should not be used to push cows. The cows that need to move ahead into the parlor platforms are in the front of the holding area and are not influenced by the pressure applied to the cows in the rear of the holding area.

Cow Restraint

There is a variety of restraint systems used for dairy cows in the dairy system. Head-locks are used as a feed barrier in a pen to allow the herdsperson to restrain the cows for herd health check or hold for sorting (**Fig. 9**). Cows should not be held longer than 1 hour in headlocks so as not to limit the cows from resting.

When a post and rail feed barrier is used in the pen, the opportunity to restrain cows is not available (**Fig. 10**). A palpation management rail can be used to restrain a group of cows for herd health treatments and pregnancy checks and can be incorporated into the traffic alley (**Fig. 11**).

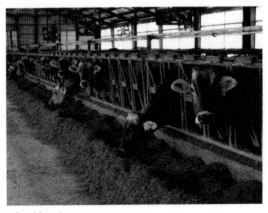

Fig. 9. Headlocks in feed barrier.

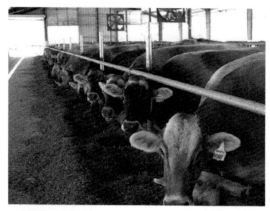

Fig. 10. Post and rail feed barrier.

HANDLING SYSTEM DESIGNS

There is a combination of cow behavior awareness, science, and art in the proper design of a handling system. Design innovations have been developed over the years by stock persons handling cattle that observed the responses of cows to a particular situation and adapted the facility design to take advantage of the response by the cattle that minimized the effort to achieve the desired goal. There are several resources for practical handling system design details for races, holding pens, and other areas mostly related to beef cattle. These designs can be adapted and integrated into the dairy farmstead facilities considering the behavior and nature of dairy cows.[36–40] The following designs have been adapted to specifically handle dairy cows on the farm.

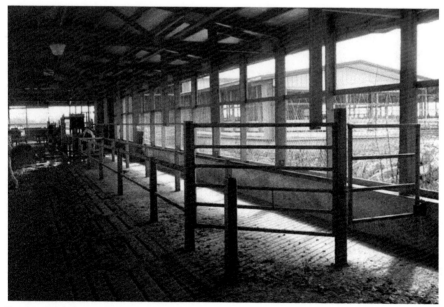

Fig. 11. Palpation management rail.

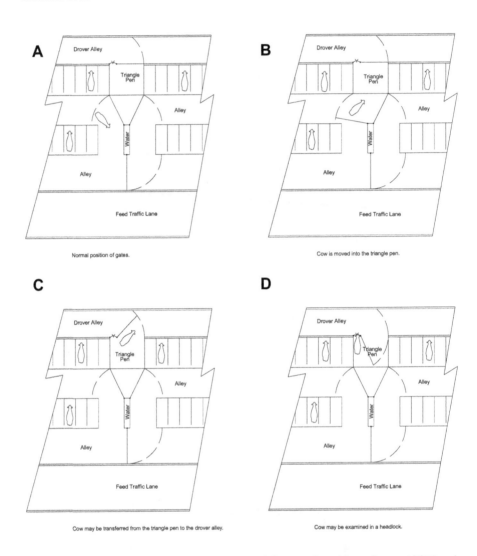

Fig. 12. Triangle pen gate entry to drover alley. (*A*) Normal position of gates. (*B*) Cow is moved into the triangle pen. (*C*) Cow may be transferred from triangle pen to drover alley. (*D*) Cow may be examined in a headlock.

Triangle Pen Entry

Fig. 12 shows a design with gates strategically located to create a pen within the main pen.[35] The stock person can isolate a cow and move it into the triangle pen and then out of the triangle pen into the drover alley with minimal effort.

Calving or Hospital Pen

Fig. 13 shows a calving or hospital pen designed for the space to hold one cow that needs special attention or requires more involved procedures. The most common area where it may be necessary to restrain a cow is in the maternity area for treatment or for calving assistance. The caregiver should have access to both sides of the cow when

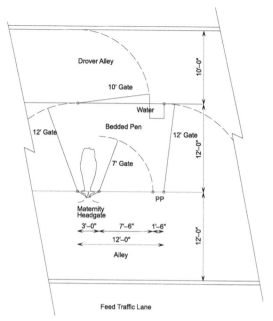

Fig. 13. Calving or maternity pen design.

restrained. Gates are strategically placed and used to direct the cow into the corner of the pen where the restraint is provided with a head gate. A maternity headlock allows the cow to be restrained while assisting calving or milking the cow for colostrum (**Fig. 14**). Another option for restraint in the maternity pen is a walk-through head gate (**Fig. 15**).

Redirection Pen (Bud Box)

The redirection box is a design that eventually was named after Bud Williams,[11] who learned how to use the design as an alternative to a crowding tub (**Fig. 16**). It takes both good design and good handling skills to use the system properly. The basic dimensions of the redirection box are 12 feet to 14 feet wide by 20 feet long. Cows

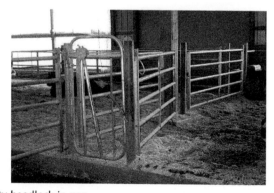

Fig. 14. Maternity headlock in pen.

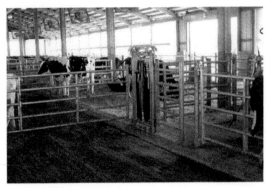

Fig. 15. Walk-through head gate in pen.

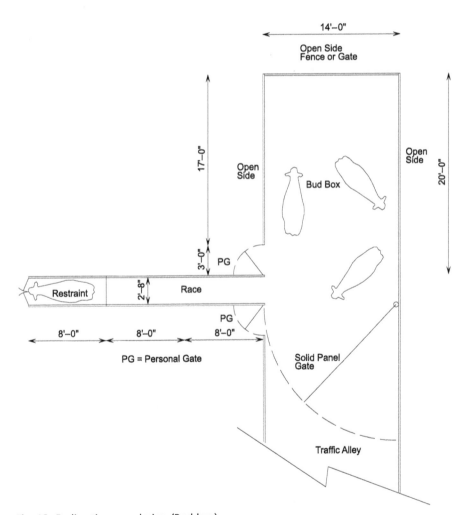

Fig. 16. Redirection pen design (Bud box).

waiting in a holding area are worked through the Bud box in small groups. The group size will be dependent on the capacity of the race leading out of the Bud box. If the race can hold 5 cows, then the group size worked into and out of the Bud box should be 5 cows.

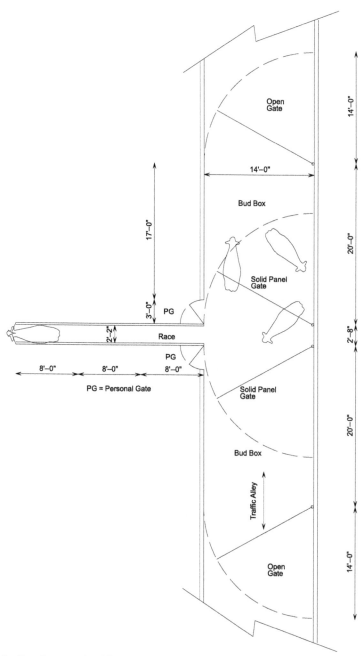

Fig. 17. Redirection pen (Bud box) in traffic alley.

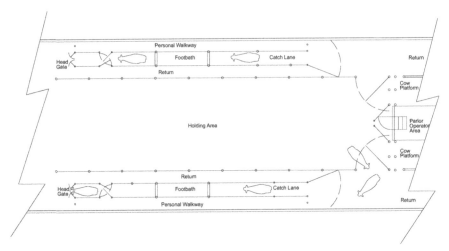

Fig. 18. Sort lane with footbath.

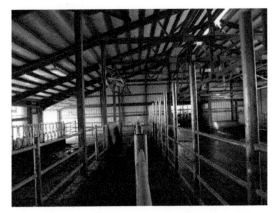

Fig. 19. Footbath in sort alley.

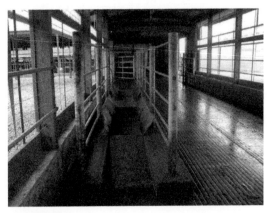

Fig. 20. Footbath in traffic alley.

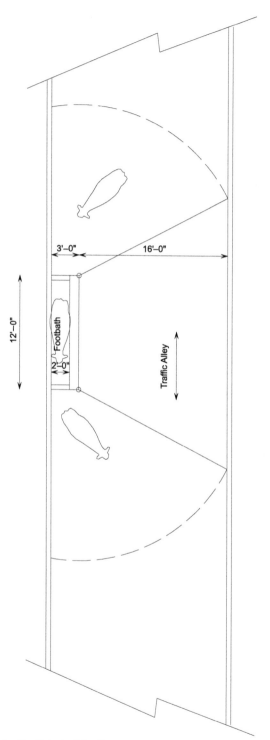

Fig. 21. Design of footbath in traffic alley.

Permanent Bud boxes can be integrated into a permanent handling system design. It can be used in a traffic alley to move cows between the pen and the milking parlor. It can also be designed into a dedicated cow handling system design space adjacent to a cow traffic alley or drover alley. **Fig. 17** shows a Bud box that can be created in a traffic lane and allows cows to be moved through the Bud box from either direction. The Bud box can feed a race used for multiple purposes.

Footbath Design and Location

The footbath design should provide the ability for the cow to get at least 2 steps of each hoof into the solution. The correct design for a footbath is readily available.[35] Length is typically 10 to 12 feet; width is 24 inches wide at the base, widening to 36 inches wide at a height of 36 inches, with a 10-inch-high step-in. In many cases, the footbath is set up in an adjacent alley next to a return alley for the parlor (**Figs. 18 and 19**). It can also be placed adjacent to the traffic alley used to move cows from the barn to the parlor (**Fig. 20**). A set of gates diverts the cows through the footbath on the scheduled day (**Fig. 21**).

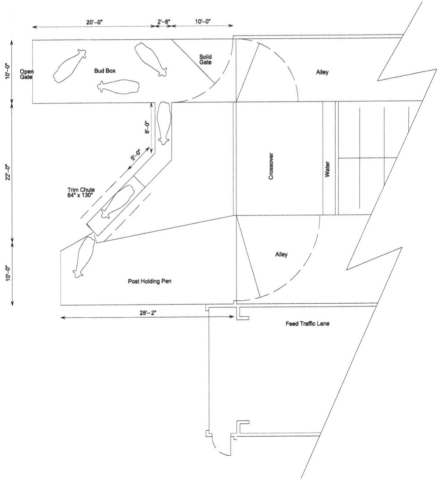

Fig. 22. Temporary redirection pen (Bud box) for trimming.

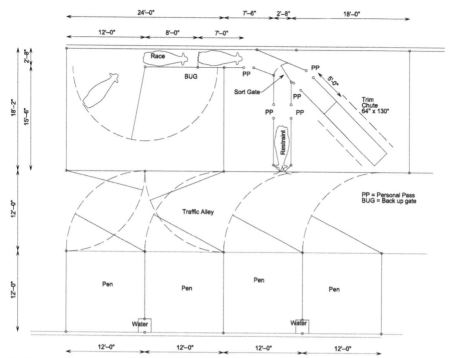

Fig. 23. Hoof trimming chute and restraint design.

Holding Area for Hoof Trimming

The capacity for holding cows and trimming the cows in a reasonable timeframe should be determined in the facility design. The holding pen should be sized to hold the number of cows that can be trimmed in less than a 2-hour period. Professional hoof trimmers can provide a quality trim to each cow and still trim between 40 and

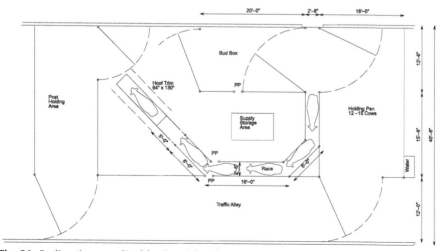

Fig. 24. Redirection pen (Bud box) and hoof trimming area design in operation at Slaktis farm in Russia.

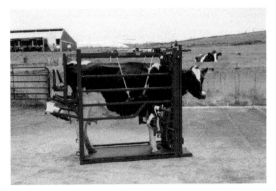

Fig. 25. Simple hoof trimming chute.

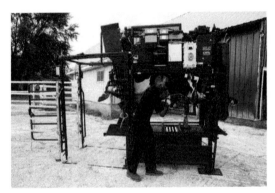

Fig. 26. Professional hoof trimming chute.

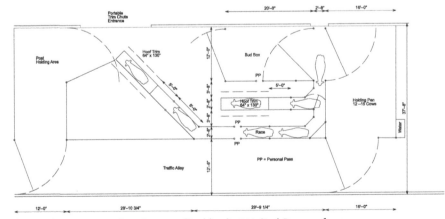

Fig. 27. Permanent redirection pen (Bud box) at United Dreams farm.

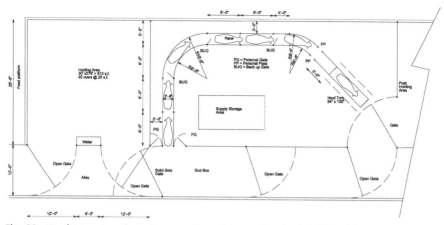

Fig. 28. Hoof trimming chute in operation at Australian Fresh Milk Holdings.

50 cows per 8-hour day or 5 to 6 cows per hour. That would make the holding area sized for approximately 10 to 12 cows. Designing an efficient handling system will pay off in lowering the time required to move cows out of the pen into the holding area and return to their pen.

A Bud box design should be sized to hold and move the number of cows that will fill the race. It should not be overfilled because it can restrict turning movement and impede free movement to the exit. The recommendation is to move 4 to 6 cows through the Bud box into a race that can hold that number of cows.

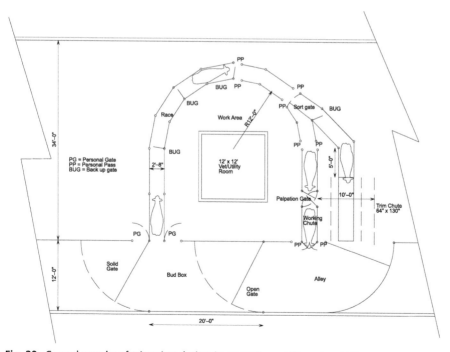

Fig. 29. Curved race hoof trimming design in operation at Riverview LLP.

Hoof Trimming Area Designs

Hoof trimming areas for smaller dairies for a scheduled trimming can be temporary setups with a portable chute brought by the trimmer. A temporary Bud box can be set up outside and on the end of the free-stall barn for periodic use by the hoof trimmer or for loading and unloading cattle (**Fig. 22**). The Bud box is placed at the end of the alley of a free-stall pen using one alley as an extension into a Bud box and set up of hoof trim chute or load out area perpendicular to the direction of the alley and Bud box. When cows are released from the trim chute, they can exit into the other alley.

   Fig. 23 shows a dedicated cow handling space that allows for the dual purposes of a permanent trimming chute and head gate. The holding area uses a swinging gate to

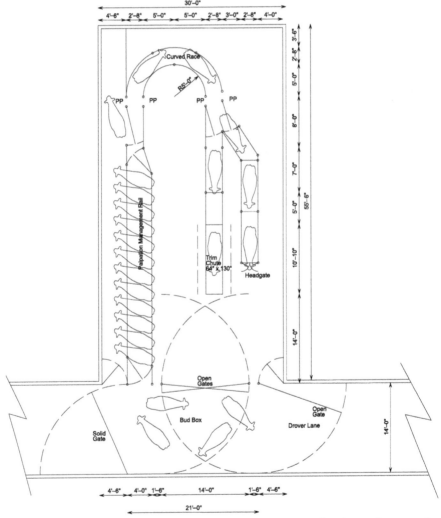

Fig. 30. Redirection pen (Bud box) with palpation management rail and curved race to trimming chute or head gate.

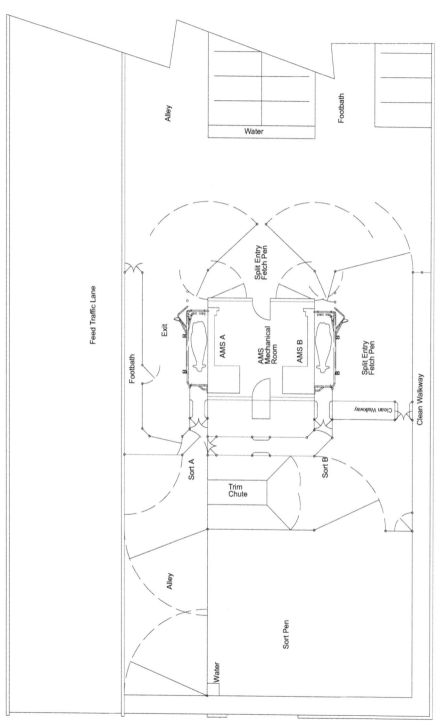

Fig. 31. Cattle handling system in an automatic milking barn.

funnel cows into the race. The race can be split to feed either a dedicated trimming chute or a head gate.

Fig. 24 shows a compact design for a larger dairy that uses a dedicated Bud box to feed a simple race and a dedicated trimming chute for as-needed trimming (**Fig. 25**). This design can be adapted both to provide an as-needed trimming chute and to allow a professional trimming chute (**Fig. 26**). The professional trimmer brings his or her own chute and can back it into the dedicated handling space. Note the gate on the Bud box entrance is hinged at the exit to create a longer race to hold an additional 2 cows (**Fig. 27**).

Fig. 28 shows a design with space for a dedicated holding area and Bud box integrated into the traffic alley. The curved race directs cows to a dedicated hoof trimming space.

Fig. 29 shows a dual purpose handling area for either restraint in a head gate for cows or a dedicated hoof trimming chute for the in-house hoof trimmer.

Fig. 30 shows a design that integrates a Bud box into the traffic alley. Three options for cow handling are integrated into the curved race design. There is a palpation management rail that also acts as a race to feed a curved race. The race can feed either a dedicated trimming chute or a head gate for cow restraint.

Handling Systems for Automatic Milking System Barns Design

Researchers and farmers are observing a marked difference in the human-cow relationship in an AMS barn.[26] Many observe a quiet barn with calmer cows. The advantage in an AMS system design is that the cow is restrained for milking and can be sorted as an individual to a cattle handling area. There should be a cattle handling area integrated into the barn design (**Fig. 31**). This cattle handling area is where treatments can be performed on an as-needed basis. Personal gates allow easy access to the pen (**Fig. 32**).

Fetch pens are used to hold a few cows that have not visited the AMS unit in the required time. Strategically located gates should be placed in the pen design to allow the stock person to easily sort a small subgroup of cows that are moved into the fetch pen.

One critical part of management for foot health in an AMS system is to integrate a cow footbath into the AMS barn design. Many farms do not want the footbath near the robot to protect it from the chemicals used. Also, when the footbath is placed at

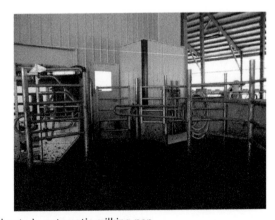

Fig. 32. Personal gate in automatic milking pen.

the exit from the AMS, cows will pass through the footbath as many times as visits to the robot. It can also slow the cows' exit from the AMS and potentially reduce visits to the AMS.

A better and more consistent treatment option is to place the footbath in an exit lane located away from the AMS unit (see **Fig. 31**). Cows can be sorted to allow them to exit the AMS or route them to the sort pen or to the footbath as programmed by the herd manager. This route also can take cows to the cattle handling area of the AMS barn design.

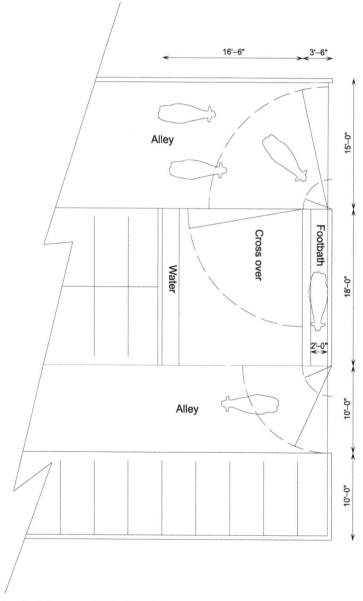

Fig. 33. Footbath in cross alley in free-stall pen.

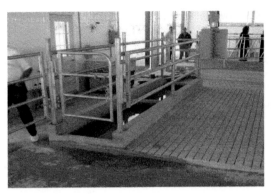

Fig. 34. Footbath at a crossover.

In some AMS barn designs the other location for the footbath is integrated into the crossover at the end of the barn opposite to the location of the AMS unit (**Fig. 33**). Gates are placed that block the normal path of the cows through the crossover and divert the cows through the footbath (**Fig. 34**). The manager moves the entire group of cows through the footbath on a scheduled basis, which is time consuming and disruptive to the daily routine of the cows and hence is not preferred.

SUMMARY

The design and management of proper handling systems for dairy cows begin with a cow handling management plan that considers the cow and the stock person's behavior. The safety of the cow and stock person is important to the cow handling management plan and design decisions. Cow welfare can be addressed in a proper cow handling system design. The 3 key components of a handling system are the skills of the stock person, the cow handling management plan, and the design of the handling facility. Good design enhances stockmanship ability and minimizes stress for cows and stock persons, lowering the risk of injury to both.

SUPPLEMENTARY DATA

Supplementary data related to this article can be found online at https://doi.org/10.1016/j.cvfa.2018.11.003.

REFERENCES

1. Grandin T. A whole systems approach to assessing animal welfare during handling and restraint. In: Livestock handling and transport. 4th edition. 2014. p. 1–13. Available at: https://www.cabi.org/vetmedresource/ebook/20143217251. Accessed December 13, 2018.

2. Jones GA, Kammel D. Large dairy herd design and systems in temperate and cold climates. In: Large dairy herd management. 3rd edition. 2017. p. 71–82. Available at: https://ldhm.adsa.org/. Accessed December 13, 2018.

3. Seabrook MF. The psychological relationship between dairy cows and dairy cowmen and its implications for animal welfare. Int J Study Anim Probl 1980;1(5): 295–8. Available at: https://animalstudiesrepository.org/acwp_habr/3/.

4. Albright JL. Human/farm animal relationships. In: Advances in animal welfare science. 1986. p. 51–66. Available at: https://animalstudiesrepository.org/cgi/viewcontent.cgi?referer=https://www.google.com/&httpsredir=1&article=1011&context=acwp_faafp. Accessed December 13, 2018.

5. Edwards-Callaway LN. Human – animal interactions: effects, challenges, and progress. In: Tucker C, editor. Advances in cattle welfare. A volume in food science, technology and nutrition. 2018. p. 72–92. Available at: https://www.sciencedirect.com/science/book/9780081009383. Accessed December 13, 2018.

6. Beaver BV, Hoglund D. Efficient livestock handling. In: The practical application of animal welfare and behavioral science. 2016. p. 1–11. Available at: https://www.sciencedirect.com/science/book/9780124186705. Accessed December 13, 2018.

7. Boivin X, Lensink J, Tallet C, et al. Stockmanship and farm animal welfare. Anim Welf 2003;12:479–92. Available at: https://www.researchgate.net/publication/232169867_Report_on_Stockmanship_and_Farm_Animal_Welfare.

8. Moran J, Doyle R. Cattle behaviour. In: Cow talk. Understanding dairy cow behaviour to improve their welfare on Asian farms. South Victoria (Australia): CSIRO Publishing; 2015. p. 37–67. Available at: http://www.publish.csiro.au/ebook/7929.

9. Grandin T. Handling methods and facilities to reduce stress on cattle. Vet Clin North Am Food Anim Pract 1998;14:325–41. Available at: https://www.vetfood.theclinics.com/article/S0749-0720(15)30257-7/fulltext.

10. Grandin T. Principles for low stress cattle handling. In: Proceedings Range Beef Cow Symposium. 1999. p. 134–44. Available at: https://digitalcommons.unl.edu/rangebeefcowsymp/134/. Accessed December 13, 2018.

11. Williams B. Stockmanship defined. Available at: www.stockmanship.com. Accessed August 9, 2018.

12. Cote S. Stress. In: Stockmanship. A powerful tool for grazing management. 2004. p. 11–6. Available at: http://www.grandin.com/behaviour/principles/SteveCote.book.html. Accessed December 13, 2018.

13. Noffsinger T, Locatelli L. Low stress cattle handling an overlooked dimension of management. 2010. Available at: https://fyi.uwex.edu/animalhusbandry conference/files/2010/03/Low-Stress-Cattle-Handling.pdf. Accessed August 9, 2018.

14. Sorge, U.S. Proper handling techniques for dairy cattle. In: Large Dairy Herd Management. 3rd edition. 2017. p. 1027–36. Available at: https://ldhm.adsa.org/. Accessed December 13, 2018.

15. Endres L, Schwartzkopf-Genswein K. Overview of cattle production systems. In: Tucker C, editor. Advances in cattle welfare. A volume in Food Science, Technology and Nutrition. 2018. p. 1–26. Available at: https://www.sciencedirect.com/science/book/9780081009383. Accessed December 13, 2018.

16. Fears R. Good stockmanship requires the right attitude. Progressive Cattleman Magazine 2014. Available at: http://www.progressivecattle.com/focus-topics/herd-health/6304-goodstockmanshiprequires-the-right-attitude. Accessed August 9, 2018.

17. Hibbard W. Definition of Stockmanship. Stockmans Journal. Available at: https://stockmanshipjournal.com/defining-stockmanship/. Accessed August 9, 2018.

18. Rapnicki P, Perala M, Hoglund D, et al. Dairy Stockmanship reconnecting cows with people. WCDS Advances in Dairy Technology 2012;24:189–200. https://wcds.ualberta.ca/wcds/wp-content/uploads/sites/57/wcds_archive/Archive/2012/Manuscripts/Jones-2.pdf. Accessed December 13, 2018.

19. Rapnicki P, Lewis J. Dairy Stockmanship. 2010. Available at: https://fyi.uwex. edu/animalhusbandryconference/files/2010/03/DairyStockmanship.pdf. Accessed August 9, 2018.

20. FAWC (Farm Animal Welfare Council). Report on stockmanship and farm animal welfare. Role and scope of stockmanship. London. 2017. Available at: https:// www.gov.uk/government/publications/fawc-report-on-stockmanship-and-farm-animal-welfare. Accessed August 9, 2018.

21. Cote S. Benefits of Stockmanship. In: Stockmanship. A powerful tool for grazing management. 2004. p. 17–9. Available at: http://www.grandin.com/behaviour/ principles/SteveCote.book.html. Accessed December 13, 2018.

22. Coleman GJ, Hemsworth PH. Training to improve stockperson beliefs and behaviour towards livestock enhances welfare and productivity. Rev Sci Tech 2014;33:131–7. Available at: https://pdfs.semanticscholar.org/a8aa/4d0b2400e49fa 5e7553760c2d3c4057db4ca.pdf.

23. Beaver BV, Hoglund D. Behavior as it relates to Handling. In: Efficient Livestock Handling. The Practical Application of Animal Welfare and Behavioral Science. 2016. p. 13–44. Available at: https://www.sciencedirect.com/science/book/ 9780124186705. Accessed December 13, 2018.

24. Grandin T. Understanding Flight zone and point of balance for low stress handling of cattle sheep and pigs. 2017. Available at: http://www.grandin.com/ behaviour/principles/flight.zone.html. Accessed August 9, 2018.

25. Albright JL. Dairy cattle behavior and welfare. 1996. Available at: https:// conservancy.umn.edu/bitstream/handle/11299/118804/1/Albright.pdf. Accessed December 13, 2018.

26. Fulwider WK. Dairy Cattle behavior facilities handling transport automation and wellbeing. In: Livestock handling and transport. 4th edition. 2014. p. 116–42. Available at: https://www.cabi.org/vetmedresource/ebook/20143217251. Accessed December 13, 2018.

27. Petrovski K. Cattle signs. In: Cockcroft PD, editor. Bovine medicine. 3rd edition. Indianapolis (IN): John Wiley & Sons, Ltd; 2015. p. 347–59. Available at: https:// www.wiley.com/en-us/Bovine+Medicine%2C+3rd+Edition-p-9781444336436.

28. Grandin T. Behavioral Principles of Livestock handling. 2017. Available at: http:// www.grandin.com/references/new.corral.html. Accessed August 9, 2018.

29. Moran J, Doyle R. Observing cow signals. In: Cow Talk. Understanding dairy cow behaviour to improve their welfare on Asian farms. South Victoria (Australia): CSIRO Publishing; 2015. p. 69–102. Available at: http://www.publish.csiro.au/ ebook/7929.

30. Cote S. Handling principles and behavioral traits. Stockmanship. A powerful tool for grazing management. 2004. p. 29–50. Available at: http://www.grandin.com/ behaviour/principles/SteveCote.book.html. Accessed December 13, 2018.

31. Beaver BV, Hoglund D. Dairy cattle handling: practical applications of science. In: The Practical Application of Animal Welfare and Behavioral Science. 2016. p. 123–58. Available at: https://www.sciencedirect.com/science/book/ 9780124186705. Accessed December 13, 2018.

32. Cote S. Techniques that help build trust. In: Stockmanship. A powerful tool for grazing management. 2004. p. 67–82. Available at: http://www.grandin.com/ behaviour/principles/SteveCote.book.html. Accessed December 13, 2018.

33. Lindahl C, Pinzke S, Herlin A, et al. Human- Animal interactions and safety during dairy cattle handling- comparing moving cows to milking and hoof trimming. J Dairy Sci 2016;99:2131–41. Available at: https://www.journalofdairyscience. org/article/S0022-0302(16)00009-6/pdf?code=jods-site.

34. Langley RL, Morgan Morrow WE. Livestock Handling—Minimizing Worker Injuries. J Agromedicine 2010;15:226–35.
35. Dairyland Initiative. Available at: https://thedairylandinitiative.vetmed.wisc.edu/. Accessed August 9, 2018.
36. Grandin T. The design and construction of facilities for handling cattle. Livest Prod Sci 1997;49:103–19. Available at: https://www.sciencedirect.com/science/article/pii/S0301622697000080.
37. Bicudo JR, McNeill S, Turner T, et al. Cattle Handling Facilities: Planning, Components, and Layouts. AEN-82. Available at: http://www2.ca.uky.edu/agcomm/pubs/aen/aen82/aen82.pdf. Accessed December 13, 2018.
38. Huhnke RL, Harp SL. Cattle Handling Safety in Working Facilities. 2016. Available at: http://factsheets.okstate.edu/documents/bae-1219-corral-and-working-facilities-for-beef-cattle/. Accessed December 13, 2018.
39. Cattle Handling and Working Facilities. The Ohio State. Bulletin 906. Available at: https://agnr.osu.edu/sites/agnr/files/imce/pdfs/Beef/CattleFacilities.pdf. Accessed December 13, 2018.
40. Borg R. Corrals for Handling Beef Cattle. 1993. Alberta Agriculture, Food and Rural Development. 7000-113 Street. Edmonton, Alberta, Canada T6H5T6. Available at: https://www1.agric.gov.ab.ca/$Department/deptdocs.nsf/all/agdex27/$FILE/420_723-1.pdf. Accessed December 13, 2018.

Printed and bound by CPI Group (UK) Ltd, Croydon, CR0 4YY

03/10/2024

01040405-0004